EAT WELL WITH ARTHRITIS

EMILY JOHNSON

To my grandmothers, for always
having open arms and open kitchens
filled with love (and, of course, food)

EAT WELL
WITH ARTHRITIS

Over 85 delicious
recipes from
Arthritis Foodie

EMILY JOHNSON

Photography by Nassima Rothacker

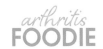

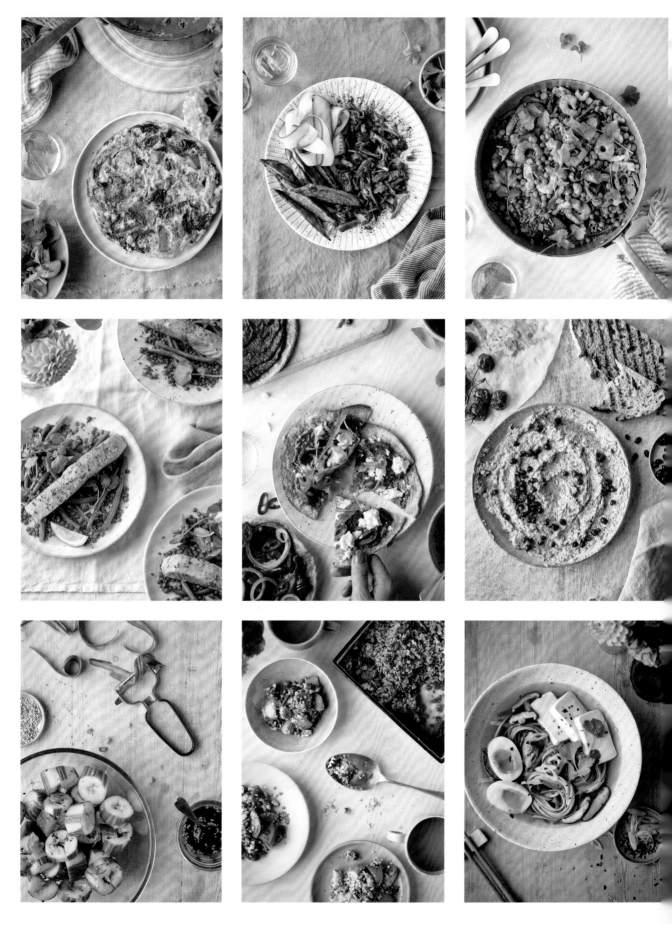

FOREWORD BY DR LAUREN FREID

Living with arthritis can feel like an overwhelming and daunting task, which is why Emily Johnson's debut book *Beat Arthritis Naturally* is fundamental to understanding how you can take ownership of your health and condition and feel better. With this, her second book, *Eat Well with Arthritis*, there is the exciting opportunity to try even more delicious anti-inflammatory recipes, with a nutritionist's approval, and learn further from two leading health practitioners. I'm delighted to be introducing it.

During my medical training, my mother was diagnosed with rheumatoid arthritis, and although medicine significantly improved her pain, allowing her to regain dexterity and strength, it was in fact the healthy lifestyle interventions in combination with the medicine that eventually restored her to her baseline. Since then, as I watched her from behind my medical texts and beyond, she has been optimising sleep, prioritising exercise, focusing on a whole food, anti-inflammatory diet, and taking steps to reduce emotional stress. Years later, she is living a healthier life with rheumatoid arthritis than she ever was prior to the diagnosis. Arthritis does not hold her back.

As a rheumatologist, and inspired by my mother, I firmly encourage healthy lifestyle approaches from the outset when seeing patients with a new diagnosis of arthritis. The goal is for my patients to live their longest, healthiest and most fulfilled lives. I am always looking for resources that can help them, and when I came across Arthritis Foodie, I knew I had struck gold. Arthritis Foodie is Emily's international health and lifestyle blog and is dedicated to living well with arthritis, and it provides invaluable support for many of my patients and resources for myself as a physician.

Beat Arthritis Naturally, and now *Eat Well with Arthritis*, use evidence-based approaches that combine traditional treatments with complementary and alternative therapies, providing a safe, healthy way to optimise the quality of life for people of all ages living with arthritis. In my experience, the best quality of life is achieved through the balanced combination of pharmacotherapy with lifestyle modifications. With these recipes, and the principles from *Beat Arthritis Naturally*, you have the opportunity to improve your health and wellbeing, and feel good.

Dr Lauren Freid

Rheumatologist,
Ventura, CA

INTRODUCTION

Eat Well with Arthritis is a gentle way to ease the door open into new ways of living and eating positively with your arthritis. Nutrition is an effective place to begin as the gut houses 70 per cent of the immune system, and it is essential to managing your physical health and mental wellbeing. But nutrition is just one part of your colourful mosaic of lifestyle habits and choices, from sleep and stress, to movement and more, blending together to create a personalised picture of your health. This picture looks different for each of us, depending on our genetics, age, sex, environment, immune health and even our daily sleeping habits, stress levels, exercise and diet. Just as our fingerprints are all different, our experience of arthritis, and how it manifests will be unique too.

Arthritis is more than a few stiff joints, or something that happens with age or the result of an old sports injury. Symptoms associated with arthritis include (but are not limited to) chronic pain and inflammation, poor sleep and fatigue, and joint swelling and flare-ups, alongside the ongoing healthcare admin of hospital appointments and blood tests, prescriptions and painkillers. It can feel overwhelming at times – and it is largely misunderstood. The most recent study of the public's perception of arthritis highlighted that people often confuse rheumatoid arthritis (RA), osteoarthritis (OA) and other joint-related conditions, with 76 per cent of Brits unable to identify a description of RA in one survey. There are over 100 different types of arthritis and related musculoskeletal conditions, affecting an estimated 350 million people globally, and it can happen to anyone at any age. (Only one third of Brits interviewed in that survey knew that it could happen to those between the ages of 16 and 24.)

When you are living with arthritis, you are not only managing that long list above, but you may also turn to healthcare professionals, family and friends or Doctor Google to find any and every idea that might help you to make your day-to-day life better. You spend (and probably have spent) hours researching, talking to others online and in person, and reading online forums, social media posts and health-blog articles to try to find the answers. And with this, it may feel as though you are adding yet another load to an already overflowing cart of stuff that you are pulling up a hill every day.

Well, I am here to take you on a downhill route and lighten the load for you at the same time, because I understand that overwhelming feeling all too well. After five years of living with arthritis, I not only felt overwhelm, but also complete despair, and I thought, 'What could I lose by giving this a go?' – 'this' being a complete overhaul of my diet and lifestyle habits, to help ease my pain and reduce arthritis flare-ups.

The first place most of us go to for help is Google (or any search engine) to look up the foods that are deemed 'good' for arthritis, and the foods that are cited as being inflammatory. Right now, as I write this, the search term 'foods for arthritis' on Google has 120,000,000 results – so many zeros that I couldn't figure out how to say the number at first, but that's 120 million different webpages listing information about the foods that may or may not (as there's a lot of misinformation around) help you manage your arthritis. And on the flip side, there are 47.5 million search results for 'foods to avoid with arthritis' and plenty of scaremongering around tomatoes (more on these later with some updated research since the first book – spoiler – they are actually very good for us).

The truth is that you could spend hours searching for the 'right' recipe or online article, and you probably will not be any closer to discovering what might help (or hinder) your journey towards feeling better. The good news is, backed by research and healthcare professionals, with *Eat Well with Arthritis* and *Beat Arthritis Naturally* we have the tools to tackle this together. The first step is understanding: understanding your condition and what you can do to feel good every day. All of the principles, research and advice in *Beat Arthritis Naturally* are reflected in this book, and woven into every recipe too. With both books, you now have access to 150 anti-inflammatory recipes, tools and tips to equip you on this road ahead.

If you are new here, *Beat Arthritis Naturally* is the foundation to taking ownership of your health and wellbeing, and learning to live with your arthritis. Both books will support you to navigate your life with arthritis. My aim is to help you to live with arthritis in a happier, healthier and more holistic way for a better quality of life. And of course, to eat well with arthritis, every day.

How did I end up writing about how to live well with arthritis?

Despite not being diagnosed with arthritis until my early twenties, I was four years old when I was hospitalised with swollen knees. I have very vague memories of sleeping on a hospital bed. After one week I was discharged, and although I was checked for juvenile idiopathic arthritis in the months following, I was signed off after no further symptoms appeared and received no formal diagnosis. It was not until years later that I was diagnosed with 'seronegative arthritis', after two years of mis-diagnosis, fatigue, frustration and feeling like my fingers were going to pop with the swelling.

My rheumatologist at the time placed me on the first rung on the ladder of medications, starting with naproxen, an NSAID (non-steroidal anti-inflammatory drug), and then sulfasalazine, a DMARD (disease-modifying anti-rheumatic drug). These had little to no effect, but then methotrexate started to reduce the swelling in my hands and the pain subsided a little too. Steroid injections also provided occasional temporary relief. But I was constantly struck with a cold, or a bug with flu-like symptoms, or flu itself,

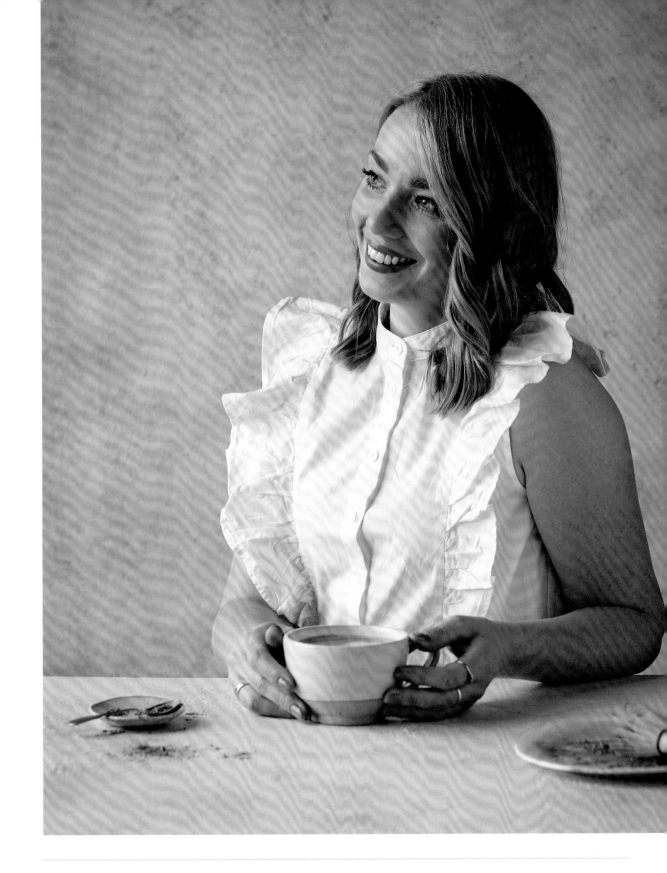

and the exhaustion remained debilitating. My lifestyle and lack of nutrition did not help, as my diet back then included a number of overly processed or preserved foods, refined carbohydrates, sugar-filled sauces and cakes, and I pushed the boundaries on caffeine and alcohol. Don't get me wrong, I did put cucumber in my tuna sandwiches, had an apple or grapes for a snack and occasionally a sliced banana on my breakfast cereal. I was not considerate about what I was eating unless I could choose from a menu and/or someone else was cooking the food for me (thank you, Mum!).

Self-care was not yet a buzzword, and even if it was, I would not have been able to tell you what it meant or how to execute it in my own life. But it's what I needed the most and I did not realise this until I started Arthritis Foodie in 2018. I became acutely aware of how important it is to take care of your body – to listen to it and be attentive to it – because we only get one. It's not just the food we put into it either. I now sing about the whole picture to anyone who will listen: food and nutrition, sleep, exercise and emotional wellbeing, as well as medicine and 'go-to' things for pain management (that work for you, your body and your condition). I documented my journey online, mainly through Instagram, and in a handwritten diary – the good and the bad – from my diet and the subsequent toilet habits, to sleep duration and potential flare-up triggers. I started to feel a small difference in my energy and pain levels after a month, but a significant and positive change after three months, and even more so after a year.

Everything that I was doing was through my own research, trial and error, and testing on myself. But I knew that the healthcare professionals who I was learning from (many have contributions in *Beat Arthritis Naturally*) were right in their approaches. And there was nothing woo-woo about it, because it was backed by science, and I was not throwing my medication in the bin. I was still taking it and I found that what I was doing complemented it. It enabled my body (and my mind) to get a hold on my arthritis and control what I could, when I could, to feel better.

The Arthritis Foodie community began asking me privately through direct messages where I was getting my information from, and how they could access it. But sadly I did not have anywhere to send them to, as there was not a pass to the inner machinery of my mind where thoughts (about beating arthritis naturally or otherwise) are produced and stored, and thank goodness there isn't. Their (your!) requests did not go unnoticed though. In 2019 I started writing the book that would become *Beat Arthritis Naturally*, but I had absolutely no idea how it would ever be published. I campaigned with a company called Publishizer, and eventually, through what can only be described as divine intervention, I met with Yellow Kite Books that December.

My wish was simple: to provide people like me with the book that I had needed when I first started living with arthritis. Using my own experiences, and the brilliant minds of rheumatologists, doctors, immunologists, nutritionists, scientists, physical therapists and health experts, it really is the book I wished I could have had in 2013, when I was 20 years old and had absolutely no idea what to do or how to feel better. Since its publication day in May 2021, it has become a bestselling book on Amazon and I have had the joy of reading countless stories and numerous online reviews on how Beat Arthritis Naturally has helped you. Every day it is empowering people all over the world to feel less alone and to find ways to manage their arthritis, pain and symptoms.

Eat Well with Arthritis blooms from my first book and is packed with colourful, nutritious and exciting new recipes for you and your loved ones to share together. It also includes insights from two brilliant healthcare professionals – Dr Deepak Ravindran and Cheryl Crow, who are doing important work in supporting many people with their chronic pain. Whether you are new here or not, I hope that the principles in my books help you to feel good and live well, for as long as possible. Thank you for being here, and thank yourself for taking these steps towards better health.

'My aim is to help you to live with arthritis
in a happier, healthier and more holistic way
for a better quality of life.'

LIVING WITH ARTHRITIS

'In fact, the only thing that's truly under our control is where, when, and how we repeatedly direct our attention – and whether we're directing it consciously.'

Dr Elizabeth A. Stanley, author and professor at Georgetown University

Before turning to your recipes, it is helpful to understand why and how they may help you on your way to feeling good. In isolation, the recipes in this book will nourish and support your body, mind and overall wellbeing – that I am sure of – but, to feel the difference even more, it is important to understand how further elements of your day-to-day life impact on you. That's why, through these pages, I will walk you through the all-important principles of living well with arthritis. As with my first book, these principles are backed up by science and research, with exciting new evidence published since I wrote *Beat Arthritis Naturally*.

In this chapter I'll explore:

- Why your arthritis is personal to you
- What the different types of arthritis are
- What helps to treat arthritis
- What doesn't help your arthritis
- How to manage your pain
- How you can adapt your kitchen to help you
- What store cupboard, fridge and freezer essentials you should have
- What easy food swaps you can do
- How to track your meals to see what triggers symptoms

Making peace with your condition, and learning everything you can to live better with it, is about taking control of your body and mindset. Some days it will be easier to do this than others. The overhaul of your habits might be hard at the beginning, but your new choices should hopefully become second nature, as you notice the difference that they are making. As Dr Stanley iterates, even if we cannot control the situation around us, what we can control and choose to do is take charge of where, when and how we direct our attention. Finally, these are all things that can be implemented alongside medication, but if you are unsure about any of the contents of this chapter or beyond, please consultant your medical professional.

'Making peace with your condition and learning everything you can to live better with it, is about taking control of your body and mindset.'

Arthritis and you

Musculoskeletal conditions are the leading contributor to disability worldwide with approximately 1.7 billion people globally living with lower back pain, neck pain, osteoarthritis and rheumatoid arthritis among others. It may afflict you when you are young or old, whether you are tall or short, male or female; it does not discriminate and occurs in all races, age groups and sexes. Osteoarthritis (OA) and rheumatoid arthritis (RA) are the most prevalent forms of arthritis, but as mentioned earlier, there are over 100 types. Whether you can pick out the name of your arthritis here or not, this book has been written with the common joint pain denominator in mind: inflammation. RA is classed as an autoimmune disease (AID) and other arthritis AIDs include juvenile idiopathic arthritis (JIA) and a category of arthritis called spondyloarthritis (this includes Ankylosing Spondylitis, Reactive Arthritis, Psoriatic Arthritis, and Arthritis related to Inflammatory Bowel Disease).

Autoimmune diseases are chronic inflammatory disorders caused by abnormal immune-system function, and research indicates that autoimmune diseases occur when a person with genetic predisposition encounters certain environmental triggers that may turn the disease process 'on'. Studies have demonstrated that up to 30 per cent of AIDs are heritable. This shows how important it is to take care of our wellbeing, from what we eat to how we move. Inflammation makes its appearance in varying ways in arthritic conditions, including gout, RA and even in osteoarthritis, which is usually perceived as simply 'something that happens as you get older', with many being told that there is very little that they can do to feel better.

Osteoarthritis is the most widespread form of arthritis, and for a long time it was considered a non-inflammatory disease that was the result of 'wear and tear'. In the last few decades (since the 1990s), it has been understood that inflammation is not only present in the majority of those living with OA, but that it is actively involved in the progression of the disease. OA may not necessarily comply with all of the classic signs of inflammation, but there is now a wealth of scientific evidence showing that inflammation plays an integral role in the development of osteoarthritis. Yet, despite the high prevalence of OA in the global population, there is no disease-modifying drug available for the management of OA, unlike other autoimmunity-based arthritic conditions like RA.

With numerous types of arthritis, and taking into account age, environment and genetics, the condition manifests differently from one person to the next. But they all involve symptoms such as joint pain, swelling and stiffness, difficultly and restriction in movement, fatigue and sleep disturbance, decline in mental wellbeing and muscle wasting. A given medicinal therapy may help one person, but that same intervention may not work for another. The journey of living with arthritis can be trial and error, but if you are taking a medication with the purpose of combatting inflammation and reducing pain, then implementing the lifestyle approaches to achieve the same effect has to be worth a try.

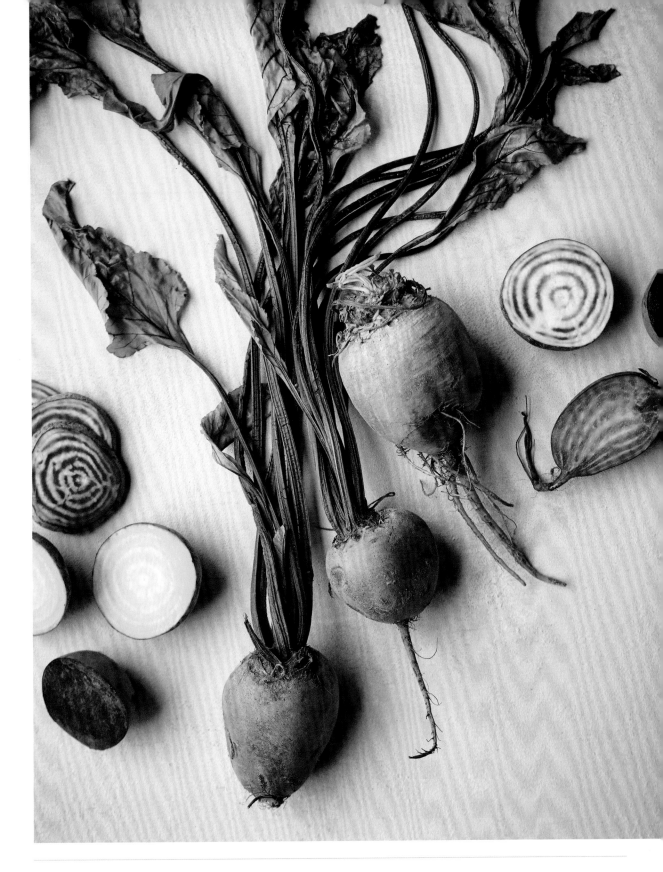

INFLAMMATION IN THE BODY

What is it? (acute and chronic)

Inflammation is often misunderstood and labelled as being 'bad' or 'not good for us', but it actually depends on what kind of inflammation it is, what the symptoms are and how long it has lasted. Acute inflammation is important to our survival as a species; in fact, life would not be possible without it. As life evolved on Earth, it was necessary for organisms to defend themselves against unwanted visitors. A highly complex system has evolved over millions of years to protect us against things like viruses, bacteria and all the other pathogens – usually without us even noticing – and this is known as the immune system.

Acute inflammation is the process by which your immune system both recognises and defends you against these unwanted visitors and repairs damage. It is visible as swelling, redness and increased temperature in the affected area. This pro-inflammatory process partially destroys the body's own tissue, which is why the process is limited in time and subsides as soon as the 'intruder' has been successfully fought off. Afterwards, the opposite of this (an anti-inflammatory process) initiates healing of the affected tissue. It is a finely tuned balance between initial pro-inflammatory activities and anti-inflammatory healing processes, which leads to a complete recovery of the affected area. To sum up, it persists for a short duration, is usually found at the area of injury or infection and is a sophisticated operation only occurring when needed.

So, when is it that inflammation can become potentially harmful to us? When inflammation happens without any obvious and typical signs, it is known as chronic low-grade inflammation. This chronic low-grade inflammation is long-lasting and can persist for weeks, months or even years. Although chronic inflammation is weaker in intensity, in time it can lead to many chronic diseases, including cancer and cardiovascular, neurodegenerative or respiratory diseases, as well as arthritis. Signs and symptoms of chronic inflammation are less obvious than the normal inflammation we see in our bodies, and include body pain; arthralgia (joint pain without inflammation); myalgia (muscle aches and pain); chronic fatigue and insomnia; depression, anxiety and mood disorders; gastrointestinal complications (gut dysbiosis) like constipation, diarrhoea and acid reflux; weight gain or weight loss and frequent infections. In conditions like arthritis, the chronic inflammation may lead to joint destruction, such as in osteoarthritis where it leads to a breakdown of the cartilage layer in joints. For more on chronic inflammation and chronic pain, head to the chapter with Dr Deepak, pages 41–45.

ACUTE VS CHRONIC INFLAMMATION

	Acute inflammation	Systemic chronic inflammation
Trigger	PAMPs (infection), DAMPs (cellular stress, trauma)	DAMPs (Exposome: a collection of environmental factors, such as stress and diet, to which an individual is exposed and which can have an effect on health, metabolic dysfunction, tissue damage)
Duration	Short-term	Long-term
Magnitude	High-grade	Low-grade
Outcome(s)	Healing, trigger removal, tissue repair	Collateral damage
Biomarkers	Il-6, TNF-α, IL-1β, CRP	Silent

DAMP	Damage-associated molecular pattern (injury, infection, unwanted visitors). DAMPs are cell-derived from the host and initiate and perpetuate immunity in response to trauma, tissue damage, tumor cells and dead or dying cells, either in the absence or presence of pathogenic infection.
PAMP	Pathogen-associated molecular pattern (a diverse set of microbial molecules that alert immune cells to destroy intruding pathogens). PAMPs are derived from microorganisms (viruses, foreign substances) and therefore drive inflammation in response to pathogenic infections.
Il-6, TNF-α, IL-1β, CRP	During acute inflammation all of these biomarkers may be elevated, and CRP is often used to diagnose forms of inflammatory arthritis.
Silent	Non canonical standard biomarkers = there is no ideal or reliable biomarker in chronic low-grade inflammation, therefore this is the name that is given to it. There are presently no standard biomarkers for indicating the presence of health-damaging chronic inflammation. (Note: this is often why it may take time to diagnose)

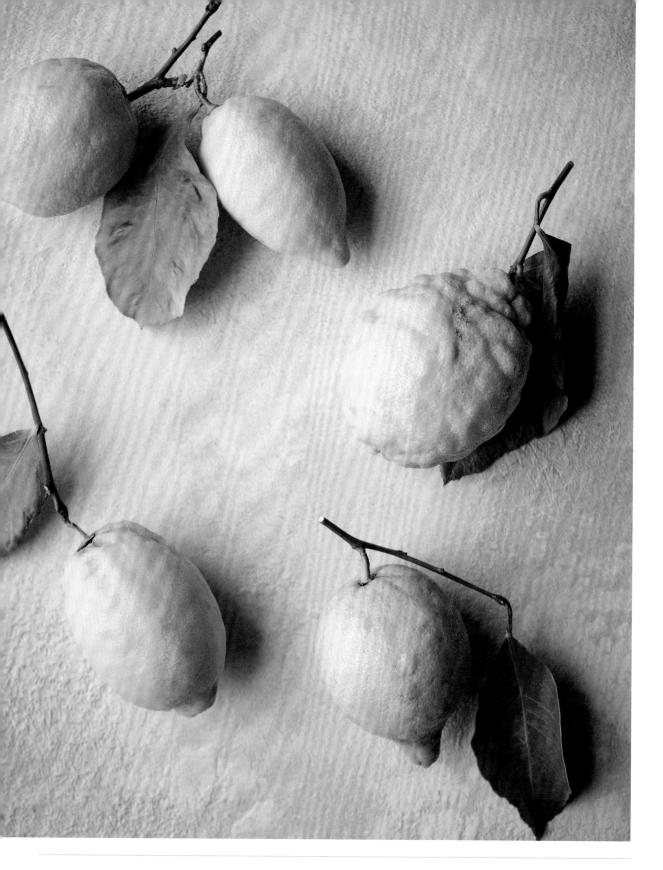

EAT WELL WITH ARTHRITIS

What may help?

Anti-inflammatory nutrition

A good place to start is the Mediterranean diet (MD), typically consisting of a high intake of vegetables, fruits, nuts, legumes and extra virgin olive oil, with moderate intakes of fish, poultry and dairy products, less red meat and a moderate amount of red wine.

It has been shown to preserve human health in myriad ways, from protecting against cardiovascular diseases, to preventing alterations in gut microbiota* (remember there's 70 per cent of your entire immune system in the gut) and exerting long-term anti-inflammatory effects. The MD is packed with polyphenols (more on these on page 52), and research has shown how plant polyphenols may have a positive impact on arthritic and inflammatory conditions, namely OA, RA and autoimmune diseases as the most researched. Studies indicates that the gut influences our feelings and communicates with the brain, and antioxidant-rich foods – found in the MD – reduce the risks of depression and cognitive decline.

The MD is a foundation of the recipe ideas in this book, but although not as researched, there are other diets that offer similar benefits, such as the Nordic diet. It's important to reiterate that we are individual human beings who will react differently, based on our genetics, gut microbiome, lifestyle, environment and immunity.

*Gut microbiota: the collection of microorganisms, including bacteria, archaea, fungi and viruses, in the gut.

Exercise and movement

Through fear of 'doing damage', many people living with arthritis tend to speculate that exercise will cause them (more) harm, but this is not the case. The European League Against Rheumatism (EULAR) 'Recommendations for Physical Activity in People with Inflammatory Arthritis and Osteoarthritis' has provided us with the first evidence-based guidelines about the quality and quantity of exercise that is beneficial specifically for people living with arthritis.

Regular exercise is demonstrated to exert anti-inflammatory effects, and regular physical activity, exercise and weight loss offer protection against a wide variety of chronic diseases associated with low-grade inflammation. Physical activity is now advocated as an anti-inflammatory therapy for patients with rheumatic diseases, and one review has demonstrated that acute exercise does not appear to worsen pain symptoms. Alongside the positive effects on mental health and wellbeing, exercise may also have a positive impact on our gut by diversifying the gut microbiota. Despite requiring more human trials, exercise may in the future provide a beneficial treatment for several chronic- and immune-based diseases, like RA, and may help to manage inflammation.

However, over-exercising can be pro-inflammatory, as can not doing anything at all. Avoiding the extremes, there is a sweet-spot in the middle – moderate or light exercise – which has beneficial anti-inflammatory effects that could help to alleviate inner inflammation. It can even help our sleep quality too, just as long as it is not right before bedtime. My favourite forms of exercise are swimming, walking and yoga. Yoga is a mind, body and soul practice and helps to increase flexibility, strength, mobility and balance, with the potential to decrease inflammation in the blood and reduce cortisol (the stress hormone), with tangible benefits for the whole body. It has been shown to reduce rheumatic disease symptoms and disability, as well as improve self-efficacy and mental health. Dr Lauren Freid, who provided the Foreword for this book, is both a rheumatologist and a yoga instructor.

Restful sleep

Getting a good night's sleep feels good and does good. Even more importantly, it's great for your immune system, with anti-inflammatory benefits. In fact, scientists are yet to find a biological function that isn't impaired by poor sleep quality, or equally doesn't benefit from good sleep quality. Humans are asleep for a third of our lives, but roughly two-thirds of adult humans are sleeping less than the necessary (and recommended minimum) of eight hours a night. Understandably, sleep disturbances are present in 67–88 per cent of chronic pain disorders, like arthritis. Poor sleep is often associated with depression too.

Immune health and sleep are bidirectionally intertwined: sleep defends and protects us when we are well, and the immune system stimulates sleep when we are unwell (I remember sleeping a lot when I first got arthritis!) Recently, emerging evidence illustrates a similar bidirectional links between sleep and inflammation, too. Sleep is the longest duration of time in which the body has low levels of inflammation, and the opportunity to heal, partly due to a reduction in stress (which impacts inflammation) and the body being in a fasted state (not eating). One study has shown that when the body is in a fasted state, it produces a substance that directly interferes with the process of inflammation connected to several disorders, including AIDs, autoinflammatory disorders, type 2 diabetes and Alzheimer's disease.

Less sleep is sure to increase our inflammation, but it is not always easy to get to sleep. Maintaining a regular sleep time and routine is key, with rituals before bed to calm, relax, and ease you into a good night's sleep, such as Epsom salts baths, reading a book or slow bedtime yoga.

Emotional wellbeing and environment

Getting into nature, connecting to our inner world and taking care of our emotional needs (as well as our physical ones) are all vital to managing inflammation levels and overall happiness. You can read about why stress impacts us further on page 23 and the ways you might be able to relieve stress and inflammation through mindful activities, and the environment around you. Your environment includes the places you are in and the people you surround yourself with. It is vital to our wellbeing to have safe spaces and in those spaces, to have people who we feel safe with. Being in nature is proven to reduce our heart rate; lower stress hormones; improve our immune system function; support our breathing;

counter stress, anxiety and depression; and increase a sense of calm and relaxation. Even indoor foliage, such as house plants and flowers, provide stress relief.

Reading, writing and drawing, are largely accessible and relatively cheap ways to feel good too. Within only six minutes, research shows that reading reduces stress levels by up to 60 per cent. Applying gratitude, specifically through positive emotional writing, also alleviates stress and anxiety, and any form of art-making has the capacity to reduce our stress levels.

Breathwork and yogic breathing, listening to music or playing it, and mindfulness and mind-body therapies (like Tai Chi, Qigong, yoga and meditation), have also all been cited as providing positive benefits and reducing stress, pain and depressive symptoms. Meditation and mindfulness help to increase awareness of your body, mind and feelings in the present moment, without judgement. New research shows how mindfulness-based meditation has been effective in reducing pain in chronic pain patients.

'Immune health and sleep are bidirectionally intertwined; sleep defends and protects us when we are well, and the immune system stimulates sleep when we are unwell.'

What hinders?

Inflammatory foods

The antitheses to the MD diet, are the standard American diet (SAD) and the Western pattern diet (WPD). They are the most inflammatory diets, characterised by a high content of meat, ultra-processed foods, processed meats, saturated fats, refined produce, sugar, alcohol, and an associated reduced consumption of fruits and vegetables, with barely any fibre. Typically the food is high in salt, sugar, additives (E-numbers), saturated or trans fats, and is largely weight gaining (obesity is associated with chronic low-level inflammation). Obesity has also been linked with an increased risk of inflammatory rheumatic diseases, such as RA, AS and psoriatic arthritis (PsA). Some of the major risk factors for inflammation-induced chronic diseases are infections, obesity, alcohol, tobacco and diet.

Inflammation and illness-inciting chemicals have been demonstrated to increase by about 70 per cent with a high-fat and low-fibre diet, but the good news is that switching to a Mediterranean-style anti-inflammatory diet for 30 days reverses the changes. One study found that those with an inflammatory diet had a 40 per cent greater risk of depression and further research found a direction connection between a poor diet (junk food, processed and unhealthy foods), and depression and anxiety. High GI foods, such as processed foods, as well as white potatoes and sugary soft drinks, are rapidly digested and cause considerable fluctuations in blood glucose and insulin levels. A diet based on high GI foods has been shown to cause and worsen inflammation whereas low GI foods, such as wholegrain breads, brown rice, legumes, quinoa and sweet potatoes are slowly digested, producing gradual rises in blood glucose and insulin levels. The MD appears to be the most science-supported diet. Naturally anti-inflammatory, it has the most potential to battle against the chronic inflammatory conditions and AIDs so prevalent in the world today.

Sedentary behaviour

Sitting is inflammatory, and one in four adults globally (28 per cent or 1.4 billion people) are physically inactive, with around 81 per cent of UK office workers spending 4–9 hours sitting at their desks each day. It's an epidemic whether or not you are living with arthritis. 'You freeze, you seize', as the saying goes, and there is truth in this. Our bodies need movement, and a lack of it results in muscle wasting, poor joint health, reduced fitness and exercise tolerance, a decrease in range of movement and flexibility, as well as a higher risk of other injuries due to poor joint stability. Exercise may be an important potential modifier of harmful pro-inflammatory markers typical to inflammation but it's not always easy when you're in pain – most people living with chronic conditions tend to exercise less, which can make symptoms worse.

Sedentary behaviour (not moving) and obesity are accompanied by low-grade inflammation. It has been demonstrated, specifically in RA, that obesity is associated with significantly higher CRP and ESR (blood markers of inflammation). Increasing sedentary behaviour results in pro-inflammatory markers, but increased levels of light, moderate and vigorous activity, induces lower inflammatory markers and higher levels of anti-inflammatory markers. It's important to go at your own pace and only do what you can, when you can, finding joy in your own movement and feeling good in your body. Be comfortable and safe when exercising. Move in a way that is right for you; find something that you enjoy and set realistic goals.

Reduced sleep

If you aren't sleeping well, then your body is not doing enough of what it needs to while you're asleep. This can cause an excess of inflammation and impact on your immune system's ability to fight against those unwanted visitors we met earlier (see page 16). Restless nights are seen as an inevitable outcome when living with arthritis, but not only does joint pain trigger a loss of sleep, but sleep disturbance worsens joint pain, fatigue, depression and anxiety, and can even accelerate joint damage. Pain can be both a cause and an effect of inadequate sleep.

Overall, chronic sleep deprivation can be viewed as a state of chronic stress impacting immune function and general health, so it's no wonder that sleep disturbance is significantly related to chronic pain intensity and function. In both pain-free individuals and those living with chronic pain, lack of sleep has been shown to contribute to the exacerbation of pain processes. Losing sleep for only one night has a significant impact on our immune system too, reducing our first line of defence (natural killer cells) against unwanted visitors by 70 per cent.

Dining close to bedtime is typically accompanied by poorer sleep, gastrointestinal reflux, worsening sleep quality and inflammation by inhibiting the anti-inflammatory fasted state. The gut needs space from you (it's not personal), so if you can avoid eating 2–3 hours before you go to bed, it should aid a better night's sleep, as may eating in a window of only 10–11 hours per day.

High stress

Stress can be triggered by your body, mind and thoughts, or your environment and is a real trigger for my inflammation and pain. Chronic stress = chronic inflammation = chronic pain. An acute stress response (perhaps when you're making a public speech or running late for an appointment), like acute inflammation, is short-lived and temporary. Severe acute stress, near-death experiences or assaults for example, can lead to mental health issues or may also worsen into a chronic state of stress, and increase bodily inflammation. Depression is four times more common among people in persistent pain compared to those without pain, and those with long-term musculoskeletal conditions are almost twice as likely to report feeling anxious or depressed compared to the rest of the population. Chronic psychological stress is connected with the body losing its ability to regulate the inflammatory response, which can lead to disease, and this excessive inflammation plays a critical role in the relationship between stress and stress-related diseases too. Living with long-term chronic pain conditions takes its toll, and it is essential to be kind to yourself and implement mindful activities to reduce your stress levels where possible. It's not easy to escape stress, but there are things we can do to manage it (see page 21).

| **Substances** | Extensive research over the last several decades has discovered that some of the major risk factors for most inflammation-induced chronic conditions are infections, obesity, alcohol, tobacco, and diet. We have already covered diet and obesity, but what is it about smoking, alcohol and caffeine that has an impact on inflammation? |

Smoking can have damaging effects on our bones and joints. The toxins associated with smoking act on the immune system, weakening our defences and promoting autoimmunity. Smoking (yourself or passively) also increases the risk of developing over 50 serious health conditions, and promotes certain AIDs, like RA or PsA. Heavy smokers have over two-and-a-half times an increased risk of the most severe form of RA; luckily after 15 years of quitting for good, the risk decreases by a third. However, if you already have arthritis, smoking can exacerbate your symptoms and disrupt the efficacy of your medication or treatments, including surgery. Speak to your healthcare provider about quitting, and they will be able to equip you with the right support to help you to do it.

Alcohol reduction or elimination is a common theme in healthy diets, including the MD where wine is enjoyed in small quantities with dinner. The WPD or SAD, on the other hand, feature a high alcohol intake which is embedded in the culture too. But unlike caffeine it's not the stimulant you might think it is. Alcohol is a sedative, but this initial sedating effect is short-lived, resulting in a fragmented and disturbed sleep in the second part of the night. And we know what happens with a lack of sleep (see page 23)! Like me, you might have noticed that alcohol aggravates your symptoms too. Heavy alcohol use can increase inflammation in the body and binge drinking especially can increase body-wide inflammation. Over-consumption may increase the risk of certain types of arthritis (if you don't already have it) and 25 conditions are entirely attributable to or associated with alcohol. Follow the recommended guidelines (or less if you're on certain types of medication), or abstain completely.

Caffeine is another enemy to sleep and alcohol's accomplice. The sleep-disruptive effects of caffeine have been well researched; it blocks the sleep-inducing activities in the brain that build up during the day and increases adrenaline production, producing a temporary increased state of alertness. We might think this alertness is temporary, but caffeine remains in your system. A large shop-bought coffee disrupts sleep significantly even when drunk six hours before bedtime, reducing the duration of sleep by an hour. Note that if you drink a caffeinated coffee at 12pm, 12 hours later in bed, a quarter of the caffeine is still affecting your brain. We need our sleep!

EAT WELL WITH ARTHRITIS

MANAGING YOUR PAIN

There are so many different things we are recommended and bombarded with to help us with our pain levels. But like many things, it is individual to you, your arthritis, comfort and pain levels. Here are some ideas for you to try that you may have already heard of, or not yet come across at all.

At home

- Heat/cold therapy
- Compression clothing
- Transcutaneous electrical nerve stimulation (TENS) machine
- Epsom salts – in a bowl or a bath
- Cannabidiol (CBD) – oral or topical
- Peppermint – oral (calming) or topical (cooling)
- Aloe vera – topical (soothing) or oral (nourishing)
- Capsaicin – topical (heat)
- Glucosamine – oral or topical

Out of home

- Acupuncture
- Massage (Swedish, hot-stone, aromatherapy, deep-tissue, shiatsu)
- Physical therapies (chiropractic, osteopathy, physiotherapy, occupational therapy, podiatry)

'It's important to go at your own pace and only do what you can, when you can. Find joy in your own movement and feel good in your body.'

Equipment and tools to help in the kitchen

Y-shaped peeler	A hand-held, Y-shaped, wide, sturdy and strong peeler is easier to use when your hands are hurting or swollen.
Avocado slicer	I had an avocado-hand mishap (I cut my hand open removing a stone from an avocado as I am heavy-handed and clumsy) and I do not want this happening to any of you. My hand was out of action for almost a month. Please use this slicer/stone remover/scooper tool!
Blender	You will use this all the time. Breville ones are not too expensive, last for years and do not take up too much room. You will be making five-minute breakfast smoothies, iced matcha lattes and cashew nut pasta sauces in no time.
Large cooking pot	Essentially, a non-stick shallow casserole dish (26 or 30cm/10½ or 12in in diameter). Make sure that it can be used on a hob, as some are for oven use only. Try to find a lightweight one if you can, too.
Pyrex oven dish	For those extra-crispy roasted vegetables or baked chocolate brownies. An essential for the kitchen.
Non-stick trays	An assortment of sizes and depths is recommended for any oven-based cooking or baking.
Measuring jug	A strong Pyrex one, with all the different units you need from litres to pints.
Weighing scales	Any will do, but I prefer digital as they provide a more precise measurement reading.
Food processor	The processor I have at home has three different set-ups: a small blender that works like a pestle and mortar, a medium-sized blender and a large food processer. The food processer has grating and peeling settings too.
Anti-fatigue mat	To help to stimulate blood circulation and reduce fatigue when standing up for long periods of time (a tip from Cheryl – more of these in the next chapter).

Go-to gadgets

The world does not always consider the arthritic hand, wrist or arm, but luckily some creative designers have. Why not let gadgets do the work for you, so that you don't have to? Or at least only with minimal effort and reduced pain. Here are some of the inventions that might help you in the kitchen:

- **Angled large-grip knives** (adaptive knife with an ergonomic handle positioned at a 90-degree angle, for example)
- **Electric tin opener**, or an under-cabinet multi jar opener
- **Silicone grips** for opening jars and bottles
- **One-cup kettle**
- **Compression gloves**
- **Automatic electric stirrers**

Utensils

Aside from the standard cutlery and wooden spoons, some tools will make your life easier when it comes to cooking.

- **Spatulas**, stirring spoons, serving spoons and a potato masher
- **Flat silicone spatula**
- **Kitchen tongs**
- **Hand-held electric whisk**

Additional essentials

- **Glass or stainless steel mixing bowls** – a range of three sizes
- **Range of pans** – griddle pan, frying pans and a wok
- **Sieve and colander**
- **Food-storage containers**

Store cupboard, fridge and freezer essentials

From week to week, recipe to recipe, the foods you are using will change, but these are the staple items that I like to have in my fridge, freezer and store cupboard as usually something can be rustled up with them. When you are in pain, struggling with a flare-up or simply not in the mood to think about cooking, having these items at the ready will help. Freezing food in batches when you can is a good idea too, and for more tips like this, see the next chapter with occupational therapist Cheryl Crow (pages 46–48). Also, please see the 'freezable' tag on the recipes to see which ones are freezer-friendly.

Fresh/frozen

- Plant milk
- Red onions
- Bananas
- Apples
- Eggs
- Avocados
- Sweet potatoes
- Courgettes
- Salmon or Chicken
- Tofu and/or Tempeh
- Carrots
- Broccoli
- Kale
- Frozen spinach
- Frozen peas
- Frozen raspberries
- Frozen blueberries
- Frozen bulk-made recipes (like mushroom soup or chickpea curry)
- Oranges

Store-cupboard essentials

If this next list is too much for you to purchase in one go, just buy items as and when you see them in a recipe. For me, it is a relief to know that I can cook absolutely anything from home by just getting in fresh ingredients from week to week and topping up the dry store cupboard – e.g. more quinoa or tins of chickpeas.

With all of the below, I choose 100 per cent whole foods wherever possible – no processing, additives or added salt and sugar. If I am able to buy organic and can afford to, then I do that too.

Oils, vinegars and sauces

- Extra virgin olive oil
- Coconut oil
- Sesame oil
- Balsamic vinegar
- White miso paste
- Apple cider vinegar
- Molasses
- Tamari (or soy sauce, if not available)
- Tahini

Beans, pulses and other tins

- Cannellini beans in water
- Chickpeas in water
- Butter beans in water
- Coconut milk
- Red kidney beans in water
- Black beans
- Chopped tomatoes
- Tomato purée

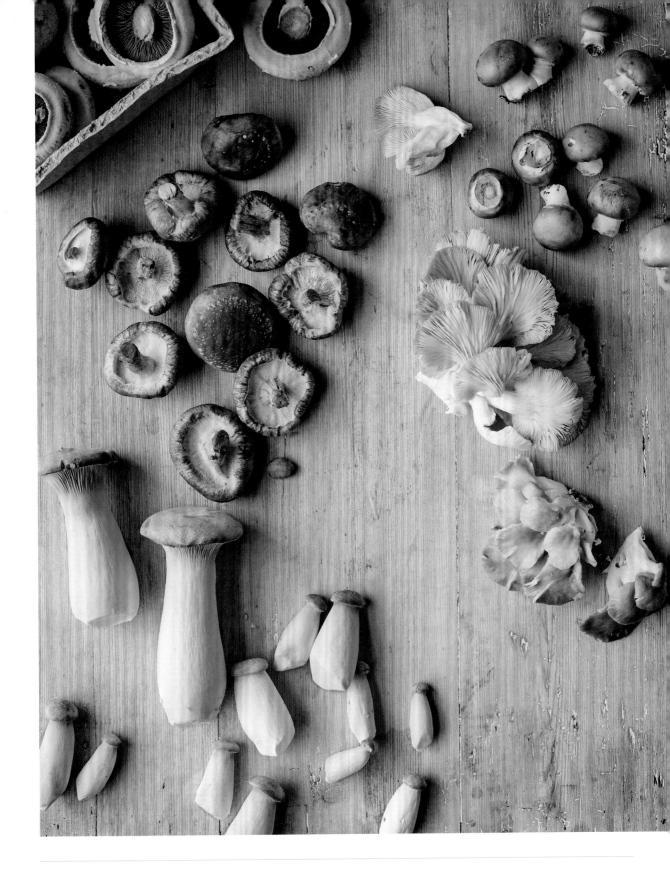

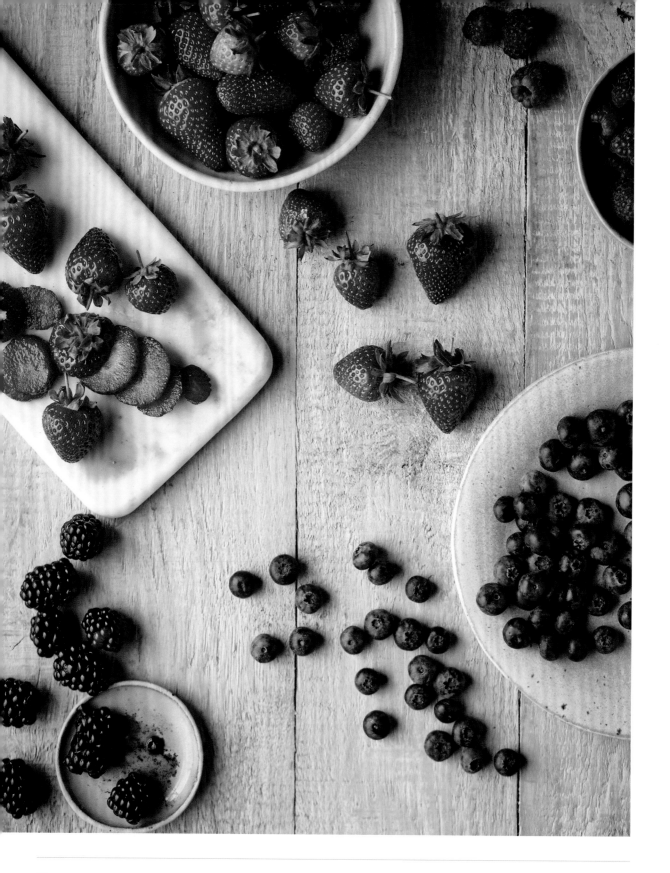

EAT WELL WITH ARTHRITIS

Dry goods	• Quinoa	• Gluten-free flours (brown rice,
	• Gluten-free pasta	buckwheat, oat, coconut, chickpea)
	(red lentil, brown rice)	• Vegetable stock cubes (I like Kallo)
	• Brown rice	• Nutritional yeast flakes
	• Red split lentils	• Polenta
	• Rice noodles	• Baking powder

Herbs, spices and powders	• Garlic cloves	• Cayenne pepper
	• Root ginger (keep	• Mild curry powder
	a piece in the freezer	• Cardamom pods/powder
	and chop from there)	• Black or brown mustard seeds
	• Turmeric root	• Cumin seeds
	• Ground turmeric	• Coriander seeds
	• Ground ginger	• Fennel seeds
	• Ground nutmeg	• Chinese five spice
	• Ground cinnamon	• Ras el hanout
	• Ground cloves	• Dried rosemary
	• Ground cumin	• Dried thyme
	• Ground coriander	• Dried parsley
	• Ground fenugreek	• Dried marjoram
	• Garlic granules	• Dried oregano
	• Onion granules	• Dried mint
	• Paprika	• Dried coriander leaf
	• Smoked paprika	• Italian herbs blend
	• Garam masala	• Bay leaves
	• Chilli powder/flakes	• Star anise
	• Chipotle chilli	• Allspice
	powder/ flakes	• Cinnamon sticks
	• Dried harissa spices	• Black pepper
	• Lacuma powder	• Sea salt
		• Moringa powder

'I became acutely aware of how important it is to take care of your body – to listen to it and be attentive to it – because we only get one.'

Oats, nuts and seeds	• Porridge oats (note: if highly sensitive to gluten, choose oats that have not been packaged in a gluten-producing setting) • Chia seeds • Ground flaxseeds • Sesame seeds • Sunflower seeds	• Pumpkin seeds • Cashew nuts (for sauces) • Walnuts • Pistachios • Hazelnuts • Mixed nuts (i.e. bags of mixed nuts for snacks – containing walnuts, almonds, Brazil nuts, pecans, cashew nuts) • Ground almonds • Flaked almonds
Sweet, savoury and teas	• Honey • Manuka honey • Maple syrup • Date syrup • Vanilla extract • Peanut butter • Almond butter • Desiccated coconut • Coconut sugar • Raw cacao powder • Cacao nibs	• Dates • Sultanas • Raisins • Dried apricots (sulphur dioxide-free) • Matcha powder • Green tea • Herbal teas (I have 30+ different ones in my cupboard, but Rooibos, peppermint and fruit teas are lovely and warming)

Easy food and drink swaps

If it is feeling overwhelming, here are some quick wins for your dinner plate – what to cut back on and what to use instead.

Foods to cut back on. . .	And could replace with. . .
Refined white, processed breads, and rolls	Sourdough bread, wholegrain and seeded wholegrain breads (not GF), oat cakes, brown rice cakes.
Refined and processed breakfast cereals	Porridge – or go to the Breakfast chapter on pages 90–109 for alternative ideas.
White rice and white potatoes	Nutrient-dense brown, red, black and wild rice, quinoa, beans, pulses and legumes, and fibre-rich vegetables (e.g. sweet potatoes).
Commercial processed baked goods: doughnuts, biscuits, cakes, cookies and chocolate bars	Make your own treats – look at the Desserts and Snacks chapters on pages 180–195 and 196–213.
Refined sugar and sugary sweets	Fresh and dried fruits, honey, maple, date or agave syrups, or try making your own snacks (pages 196–213).
Deep-fried foods and trans-fat fried crisps (or chips)	There is no replacement for junk food other than wholesome food, for savoury alternatives, try olives, Crispy Kale (page 211), hummus (page 206), sliced apple with peanut butter, or flavoured nuts (page 210).
Pizza	If you are craving pizza, try the recipe on page 166. You could also have an omelette as your 'pizza' base and top accordingly.
Pasta	Reduce your intake of refined flour by replacing it with wholegrain or brown-rice-noodle dishes, or using brown rice/quinoa/spelt/buckwheat pastas.
Pre-prepared meals, like soups or sandwiches	Be cautious of any additives – only some brands are fresh and transparent about their ingredients – otherwise try the soup and lunch recipes on pages 110–133.
Dairy products	See how you feel with dairy, but certain fermented dairy like kefir, feta cheese, or natural Greek yoghurt has anti- rather than pro-inflammatory effects (due to the breakdown in lactose and high probiotic content).
Alcohol	Organic red wine, alcohol-free lookalikes, or abstention – just be wary of your sugar intake and balance with H_2O.
Fizzy drinks	Add fresh fruit and herbs to water for a delicious refresher or use fruity tea leaves to make iced tea.

TRIGGER TRACKER

A Trigger Tracker is a food diary, a symptom notebook and a tracker for how you are feeling. I hope that some of you may have already thought to do this, but if not, then let me help you to start. Keeping track of the food we eat, our stress levels, the medication we take, and the amount of exercise that we are managing to do (or not do), on top of everything else life may throw at us, can prove to be difficult. It might seem a daunting task to keep track, stay on track and keep tracking whether or not you are on track. Let me break it down for you.

Steps to Your Trigger Tracker

Step 1	Decide what to track (this book will help!).
Step 2	Ensure you listen to your body and stay on a healthy path (eating well and taking care of yourself).
Step 3	Be consistent with writing down how you are feeling from day to day. (Set an alarm to remind yourself at the same time each day, for example.)
Step 4	Review and check in with yourself to see what seems to be helping, what might not be and what could be improved.
Step 5	Stick to it for at least 6–12 weeks, with 12 weeks being the optimal amount of time to notice any changes.

Doctor, yoga instructor and rheumatologist Lauren Freid advises her rheumatology patients to keep journals, tracking food alongside their arthritic symptoms of pain, swelling, stiffness and fatigue. This way, both her and her patients are able to identify patterns, lifestyle habits and dietary triggers that may be intensifying the symptoms of their condition. Not everyone has the same trigger(s). For me, stress, lack of sleep and certain dairy products have an impact on my symptoms. Alcohol used to really affect me the day after drinking it, but I do not drink enough alcohol, or regularly enough, for it to do this now (I drink on special occasions, or when the mood strikes, but very rarely). Whereas, for a friend of mine, her most notable triggers are red meat and alcohol. The only way to know what will be triggering your arthritis is to put in the work, using the template below as a place to begin. This way, you potentially avoid flare-ups of pain, making choices that work for you physically and mentally too (because we all know how pain can impact our mental wellbeing). Being informed about how your body and arthritis operates allows you to make healthier choices in the future. Eventually, these choices will become second nature, as you realise the difference that they make to your wellbeing.

A Trigger Tracker notes what you eat and when, as well as stress, medication, sleep, exercise and alcohol consumption. You note any symptoms you experience along the way. For additional support, you could work with a dietitian or nutritionist, if you have the time and financial ability to do so. I recommend recording how you feel the day after, for example on Thursday write down Wednesday's date and how you are feeling off the back of it, reflecting on what you ate and did on Wednesday. Once you have completed 12 weeks, repeat the process. If you can extend the 9 weeks to 12 before reintroducing anything, then do!

Week 1	Cut out all potential triggers and inflammatory substances, lifestyle behaviours and potential stressors. Start eating, and living, in an anti-inflammatory way.
Weeks 2–8	Continue as you have been doing.
Week 9	On one day of the week only, in one time window of 2 hours (e.g. breakfast, lunch or dinner), reintroduce one 'inflammatory' product and review. (You can also start this process after week 12, if you have more time to devote to this.)
Week 10	On one day of the week only, in one time window of 2 hours (e.g. breakfast, lunch or dinner), reintroduce one 'inflammatory' product and review.
Week 11	On one day of the week only, in one time window of 2 hours (e.g. breakfast, lunch or dinner), reintroduce one 'inflammatory' product and review.
Week 12	On one day of the week only, in one time window of 2 hours (e.g. breakfast, lunch or dinner), reintroduce one 'inflammatory' product and review.

On the next page is an example of a Trigger Tracker in use - you'll see I've filled out a few entries for week 2 and for week 10. Have a go at creating your own using the headings I've used. You can download a Trigger Tracker template free from my website if you'd like to, too. And, remember to use the tracker every day!

Trigger Tracker Template

WEEK/DATE	Breakfast	Lunch	Dinner	Drinks	Snacks
WEEK 2 **Saturday**	Indulgent Chocolate Porridge	Spiced Sweet Potato Soup	Salmon and Puy Lentils with Orange Dressing	Matcha tea Water [3–4 litres*]	Banana Cacao and Coconut Energy Balls
WEEK 2 **Sunday**	Cinnamon Toast Overnight Oats	Spiced Sweet Potato Soup	One-Pot Chicken and Prawn Jambalaya	Green tea Water [3–4 litres*]	Apple Sweet Cinnamon Mixed Nuts
WEEK 10 **Monday**	Bakewell Tart Overnight Oats	Mushroom Noodle Soup	Harissa Lentil Pot	Orange and Cinnamon Warmer Water [3–4 litres*]	Apricot Chia Seed Bites
WEEK 10 **Friday**	Breakfast Granola Bowl	Harissa Lentil Pot leftovers	Grandad Speight's Nasi Goreng	Vanilla Date Hemp Seed Smoothie Water [3–4 litres*]	Coconut Banana 'Cookie' Bites

Exercise (amount and quality) (1–10)	Sleep (duration and quality) (1–10)	Stress (0 = no stress, 10 = high stress)	Alcohol consumption (0 = no alcohol, 10 = more than the recommended units)	Medications Yes/No (write yes if taken them that day)	How do you feel today – pain levels, gut health, swelling, stiffness symptoms? (1–10)	Any potential triggers today? New inflammatory substance introduction?
5, long walk	7, not much sleep	1	0	Yes	6, medium pain levels	No
0, no exercise today	8, fatigued today	5	0	No	7, slightly more than yesterday	No
3, short walk	4, okay sleep	3	0	No	4, not too bad	No
6, light yoga stretches	4, okay sleep	7	7, slightly more than average amount	No	6, a bit sore	Alcohol – glass of white wine last night

0 = extremely good, 10 = very poor, unless otherwise stated
*Water measurement, 1 litre = 35 ounces = 4¼ cups = 1¾ pints

HOW TO NAVIGATE LIFE WITH CHRONIC PAIN

'It's not about getting over things,
it's about making room for them. It's about
painting the picture with contrast.'

Brianna Wiest, author

After reading Chapter 1, you are hopefully now aware of the myriad things that you can do to feel better from day to day. With food being a big part of this, the feel-good, anti-inflammatory recipes in this book will hopefully be recipes that you will go to frequently. But I know what you may have already been thinking. 'How will I be able to cook these recipes without triggering more pain?', or 'What if I am struggling and I need to make something nourishing to eat?'.

Cooking may seem like an overwhelming and daunting task, and even more so when you are living with arthritis. There will be some days when you have the energy to do it, and others when your inner battery is depleted and it is the last thing you can face. Perhaps there will be days when you feel excited by a new recipe, and other days when heating up your leftovers or asking for help is the only way you will actually get fed that evening.

The only thing that ensures that I eat well with arthritis is preparing and planning ahead as much as possible, and ensuring that I have plenty of the Arthritis Foodie 'essentials' listed on page 28 to be able to rustle something up quickly when I need to. Whether it's keeping those essentials stocked up, cooking a big batch of food to either eat during the week or place in the freezer for a later date, or making three jars of overnight oats all at once, so that I know that I have my breakfast sorted for three days in a row. Preparing and planning ahead is what Future Emily consistently thanks Past Emily for. Not only does it save time, but it also saves hassle, stress, and money.

But, what about the day-to-day challenges of living with your arthritis, pain and symptoms? And when you are in the kitchen itself preparing and planning ahead? It can be challenging at times, but the more I have noticed the difference eating well with arthritis has made on my life, the more willing and happier I am to be in the kitchen, because the food makes me feel good and does good. I now get joy from making it (as well as eating it!). If you are new to this journey however, and/or only just beginning to navigate your condition, it may still seem perplexing. That's why I have invited two brilliant minds to contribute to this section of the book. They have kindly provided their expertise in the realms of chronic pain and occupational therapy so that you can understand how to take care of your body (and chronic pain) in the best possible way, inside and outside of the kitchen.

About Your Experts

Dr Deepak Ravindran, NHS Consultant and author

Dr Deepak Ravindran has over 20 years of experience in acute and chronic pain management and is the author of *The Pain-Free Mindset: 7 Steps to Taking Control and Overcoming Chronic Pain*. He has been a consultant in pain medicine since 2010, and is the clinical lead for pain medicine and the Long Covid service at the Royal Berkshire Hospital, Reading. He is one of the few consultants in the UK to possess a triple certification in musculoskeletal medicine and pain medicine, and is a diplomate with the British Society of Lifestyle Medicine. Dr Deepak believes in a multidisciplinary approach to pain conditions, and helps people to overcome their pain, and to improve their quality of life both in the NHS and through his private practices.

Cheryl Crow, Occupational Therapist, and Founder of 'Arthritis Life'

Cheryl Crow has been an occupational therapist for the last 14 years and has lived with rheumatoid arthritis for 20 years. She is well known for her educational (and entertaining) videos featuring arthritis life hacks, product demonstrations and insights into the psychosocial aspects of life with an invisible chronic condition. Having lived with arthritis herself, she has a wealth of knowledge on how helpful the profession of occupational therapy is to those with arthritis and uses it to help people through her channel 'Arthritis Life'.

'Exercise may be an important potential modifier of harmful pro-inflammatory markers typical to inflammation but it's not always easy when you're in pain.'

How to Overcome Your Pain: What is Pain, and How Can You Manage it for a Better Quality of Life?

WITH DR DEEPAK RAVINDRAN

—

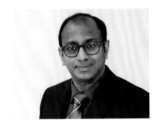

© Rob Cao

Whether it's arthritis, back pain, or pain from an injury, many people all over the world are having to share their life with pain. There is a chronic pain epidemic with estimates that globally 20 per cent of adults, or 1 in 5 people, live with chronic pain, and 10 per cent of adults are newly diagnosed with chronic pain each year. Around 19 per cent of European adults and 20.4 per cent of US adults are living with chronic pain, and it can have a significant impact on your overall health, physical, mental and emotional wellbeing.

Having explored this topic in *Beat Arthritis Naturally*, I thought it was important to delve a little deeper and speak with UK-leading pain consultant and author Dr Deepak Ravindran, to gain even more insight into our pain, how it manifests and what you can do to help reduce it, with some real-life arthritis case studies from his previous NHS patients. For numerous pain relief tips, see Chapter six of *Beat Arthritis Naturally*.

'Aided by good support and lifestyle measures that can reverse the effect that stress and inflammation can have on the nervous and immune systems, there is a very good chance that you can overcome your pain.'

Dr Deepak Ravindran

Emily: Why do you work with people living with chronic pain?

Dr Deepak: Pain is often the most common reason for people to seek help and requests from healthcare, from primary care and general practice to a hospital appointment or accident and emergency. But there is a bigger picture to pain, and I saw the importance of helping patients to access more ways to manage their pain than was originally thought possible.

Emily: Pain is a huge topic, and you explain it so well in your book. Nociception and pain are not the same, how?

Dr Deepak: 'Nociception' is a new word for your readers to learn, it has been around for a little while in the medical language and literature, but it has been frequently misunderstood. It is a phenomenon that occurs in all of us. But we've always confused it with the term 'pain'.

We should use the term 'nociception' when somebody is hurt, and chemicals are released at the site of the injury. This may be a surgery, a heart attack, a road traffic accident, or an arthritis flare-up where there is swelling, redness and heat in the joint. All of these incidents are going to release chemicals at the site of the injury, and this creation of chemicals is called nociception.

Nociceptive signals then travel in the nerves to the spinal cord, and then to the brain. We used to talk about 'pain pathways', but in fact, nociceptive signals travel in the same nerves that are carrying every other sensation that we feel And, when these signals reach the spinal cord and the brain, they are then processed. This processing happens in the brain based on various predictions, and if it decides that it must bring out a protective response, that's when we get the experience of pain.

In acute pain, when you have surgery, this nociception may be responsible for almost all of the pain experience. However, if you have chronic pain or persistent pain beyond three months and there are not enough chemicals being released or there's no obvious swelling, or the blood tests don't show any sign of infection, it is likely that nociceptive signals form a very small percentage of the pain experience. The rest is going to be determined by the processing that occurs in the spinal cord, bringing about the pain perception and bio-psycho-social model of pain (an approach that considers the interconnection between biology, psychology, and socio-environmental factors). So that is why 'nociception' and 'pain' are two separate phenomena.

Emily: How is pain connected to inflammation?

Dr Deepak: This is a big topic, but you can probably take it apart in small layers. The first part of our understanding of inflammation is based on four characteristics:

- Redness (rubor)
- Heat (calor)
- Swelling (tumour)
- Pain (dolor)

With acute inflammation, these chemicals get released at the site of the injury or inflammation. In the last 10 to 20 years, we have now come to understand that with chronic pain, or when pain has been beyond three months, some kind of an inflammatory process also occurs to account for the severity, or the manifestation, of the pain.

Meaning that the emotion or sensation of pain also occurs because there is a level of inflammation. The only difference is that the inflammation is not something that is accompanied by the redness or the swelling, or anything that you notice when you have an acute injury.

In an acute injury, we know that the immune system is pushing out all these inflammatory cells that make all these changes happen, and we can accept that those changes are painful, because these kinds of acute inflammatory chemicals bring about the nociception.

After travelling to the brain, these signals jump from one nerve to another, and at these junctions (synapses), they are also monitored by representatives of the immune cell. When these immune cells detect a high number of signals coming through from an acute pain or injury, they will change shape, and they start to amplify or dampen the signals depending on whether protection is needed or not.

And so, in the brain and in the spinal cord, at each of these junctions, these representatives of the immune cell (called the microglia) are actually deciding whether or not they have to be a Dr Jekyll (fighting off viruses, and other foreign invaders, removing cellular debris to facilitate wound repair) or a Mr Hyde (releasing inflammatory cytokines that amplify the inflammatory response). If they are in the Mr Hyde mode, they cause a low-grade inflammation, which will amplify all of the signals that are coming from an injured part. And the problem is that in some people, even though the acute inflammation may have gone down, or their knee is not that swollen any more, these Dr Jekyll and Mr Hyde cells haven't gone back to normal. They stay hyper vigilant and looking out for action, and they are ready to protect at the slightest pin drop.

And because they are recalibrated differently, the system stays in a pain experience. These are the people who are left with chronic pain, even though they have nothing acute to show for it (for example, a blood test does not show any signs of it there). But there is still a form of neuro-inflammation ongoing in their junctions in the spinal cord and in the brain. And that is the prevailing theory of central sensitivity, and why chronic pain may be persistent in some people because of this change.

Emily: How is pain connected to food? Why does eating in an anti-inflammatory way matter?

Dr Deepak: This has been one of the most important game changers for me, Emily, and that is why I'm so pleased to connect with you. I have seen living examples of how eating well can make such a difference to pain levels, and it is something that is still very alien for a lot of the mainstream medical minds to wrap their heads around.

To me it is the underlying mechanism. As I mentioned, we understand that central sensitisation is a very real phenomenon, driven largely by these microglial cells. And these microglia, along with other kinds of immune cells, are responsible for nourishing and looking after the nerve cells normally, but when they get hit by an inflammatory response, outside in the form of an injury, or it can come from inside, then it will trigger the immune cell, and that information travels back to the brain through the vagus nerve, and these microglia then are activated. This activation puts them into a Mr Hyde-like mode where they start to express more chemicals, causing the furthering or the amplification of the sensitivity. And this is a phenomenon or the underlying principle of how foods can actually become inflammatory and can worsen the pain in some people.

And when I say 'inside', the gut is the main focus of the inside. What we eat has a huge impact and implication because around 70 per cent of our immune system resides in the gut. Therefore, if you eat a food that is potentially considered as threatening or inflammatory, it's going to trigger the immune cell, and that information travels back to the brain through the vagus nerve, and these microglia get activated.

I have patients who are able to say that they've been able to manage their fibromyalgia, chronic pain or their arthritis pain to a great extent, but then if they have days where they end up eating a load of doughnuts, or ultra-processed foods, that within 24 hours, or sometimes in eight hours, they can feel that their joints get much more painful, that their migraines come back again, or that they feel bloated and their tummy is painful and their IBS acts up. Then it takes a couple of days or a week for them to get back to where they were. And that's how food and nutrition is now a very important consideration when it comes to managing or overcoming your chronic pain. But inflammation can be activated not just by what we eat, but also by lack of sleep, stress, sedentary behaviour and more.

Emily: How important is self-management of your own wellbeing, condition and pain?

Dr Deepak: When living with a chronic condition, you have to put in place simple and important lifestyle measures, because seeing your doctor or a specialist can prove to be difficult. There are often long waiting lists for consultant-led appointments and/or surgical procedures.

For most people living with chronic pain, they may see a healthcare professional for a total of five hours in a year, and for the remaining 8,755 hours are left to their own devices. You need to know what to do for yourself. It can be very overwhelming, so start with something that you're most comfortable with, but you have to start somewhere.

It's so important to have the ability and the confidence to self-manage, and once you do have the confidence, there are so many tools for improving your day-to-day wellbeing.

Emily: How many patients living with chronic pain and/or arthritic conditions have seen a difference in their symptoms after following the plans you have put in place for them?

Dr Deepak: One patient who has osteoarthritis had gone up to 25 stone and was struggling significantly with her weight, as well as being on a high dose of opioids. The opioids were causing side effects and constipation. The biologics hadn't worked, but she didn't have any active arthritis. She reached a point where the constipation was causing a couple of hospital admissions, and at one of those admissions she felt that she was at rock bottom.

This was a pivotal point for her, and she decided that she would make changes to her lifestyle. At the beginning she started to take up walking as her physical activity and change her dietary habits. Whenever she felt a flare-up of pain, and she knew she had been told that there was no damage she could do if she continued to walk, she chose to sometimes walk through the pain and other times, slightly pace herself, but keep being active.

As she reduced her medication as well, and decreased her consumption of processed sugary foods, her pain got a bit better. She began to eat in a more plant-based way, not completely vegetarian or vegan, but it was more healthy, unprocessed food cooked at home, and that was what she feels made the difference. In four to six weeks, she started to notice that the pain wasn't as intense as it used to be, which made her more confident that she was on the right track. And you know, three years down the line, she is as functional as she can be, and last year she finally gave up her 10 or 15 years of Blue Badge ownership and came off the unemployment rolls having started a job. This was after 15 years of persistent pain, osteoarthritis and fibromyalgia. She's taken up wild swimming alongside the other things, and she's been able to lose eight or nine stone.

Once you have made those lifestyle changes, you look back at what you used to do and you don't want to do it any more, because you feel so good when you are making a positive lifestyle change.

Cooking Without Pain: Best Life Hacks, Tools and Adaptations for the Kitchen

WITH CHERYL CROW

—

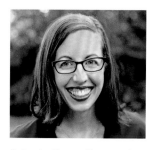

© Jessica Keener Photography

The kitchen can be a source of joy and camaraderie, but for people living with arthritis it may also be a source of pain. From twisting jars open and slicing up your vegetables to lifting heavy items out of the oven or standing over the countertop for long periods of time, there's no denying that cooking tasks may be tiresome on the delicate joints in our hands, wrists and elbows in particular.

The good news is that there are many gadgets, adaptations and alternative approaches to minimise joint pain and strain and increase joy in the kitchen. I've teamed up with occupational therapist Cheryl Crow, who also lives with rheumatoid arthritis, to take a look at the best life hacks, tools and adaptations for the kitchen.

'The small changes you make really can add up over time. Celebrate the small ways that you can do things differently in the kitchen, at work, or in social settings to protect your joints and prevent further pain.'

Cheryl Crow

Emily: For someone who has never heard of it before, please describe what occupational therapy is?

Cheryl: If I could rename the profession, I would name it 'Life Skills Therapy', because 'occupations' in this context are meaningful activities of daily living. The American Occupational Therapy Association had a really great tagline: 'Occupational Therapy: Skills for the Job of Living'. This ranges from the most basic everyday self-care activities, such as taking a shower, getting dressed, or cooking at home, but there is also support for more potentially challenging tasks from work responsibilities to finances, relationships, childcare and recreational activities.

If you have an illness, injury or disability, occupational therapists specialise in helping you to develop the skills needed to complete your everyday activities or find alternative ways to do them with more independence, whether at home, in social settings or in the workplace.

An example for someone living with arthritis could be that their hands are weak, and they are struggling with their daily tasks, so as an occupational therapist I would try to strengthen their hands, or if it is not possible for them to regain strength, then I'd look at what 'work arounds' or adaptations we could make. We enable people to live better alongside their condition, more independently and joyfully.

Emily: How important is occupational therapy in the management of arthritis and chronic pain?

Cheryl: We really personalise the treatment to the individual. For instance, if there are five people who are living with arthritis, the treatment is going to be totally different for each person, dependent on the type of arthritis that they have, its severity, and what their daily life looks like.

What's difficult for you in your life that you want to make better? And what is going well, too, so that we can keep building on that? We take a holistic lens and look at the mental health of the individual as well, taking the 'bio-psycho-social' approach to their pain. As we know, you may struggle with feeling low and being depressed when you live with chronic pain. So, we would also integrate mental coping strategies, taking a look at the bigger picture of 'How do I live a good life with this condition? How do I accept it? And how do I commit to living well, and the best life I can with it?'.

Emily: How can people set their kitchen up for success, joint protection and pain prevention?

Cheryl: So, when it comes to kitchen life hacks, and most home life adaptations, they fall into three categories:

Number one – adding a new 'life hack', gadget, adaptive or assistive device to your life.
This could be an object such as an electronic tin or jar opener, or an adaptive knife. As you mention in your recipes, Emily, a food processor is a brilliant piece of kitchen equipment, which you can use to blend soups, grate carrots and more. I have an adaptive knife with an ergonomic handle positioned at a 90-degree angle, it helps those with weaker grip strength and thumb pain in particular. I have also just started using an under-cabinet multi-jar opener, instead of a hand-held one, which simply sticks underneath your upper kitchen cabinet. You just hold the object with two hands and then twist the jar, taking the stress off your fingers and hands.

Number two – changing how you interact with the objects that you have to protect your joints.

Joint protection means modifying how you interact with things, so that you protect your joints from strain or pain. The most tender areas of hand arthritis are typically in the thumbs, fingers and wrists. So, try to distribute the weight across multiple joints. As an example, if you are holding a tin of food, hold it with two hands, or if you are carrying a heavy box try to hold it close to your core, so that you are able to stabilise it with your larger joints.

Number three – working around the problem, and finding an alternative way to complete a task.

Some examples of this in the kitchen would be:

- Instead of having to modify how you hold your knife, or using an adaptive knife, can you order pre-chopped vegetables? Or try different ways to grasp a regular knife that reduces strain on the thumb joint, or ask for help instead.

- Rather than going to the grocery store, buying everything and physically putting it into the bags, then driving, walking or catching public transport home, then carrying it into the house, you could order a grocery delivery instead to save your joints a lot of stress.

- If you are standing over the countertop for long periods of time, you could use an anti-fatigue mat (I use one of these) or conserve your energy by sitting on a stool instead, or taking rest breaks. Additionally, make sure you have a good night's sleep before a day when you know you're going to be doing a lot of cooking, and wear supportive indoor shoes (a clean old pair of trusty trainers, for instance).

MY FAVOURITE HACKS AND TOP TIPS

It's so interesting that Cheryl also brought up the division of tasks and taking breaks in between them. Every week I do meal prep, because I don't always have the energy to cook every night. I'll make one big pot of something, and have it over the course of a few days, or even freeze some for a day when defrost-cook is a helpful option. When making things in bulk, I often chop the vegetables in the morning and place them in the fridge, so that in the evening I am able to throw them together and start cooking. Planning and preparation are so helpful. It might be extra brain effort to plan it initially, but then there is no need to think about it for the rest of the week.

Freeze your foods	Including herbs (or crushed garlic) in ice-cube trays, freezing meal prep (use flat freezer bags to save space), buying frozen (or freezing) fruits (berries, sliced banana, mango pieces) and vegetables (peas, sweetcorn, spinach).
Purchase pre-chopped foods	Especially those that may be heavy or particularly tricky, like butternut squash.
Use a food processor	For a helping hand – I never hand grate, unless it's for a bit of orange zest – I use the grating setting on my food processor, which helps so much.
Store and organise items	More efficiently – for example, pouring large heavy items like olive oil into smaller containers and placing the most frequently used items in easily accessible places.
Sitting	At the dining table/kitchen table or at countertop if chopping and preparing for long periods of time.
Break up the task/recipe	into smaller parts, such as chopping things in the morning (my mum calls this having a 'kitchen fairy').
Asking for help	When you need it and being kind to yourself.

See pages 26–7 for helpful cooking equipment and gadgets and pages 28–32 for essential foods (fresh, frozen and store cupboard).

ANTI-INFLAMMATORY COMPONENTS

'Nothing in life is to be feared, it is only to
be understood. Now is the time to understand
more, so that we may fear less.'

Marie Salomea Skłodowska–Curie, physicist,
chemist and pioneer in the study of radiation

Keeping up with food trends and diets is impossible so, don't worry, I am not about to tell you some new-found way to keep your inflammation at bay with a pineapple-apple-cider-vinegar-honey-turmeric-syrup that you squeeze onto your porridge every day. The key is getting back to basics: simple, nourishing and science-backed anti-inflammatory foods that we already are aware of and know are good for us, which can largely be found in the Mediterranean diet (MD). And no, this does not equate to lots of artisan breads (sorry, you will thank me later!), but rather a heavy focus on plant-based foods, packed with protein and fibre, phytonutrients (and polyphenols), vitamins and minerals, healthful fats, and a limited consumption of meat and animal produce.

In this chapter, I have compiled a table of key anti-inflammatory ingredients and listed which recipes you can find them in. You'll learn why and how these ingredients are anti-inflammatory, and the all-important vitamins, minerals, nutrients and phytochemicals that reside within them. I also share how they may ease chronic inflammation, help the immune system and reduce pain. In recent decades, more and more research has surfaced about the gut microbiome, and its effects on human health and disease. However, there remains a need for more human clinical evidence, as results are not always substantial, partly because every person's body, gut, immune system, genetics, lifestyle and eating habits are different – because we are all different.

There is a new science, which I briefly touched upon in my first book, that explores the connection between the food we eat and our genes. Nutrigenetics, nutrigenomics and epigenetics look at how food interacts with our DNA and, alongside other lifestyle factors, has the potential to change the expression of our genes, and even prevent chronic disease in future generations. Our genes go unchanged, but we can alter their output (how they operate within us) with the input they receive (from our food or environmental factors). This is also why nutrition is most effective when it is personalised – it's up to you to discover what works best for you, but you are in the best place to begin.

As inflammation and autoimmunity are the key focus of this book, I have pulled out nutritional compounds from each of the recipes that have been scientifically linked to reducing inflammation, helping our immune system and/or anti-arthritic benefits. There are numerous different types of nutrients and plant-based compounds that are able to assist in keeping our inflammation and inflammatory responses in check. However, it's a lot more varied and complex than we think, and the gut microbiome is affected by a multitude of factors. Poor gut health is usually accompanied by poor health elsewhere, reflected in a low-fibre and nutrient-poor diet, lifestyle factors like an irregular sleep pattern, being sedentary and stressed, as well as alcohol, smoking and medications. The emphasis is on keeping your gut happy, with more than one way to do so.

What are phytonutrients?

You have likely heard of turmeric, but its plant compound and phytonutrient (that arguably does all the hard work) is called curcumin. Curcumin is one of 25,000 phytonutrients from different phytochemical classes, all of which have been found largely in plants, from fruits and vegetables to nuts and seeds, legumes and whole grains to herbs and spices. These naturally occurring bioactive compounds have been shown to support and be beneficial to human health in numerous ways. Phytonutrients maintain and modulate immune function to prevent specific diseases, with the potential to be utilised within treatments in the future (to help chronic inflammation in conditions like ours), but more research is needed, as well as methods to increase their bioavailability.

The largest group of phytonutrients are polyphenols, which can be subclassified into four main groups: flavonoids (including eight subgroups), phenolic acids (such as curcumin), stilbenoids (such as resveratrol) and lignans. As of now, 8,000 different types of polyphenols have been identified in plants, and they have probably existed in the plant kingdom for over a billion years. They have an array of biological properties: antioxidant (fighting inflammatory by-products called free radicals), anti-inflammatory, cardioprotective (for good heart health) and antimicrobial (fighting against harmful microorganisms). In the field of nutrigenetics, polyphenols have a huge impact on our human cells, interacting with our DNA. Increasingly, studies are demonstrating how regular consumption of polyphenols has been associated with a reduced risk of a number of chronic diseases.

'They have an array of biological properties: antioxidant (fighting inflammatory by-products called free radicals), anti-inflammatory, cardioprotective (for good heart health) and antimicrobial (fighting against harmful microorganisms).'

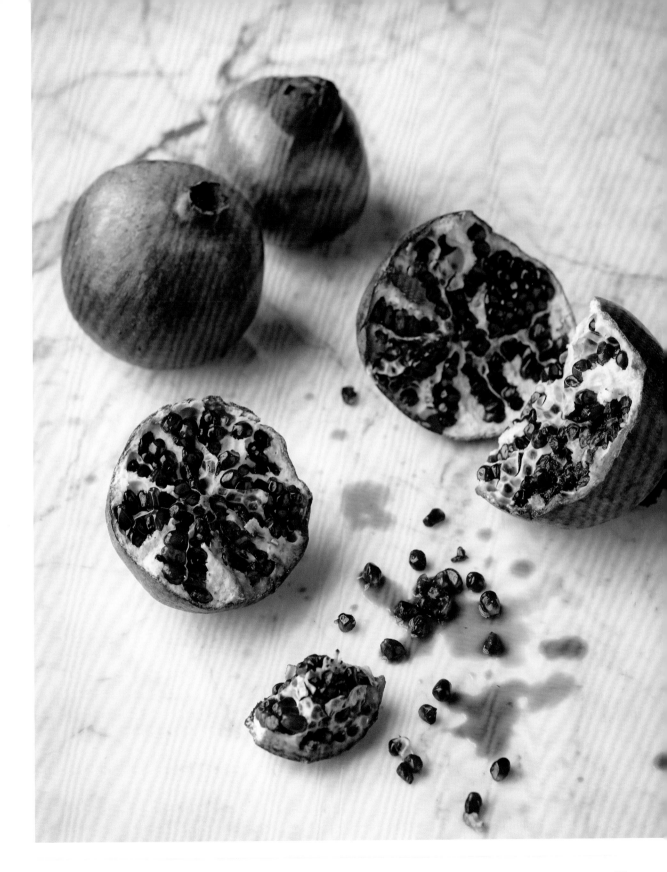

AN A–Z OF ANTI-INFLAMMATORY COMPONENTS

INGREDIENT	RECIPE(S)	CATEGORY
Almonds (including almond butter)	Breakfast Granola Bowl (page 108), Bakewell Tart Overnight Oats (page 101), Apricot and Almond Baked Oats (page 104), Bang Bang Cauliflower Salad (page 126), 'Fakeaway' Katsu Curry, or Katsu Curry Salad (page 160), No-Bake Ginger and 'Caramel' Slices (page 188), Almond Butter Brownies (page 191), Vegan Chocolate Tiffin (page 189), Cacao and Coconut Energy Balls (page 203), Sweet Cinnamon Mixed Nuts (page 210), Homemade Almond Mylk (page 229)	Nuts and Seeds
Anchovies	Creamy Caesar Salad (page 172)	Grains and Proteins
Apples	'Fakeaway' Katsu Curry, or Katsu Curry Salad (page 160), Apple and Berry Bake (page 182), Pick N Mix Chocolate Fruit Yoghurt (page 194), Green Dream Juice (page 222), Bold Beetroot Juice (page 223), Anti-Inflammatory Power Juice (page 223), Golden Delicious Green Smoothie (page 218), Sunshine Juice (page 222), Turmeric Kick Juice (page 219)	Fruit
Apricots (try to get sulphite-free dried apricots if you can)	Apricot and Almond Baked Oats (page 104), Moroccan Salmon with Fresh Mint Quinoa Salad (page 122), Hasselback Potatoes with Chilli Apricot Chutney and Cashew Cheese (page 163), Pick N Mix Chocolate Fruit Yoghurt (page 194), Apricot Chia Seed Bites (page 202), Chilli Apricot Chutney (page 237)	Fruit
Asparagus	Creamy Mushroom Butter Beans with Asparagus (page 120)	Vegetable
Aubergine	Aubergine Dip Topped with Pomegranate Seeds (page 198)	Vegetable

EAT WELL WITH ARTHRITIS

NOTABLE ANTI-INFLAMMATORY COMPONENT(S)	THE SCIENCE AND ANTI-INFLAMMATORY BENEFIT
Magnesium, monounsaturated fatty acids (MUFAs)	A 2010–2017 study concluded that daily MUFA intake via the Mediterranean diet (MD) might suppress disease activity in rheumatoid arthritis patients. In contrast to inflammatory high-saturated-fat diets and Western diets, high-MUFA diets are anti-inflammatory, with studies demonstrating that people who eat a MD high in MUFAs have significantly lower inflammatory markers (such as CRP and IL-6) in their blood.
Selenium, polyunsaturated fatty acids (PUFAs – omega-3)	There is extensive evidence that omega-3 PUFAs can mediate anti-inflammatory effects and the combination of polyphenols and fish oils have demonstrated both antioxidant and anti-inflammatory effects.
Flavonoids, such as quercetin	Quercetin is able to modulate inflammation and has been shown to be effective against chronic diseases like arthritis and psoriasis. In one study, RA patients took quercetin as a supplement for 8 weeks and had reduced markers of inflammation compared to those who took a placebo, plus reduced morning joint stiffness and pain, and after-activity pain. The anti-inflammatory activity of flavonoids is also known to have a role in reducing pain and inflammation in joints. Apples are rich in flavonoids, such as procyanidin and condensed tannins. In one animal study, it was shown that the supplementation of condensed tannins from apples delayed arthritis symptoms. Further analysis and clinical trials are needed, but so far, the indications are hopeful.
Carotenoids, β-cryptoxanthin/ beta-cryptoxanthin, vitamin A, vitamin C	Polyphenolic compound beta-cryptoxanthin exerts anti-arthritic actions and studies suggest that it may be useful in blocking the progression of rheumatoid arthritis and osteoarthritis.
Quercetin, kaempferol, rutin	Green asparagus spears are a good source of phytochemical antioxidants, and research has shown that rutin and other phenolic compounds in asparagus spears appear not to degrade when heated.
Quercetin, kaempferol, rutin	Nightshade vegetables like aubergines contain really nutritious components, so it is not advisable to cut them out unless you really think you are being affected by them. If possible, use the Trigger Tracker on page 36 to see if they affect your symptoms. Aubergines are packed with dietary fibre, vitamins, and polyphenols with antioxidant and anti-inflammatory properties.

Avocado	Mexican-Style Salad Bowl (page 112), Moroccan Salmon with Fresh Mint Quinoa Salad (page 122), Brown Rice 'Sushi' Nori Bites (page 128), Honey Mustard Chicken or Tofu Salad (page 170), Creamy Caesar Salad (page 172), Italian-Style Chicken with Sweet Potato Wedges (page 178), Almond Butter Brownies (page 191)	Fruit
Bananas	Carrot (and Courgette) Loaf Cake (page 187), Coconut Banana 'Cookie' Bites (page 201), Vanilla Date Hemp Seed Smoothie (page 218), Golden Delicious Green Smoothie (page 218), Mint Choc Chip Smoothie (page 230)	Fruit
Basil	Breakfast Savoury Muffins (page 92), Italian-Style Chicken with Sweet Potato Wedges (page 178), Katy's Quinoa-Base Pizza (page 166), Saucy Vegan Pesto (page 239), Walnut Vegan Pesto (page 239)	Herbs and Spices
Beans: butter beans, cannellini beans, kidney beans	Creamy Mushroom Butter Beans with Asparagus (page 120), Creamy Caesar Salad (page 172), Italian-Style Chicken with Sweet Potato Wedges (page 178), Roasted Vegetables with Tuscan White Bean Dip (page 130), Vegan Chilli (page 156), Sea Bass with Infused Quinoa (page 139), Spicy and Warming Dahl (page 158)	Grains and Proteins
Beetroot	Roasted Beetroot Hummus (page 207), Bold Beetroot Juice (page 223)	Vegetable

Monounsaturated fatty acids (MUFAs), fibre, protein, prebiotics, magnesium, carotenoids, vitamin C, vitamin E, vitamin B6, potassium and folate	Avocado helps to slow the release of glucose, which in turn helps reduce the blood sugar spike that can often trigger inflammation. The Mediterranean diet is high in MUFAs (present in avocados) and in one recent study, the MD combined with exercise improved pain, knee range of motion (ROM), and weight reduction more than exercise alone in RA patients.
Ferulic acid, fibre/prebiotics, quercetin, kaempferol	Bananas are rich not only in carbohydrates, dietary fibres, certain vitamins and minerals, but also in many health-promoting bioactive phytochemicals, with antioxidant properties and anti-inflammatory benefits. As a banana ripens, its natural sugar content and antioxidant activity increase. However, eating it less ripe enhances its prebiotic properties. Both may be good for reducing inflammation in the gut.
Rosmarinic acid, quercetin, rutin	Basil benefits that have been identified include the strengthening of the immune system, plus alleviating stress and anxiety, and enhancing memory. Rosmarinic acid (one of the main phenolic compounds in sweet basil) has pharmacological properties boasting antioxidant, antiviral, antimicrobial and anti-inflammatory effects.
Quercetin, kaempferol, folate	Legumes and beans are recognised as both a vegetable and as a meat alternative because of a nutrient profile that is high in protein, iron and zinc. Beans are a low glycemic source of complex carbohydrates, vitamins, minerals, protein, fibre and phytochemical compounds with a multitude of bioactive properties. The dietary inclusion of pulses, beans and legumes is beneficial to improving disease conditions such as gut microbial diversity, and chronic low-grade inflammation. Butter beans, though white (darker beans are a richer source of phytochemicals, see Black beans on page 58) are still rich in vitamins and minerals, which are important for overall health. A source of potassium, magnesium, folate (see Pecans on page 72), iron, and zinc, they also contain calcium.
Nitrates, vitamin C	The body converts nitrates into nitric oxide – a compound that relaxes and dilates blood vessels, turning them into superhighways for your nutrient- and oxygen-rich blood. While rheumatoid arthritis affects the body's joints, rheumatoid vasculitis is a condition in which blood vessels become inflamed. When blood vessels become inflamed, they may become weakened and increase in size, or become narrowed, sometimes to the point of stopping blood flow. Beetroot supplementation has been shown to improve thumb blood flow, and anti-inflammatory status, in people with Raynaud's disease (often associated with arthritic conditions such as RA, scleroderma, lupus or Sjogren's syndrome).

Bell pepper	Breakfast Savoury Muffins (page 92), Mexican-Style Salad Bowl (page 112), Ready-To-Go Jar Noodle Pot (page 119), Spicy Tahini Prawn 'Submarines' (page 125), Bang Bang Cauliflower Salad (page 126), Brown Rice 'Sushi' Nori Bites (page 128), Roasted Vegetables with Tuscan White Bean Dip (page 130), Plant-Packed Chow Mein (page 138), One-Pot Chicken and Prawn Jambalaya (page 140), One-Pot Harissa Tempeh Stew (page 143), Grandad Speight's Nasi Goreng (page 144), One-Tray Roast Chicken with Vegetables (page 150), Sticky and Sweet Mixed Veg Stir-Fry with Cashew Nuts (page 152), Vegan Chilli (page 156), Honey Mustard Chicken or Tofu Salad (page 170), Goan Prawn and Cod Curry (page 176), Italian-Style Chicken with Sweet Potato Wedges (page 178), Hummus Accompaniments/Crudités (page 207), Mango Salsa (page 235)	Vegetable
Berries: blackberries, blueberries, strawberries (for Raspberries, see page 72)	Lemon and Berry Muffins (page 107), Pick N Mix Chocolate Fruit Yoghurt (page 194), My Fair Lady Pancakes (page 98)	Fruit
Black beans	Mexican-Style Salad Bowl (page 112)	Grains and Proteins
Black pepper	Most recipes, excluding Desserts and Drinks, Juices and Smoothies	Herbs and Spices
Butternut squash	Butternut Squash and Leek Risotto (page 175), Vegan Chickpea Curry (page 169)	Vegetable

Vitamin C, quercetin, carotenoids (lycopene and more)	Red peppers are richer in potassium, folate and vitamin C than yellow or green varieties. Immature green peppers have a very high phenolic content while green, immature red and ripe red peppers showed 4–5 times less. Another study showed red peppers have nine times more lycopene than green varieties. For more detail on lycopene, see Tomatoes on page 76.
Resveratrol, quercetin, vitamin C	Berries are beneficial to health with their phytochemical and vitamin content and a wide diversity of health advantages for the digestive system, suggesting berries can serve as a strong support to established treatments for a variety of gastrointestinal and immune-related illnesses. A well-balanced gut microbiome is important for health and wellbeing, whereas an imbalanced microbiome can cause inflammation. Studies have demonstrated that berries can provide a general strengthening of the adaptive immune system and a reduction in overall inflammatory status. In general, whole berries demonstrate more beneficial health effects than extracted individual berry components. This is exemplified by quercetin, as vitamin C in the berries can stabilise quercetin and therefore enhance health-related quercetin effects. Strawberries contain the most vitamin C in this section of berries. However, if you can access blackcurrants (not easy to find here in the UK), they contain 226 per cent of the RDA per 100g.
Magnesium, polyphenols	Generally, darker beans, such as black beans, are a richer source of phytochemicals, with a higher antioxidant capacity and a more diverse mix of polyphenols, compared to lighter beans. Black beans are a dietary source of total polyphenols, and specifically, dietary anthocyanins, which have been associated with improvements in inflammation. Magnesium deficiency can cause inflammation in the body. A 1-cup (172g) serving of cooked black beans contains 120mg of magnesium (30 per cent of the RDA), and magnesium has a wide range of health benefits. See more on Spinach (page 74).
Piperine	Several studies have indicated the anti-inflammatory activity of piperine, including promising anti-inflammatory effects against arthritis by suppressing inflammation and cartilage destruction. Some studies have shown that it can inhibit monosodium urate crystal-induced inflammation and could be a possible treatment of gouty arthritis. Moreover, it helps the absorption of curcumin, which has low bioavailability (how much of a nutrient in food is able to reach our circulation in order to have an effect). When piperine is combined with curcumin, it has been shown to increase the bioavailability of curcumin by 2,000 per cent.
Carotenoids (high in beta-carotene and lutein)	Research has shown that butternut squash is beneficial in combating macular degeneration and boosting heart health and immune function due to a quite high level of carotenoids, which are able to convert to vitamin A in the body. Carotenoids are associated with different physiological processes including vision, the absorption of iron, the functioning of the immune system and combatting inflammation.

Cabbage	Spicy Tahini Prawn 'Submarines' (page 125), Mushroom Noodle Soup (page 136), Plant-Packed Chow Mein (page 138), Grandad Speight's Nasi Goreng (page 144), 'Fakeaway' Katsu Curry, or Katsu Curry Salad (page 160)	Vegetable
Cacao powder and cacao nibs (raw)	Indulgent Chocolate Porridge (page 96), Date, Cacao and Banana Chia Pot (page 109), Vegan Chilli (page 156), Matcha and Berry Compote with Pistachio Crumb and Chocolate Sauce (page 184), No-Bake Ginger and 'Caramel' Slices (page 188), Almond Butter Brownies (page 191), Vegan Chocolate Tiffin (page 189), VJ's Black Cherry Ice Cream (page 195), Pick N Mix Chocolate Fruit Yoghurt (page 194), Coconut Banana 'Cookie' Bites (page 201), Cacao and Coconut Energy Balls (page 203), Mint Choc Chip Smoothie (page 230), Chocolate Sauce (page 235)	Pastes and Powders
Capers	Creamy Caesar Salad (page 172)	Vegetable
Carrots	'Carrot Cake' Overnight Oats (page 101), Ready-To-Go Jar Noodle Pot (page 119), Moroccan Salmon with Fresh Mint Quinoa Salad (page 122), Spicy Tahini Prawn 'Submarines' (page 125), Roasted Vegetables with Tuscan White Bean Dip (page 130), Mushroom Noodle Soup (page 136), Plant-Packed Chow Mein (page 138), One-Tray Roast Chicken with Vegetables (page 150), Vegan Chilli (page 156), Vegetable-Packed Shepherd's Pie (page 164), 'Fakeaway' Katsu Curry, or Katsu Curry Salad (page 160), Carrot (and Courgette) Loaf Cake (page 187), Hummus Accompaniments/Crudités (page 207), Bold Beetroot Juice (page 223), Anti-Inflammatory Power Juice (page 223)	Vegetable
Cashew nuts	Cinnamon Toast Overnight Oats (page 100), Salmon Fishcakes and Cashew Parsley Sauce (page 116), Grandad Speight's Nasi Goreng (page 144), Sticky and Sweet Mixed Veg Stir-Fry with Cashew Nuts (page 152), Hasselback Potatoes with Chilli Apricot Chutney and Cashew Cheese (page 163), Creamy Caesar Salad (page 172), Matcha and Berry Compote with Pistachio Crumb and Chocolate Sauce (page 184), No-Bake Ginger and 'Caramel' Slices (page 188), Vegan Chocolate Tiffin (page 189), Pick N Mix Chocolate Fruit Yoghurt (page 194), Sweet Cinnamon Mixed Nuts (page 210), Cacao and Coconut Energy Balls (page 203), Cashew Parsley Sauce (page 236), Cashew Cheese (page 237)	Nuts and Seeds
Cauliflower	Bang Bang Cauliflower Salad (page 126)	Vegetable

Kaempferol, vitamin C, sulforaphane	Cabbage has high levels of flavonoids and anthocyanins, which possess antioxidant properties and can increase the levels of antioxidant enzymes, leading to protection from free radicals. In one study, cabbage leaf juice was shown to lower the pro-inflammatory activity of TNF-α (a blood marker for inflammation). The outer leaves of Chinese cabbage have the highest levels of antioxidant capacities and polyphenolics.
Resveratrol	Research has shown resveratrol demonstrating joint protective effects. In one clinical study, 50 per cent of RA patients received resveratrol daily alongside their conventional treatment for 3 months, and other patients just received their regular treatment. The resveratrol-treated group showed a significant drop in the major clinical markers of RA.
Rutin, kaempferol, quercetin and quercetin derivatives	In traditional medicine, different parts of the caper plant have been used for the treatment of various human diseases, such as rheumatism. Caper flavonoids are known to have anti-inflammatory properties, and caper extract has even been shown to have a greater joint protective effect than indomethacin* in one lab-based study, but there has yet to be human trials in this area. They're also packed with quercetin (see page 73) and have one of the highest polyphenol contents of any food, varying from 10,720 to 3256mg per 100g. *Indomethacin is a non-steroidal anti-inflammatory drug (NSAID), NSAIDs are medicines that are widely used to relieve pain, reduce inflammation and bring down a high temperature.
Carotenoids (high in beta-carotene, but also contains lutein and lycopene)	The phytonutrient carotenoids in carrots have been shown to help with inflammatory arthritis. Carotenoids are associated with different physiological processes including vision, the absorption of iron, the functioning of the immune system and combatting inflammation. For more detail on lycopene, see Tomatoes on page 76.
Polyphenols, zinc, magnesium, monounsaturated fatty acids (MUFAs)	Cashew nuts are rich in heart-healthy MUFAs, which have been found in some studies to reduce inflammation. Cashew nuts also contain carotenoids and polyphenols, two categories of antioxidants that may help reduce inflammation, but more cashew-specific research is needed. Overall, they possess anti-inflammatory and antioxidative benefits.
Sulforaphane, vitamin C	Sulforaphane has been shown to have anti-inflammatory and anti-arthritic effects in some studies, including relating to rheumatoid arthritis, and promising anti-inflammatory properties for osteoarthritis treatment, but more research is needed.

Cherries	VJ's Black Cherry Ice Cream (page 195), Pick N Mix Chocolate Fruit Yoghurt (page 194)	Fruit
Chia seeds	Cinnamon Toast Overnight Oats (page 100), Bakewell Tart Overnight Oats (page 101), Apricot and Almond Baked Oats (page 104), Date, Cacao and Banana Chia Pot (page 109), Layered Mango and Passion Fruit Dessert (page 192), Apricot Chia Seed Bites (page 202), Raspberry Jam (page 234)	Nuts and Seeds
Chickpeas	Bang Bang Cauliflower Salad (page 126), One-Pot Harissa Tempeh Stew (page 143), Honey Mustard Chicken or Tofu Salad (page 170), Creamy Caesar Salad (page 172), Vegan Chickpea Curry (page 169), No-Bake Ginger and 'Caramel' Slices (page 188), Plain Hummus (page 206), Roasted Beetroot Hummus (page 207), Sweet Roasted Pepper Hummus (page 207)	Grains and Proteins
Cinnamon	Breakfast Granola Bowl (page 108), My Fair Lady Pancakes (page 98), Cinnamon Toast Overnight Oats (page 100), Carrot Cake Overnight Oats (page 101), Apricot and Almond Baked Oats (page 104), Moroccan Salmon with Fresh Mint Quinoa Salad (page 122), Spiced Sweet Potato Soup (page 132), Spicy and Warming Dahl (page 158), Apple and Berry Bake (page 182), Carrot (and Courgette) Loaf Cake (page 187), No-Bake Ginger and 'Caramel' Slices (page 188), Vegan Chocolate Tiffin (page 189), Sweet Cinnamon Mixed Nuts (page 210), Coconut Banana 'Cookie' Bites (page 201), Apricot Chia Seed Bites (page 202), Orange and Cinnamon Warmer (page 216), Chilli Apricot Chutney (page 237)	Herbs and Spices
Citrus fruit (oranges, lemons, limes)	Most recipes	Fruit

Quercetin	Consumption of sweet or tart cherries can promote health by preventing or decreasing oxidative stress and inflammation. Cherries are beneficial for those suffering from gout, a type of arthritis that affects over 3 million people in the US, as they help to lower the amount of uric acid in the body. Cherries have antioxidant and anti-inflammatory properties, so many with gout try drinking cherry juice to help their symptoms and prevent flare-ups. In one study, cherry intake over a 2-day period was associated with a 35 per cent lower risk of gout attacks compared with no intake.
Polyunsaturated fatty acids (PUFAs – omega 3), zinc, magnesium, calcium, genistein, kaempferol, quercetin	Chia seeds are the richest plant source of omega-3, as well as being packed with antioxidants, and with more calcium by weight than milk. As a complete protein, chia seeds contain all nine essential amino acids that cannot be made by the body. They can hold up to ten times their weight in water, which is why they make an excellent substitute for egg for vegans (see page 88).
Zinc, iron, B vitamins	Pulses like chickpeas are full of gut-nourishing fibre, prebiotics and plant protein. See Black Beans on page 58 for more information.
Cinnamaldehyde	In a recent study, cinnamaldehyde has shown potential therapeutic properties against RA. In another study, cinnamon consumption improved clinical symptoms and inflammatory markers in RA patients. Cinnamon may also have therapeutic importance in different autoimmune disorders, but more clinical trials are needed.
Vitamin C, flavonoids such as quercetin, carotenoids	Vitamin C is well-known for its antioxidant properties and helps protect cells from damage. Carotenoids, including beta-cryptoxanthin, are converted to vitamin A in the body. In some trials, orange juice has been shown to reduce inflammation. Citrus can also help your body absorb iron, a mineral that's important for the immune system and helps your body produce red blood cells, which is why when citrus is consumed with iron-rich foods – like leafy greens, fish, poultry, and meat – it improves our uptake of this important mineral (as with many of the recipes in this book!). There is also some evidence on the role of specific fruit polyphenols, such as quercetin and citrus flavonoids, in alleviating RA symptoms. A particular flavonoid, nobiletin, that is present in orange and a number of citrus fruits, has been shown to have anti-inflammatory effects, and another, naringenin, may have a therapeutic role in alleviating inflammatory pain, but more clinical trials are required.

Dates	Carrot Cake Overnight Oats (page 101), Date, Cacao and Banana Chia Pot (page 109), Cacao and Coconut Energy Balls (page 203), Homemade Almond Mylk (page 229)	Fruit
Extra virgin olive oil	Most recipes, excluding Desserts and Drinks, Juices and Smoothies	Oils and Syrups
Fish: salmon, sea bass	Creamy Caesar Salad (page 172), Mexican-Style Salad Bowl (page 112), Salmon Fishcakes and Cashew Parsley Sauce (page 116), Moroccan Salmon with Fresh Mint Quinoa Salad (page 122), Salmon and Puy Lentils with Orange Dressing (page 148), Sea Bass with Infused Quinoa (page 139)	Grains and Proteins
Flaxseeds	Carrot Cake Overnight Oats (page 101)	Nuts and Seeds
Garlic	Most recipes, excluding Desserts and Drinks, Juice and Smoothies	Herbs and Spices
Ginger	Most recipes	Herbs and Spices
Hazelnuts	Date, Cacao and Banana Chia Pot (page 109), Pick N Mix Chocolate Fruit Yoghurt (page 194)	Nuts and Seeds

Polyphenols, flavonoids and carotenoids	Dates are high in fibre with a low GI and so work well as a sugar replacement in desserts, smoothies and breakfasts. Dates filled with nut butter are one of my favourite snacks, and the nut butter helps slow the release of the sugars.
Hydroxytyrosol, monounsaturated fatty acids (MUFAs), oleocanthal	Both the American Food and Drugs Administration (AFDA) and the European Food Safety Authority (EFSA) recommend daily consumption of extra virgin olive oil, as it has shown to improve symptoms, and prevent and delay the onset of immune-inflammatory diseases, including arthritis. Try to avoid lower quality olive oil (refined olive oil) if you can, as it loses antioxidant and anti-inflammatory capacities through overprocessing. Uncooked extra virgin olive oil is the best form to consume it in, which means getting it into salad dressings. In a recent study, oleocanthal has been shown to help prevent the inflammatory effects of autoimmune and inflammatory disorders, including rheumatoid arthritis. In a separate study, it has shown to possess similar anti-inflammatory properties to ibuprofen.
Selenium, polyunsaturated fatty acids (PUFAs – omega-3), vitamin D	There is extensive evidence that omega-3 PUFAs can mediate anti-inflammatory effects, and the combination of polyphenols and fish oils have demonstrated both antioxidant and anti-inflammatory effects.
Zinc, magnesium, polyunsaturated fatty acids (omega-3)	Flaxseeds are high in fibre and omega-3 fatty acids, as well as phytochemicals called lignans, plus zinc and magnesium. There is extensive evidence that omega-3 PUFAs can mediate anti-inflammatory effects, and as discussed previously, fibre is great for the gut and, in turn, our immune system.
Allicin, lutein, vitamin C	Allicin is an unstable compound that is only briefly present in fresh garlic after it's been cut or crushed. It also decreases when the garlic is heated. If it is activated 10 minutes before cooking by being crushed, minced or sliced, then it keeps all of its health benefits. One study suggests that the consumption of garlic may give some relief from the inflammatory symptoms of osteoarthritis. Another study looked at how garlic compounds are anti-inflammatory and appear to enhance the functioning of the immune system, but more human studies are needed.
Gingerol	The polyphenolic compound 6-gingerol, derived from the root of ginger, displays similar biochemistry to that of curcumin (see Turmeric on page 76). A range of trials have revealed the beneficial properties of gingerols against OA, RA and gout: reducing chronic inflammatory responses and protecting bone cartilage from damage in knee joints, suppressing joint swelling, as well as anti-inflammatory activity, plus preventing both joint inflammation and destruction. In one study with OA and RA patients, powdered ginger was used for a 3-month to two-and-a-half-year period and more than three-quarters of RA patients experienced a remarkable relief in pain and swelling. Other studies have shown that it can also reduce OA symptoms, decreasing pain and inflammation. Amongst 261 patients with OA, around 95 per cent claimed to have had a reduction in pain when supplementing with an extract of ginger.
MUFAs, PUFAs (omega-3), calcium, magnesium, copper, folate, fibre, vitamin E	Hazelnuts have been linked to reduced inflammation due to their high concentrations of healthy fats like omega-3, plus antioxidants and phytonutrients. One study showed that eating 40g of hazelnuts may reduce the inflammatory response, but further studies are required.

Hemp seeds	Vanilla Date Hemp Seed Smoothie (page 218)	Nuts and Seeds
Herbs: marjoram, mint, oregano, rosemary, sage, thyme	One-Tray Roast Chicken with Vegetables (page 150), Mexican-Style Salad Bowl (page 112), Moroccan Salmon with Fresh Mint Quinoa Salad (page 122), Smashed Cucumber Sesame Seed Salad (page 204), Orange and Cinnamon Warmer (page 216), Green Dream Juice (page 222), Golden Delicious Green Smoothie (page 218), Mint Choc Chip Smoothie (page 230), Mango Salsa (page 235), Easy Frittata (page 115), Creamy Mushroom Butter Beans with Asparagus (page 120), Moroccan Salmon with Fresh Mint Quinoa Salad (page 122), Sea Bass with Infused Quinoa (page 139), Roasted Vegetables with Tuscan White Bean Dip (page 130), Plant-Packed Chow Mein (page 138), One-Pot Chicken and Prawn Jambalaya (page 140), Vegan Chilli (page 156), Butternut Squash and Leek Risotto (page 175), Italian-Style Chicken with Sweet Potato Wedges (page 178)	Herbs and Spices
Honey, especially Manuka honey	Apricot and Almond Baked Oats (page 104), Plant-Packed Chow Mein (page 138), Apple and Berry Bake (page 182)	Oils and Syrups
Kale	Creamy Mushroom Butter Beans with Asparagus (page 120), Sea Bass with Infused Quinoa (page 139), Creamy Caesar Salad (page 172), Honey Mustard Chicken or Tofu Salad (page 170), Vegan Chickpea Curry (page 169), Cheese and Onion Crispy Kale (page 211), Salt and Vinegar Crispy Kale (page 211), Smoky Paprika Crispy Kale (page 211)	Vegetable
Lentils	One-Pot Harissa Tempeh Stew (page 143), Salmon and Puy Lentils with Orange Dressing (page 148), Spicy and Warming Dahl (page 158)	Grains and Proteins
Lucuma powder	VJ's Black Cherry Ice Cream (page 195)	Pastes and Powders

Polyunsaturated fatty acids (PUFAs – omega-3), vitamin E, potassium, sodium, magnesium, calcium, iron, and zinc	Hemp seeds have high nutritional value, with almost as much protein as soybean. They are rich in vitamin E and minerals such as phosphorus, potassium, sodium, magnesium, sulfur, calcium, iron and zinc. Trials using daily consumption of gamma linolenic acid (GLA), present in hemp seed oil, for up to 12 months have shown progressive improvements in symptoms of RA, but more research is required.
Carnosol, carnosic acid	Polyphenols carnosol and carnosic acid are the two major components of the culinary herbs sage, rosemary, thyme, marjoram and oregano, and they all derive from the same family (which also includes basil, mint and lavender). There is numerous research analysing the potential of these herbs to fight inflammation, as they have been found to have anti-inflammatory and antioxidant properties. In studies, carnosol has shown to effectively prevent pro-inflammatory mediators of cartilage breakdown, and carnosic acid to reduce cartilage degeneration. Two further studies showed how carnosol might act as a potent antioxidant and regulate the oxidative stress associated with OA with strong effects on inflammatory mediators. In one study of RA, carnosic acid reduced the manifestations of arthritis and reduced pro-inflammatory cytokines, and in another, rosemary-derived carnosic acid was shown to be a promising natural compound for the treatment of RA. More clinical studies are required to further determine and quantify its effects on human diseases.
Antioxidants, methylglyoxal (MGO)	Honey has health-promoting antioxidant, antibacterial and anti-inflammatory properties. Due to its natural antioxidants, including mostly phenolic compounds, honey has the capacity to serve as an important source of antioxidants, and its low glycemic index means that it does not raise blood sugar levels too high. Honey has the potential to decrease inflammatory responses and could be potentially useful for anti-inflammatory treatment (dependent on the type and quality). If you can find honey locally with minimal processing, then this would be a great option. Manuka honey, in particular, is a medical-grade honey known worldwide for its antimicrobial and anti-inflammatory potential.
Kaempferol, quercetin, vitamin C, vitamin K, sulforaphane, carotenoids (lutein, beta-carotene), calcium, folate	Kaempferol has the potential to be beneficial to the body in defending against inflammation and infection, and some studies suggest its potential future use in the prevention and treatment of inflammatory diseases, such as RA, SLE, AS and even OA. In a preclinical study, kaempferol relieved the frequency and severity of arthritis, and has also been shown to exert potential anti-OA effects. However, further studies and human clinical trials are needed.
Kaempferol, quercetin, iron, magnesium, folate, calcium, vitamin C and vitamin B6.	Lentils are packed with dietary fibre and, in particular, black gram or urad dal has plenty of protein (25g per 100g) and is rich in antioxidant compounds and nutrients. It is also an excellent source of copper, zinc, potassium (983mg per 100g) and phosphorus. Most significantly, it has a great amount of iron, about 37 per cent of your RDA in one cooked cup, but it is non-heme iron, so is better absorbed when eaten with vitamin C, found in many of the ingredients you will find black gram in, such as spinach, tomatoes, oranges, limes and bell peppers.
Vitamin C, polyphenols and carotenoids	Lucuma powder has a maple syrup taste and can be used to sweeten a smoothie or ice cream, and can be a sugar alternative in baking. Unlike other alternative sweeteners like agave syrup or honey, lucuma does not cause the blood sugar to spike. This is partly due to its high fibre content – around 2g per tbsp – which helps with digestion and feeds gut bacteria. It is also high in polyphenols and carotenoids, antioxidants known for their anti-inflammatory properties.

Maca powder	Date, Cacao and Banana Chia Pot (page 109)	Pastes and Powders
Mango	Layered Mango and Passion Fruit Dessert (page 192), Turmeric Kick Juice (page 219), Mango Salsa (page 235)	Fruit
Matcha powder	Matcha and Berry Compote with Pistachio Crumb and Chocolate Sauce (page 184), Calm and Energising Matcha (page 226)	Pastes and Powders
Miso paste	Ready-To-Go Jar Noodle Pot (page 119), Vegetable-Packed Shepherd's Pie (page 164), Plant-Packed Chow Mein (page 138), Creamy Caesar Salad (page 172), Butternut Squash and Leek Risotto (page 175)	Pastes and Powders
Moringa oleifera powder	Golden Delicious Green Smoothie (page 218)	Pastes and Powders
Mulberries	Lemon and Berry Muffins (page 107)	Fruit
Mushrooms	Creamy Mushroom Butter Beans with Asparagus (page 120), Spicy Tahini Prawn 'Submarines' (Suki Rolls) (page 125), Mushroom Noodle Soup (page 136), Plant-Packed Chow Mein (page 138), One-Pot Harissa Tempeh Stew (page 143), Grandad Speight's Nasi Goreng (page 144), Vegan Chilli (page 156), Vegetable-Packed Shepherd's Pie (page 164), Katy's Quinoa-Base Pizza (page 166)	Vegetable

Flavonoids, sulforaphane, quercetin	Maca powder is packed with a number of vitamins and minerals, such as potassium and calcium, plus it is also a good vegan source of iron. One 5g teaspoon provides almost 5–10 per cent of the RDA and about 20 per cent of the RDA of copper. Maca powder can easily be added to smoothies, desserts or drinks.
Mangiferin, quercetin	Mango is rich in polyphenols, carotenoids and vitamin C, and a good source of dietary fibre, which have all exhibited anti-inflammatory properties. Several studies have demonstrated that the prebiotic effects of mango polyphenols and dietary fibre have the potential to lower intestinal inflammation.
Epigallocatechin Gallate (EGCG)	Matcha has a lower caffeine content than coffee, and the caffeine is also accompanied by L-theanine, which may enhance concentration. With L-theanine, the caffeine is released slowly in the body, allowing for alertness without the jitters, creating a calming effect and alleviating stress. L-theanine stimulates alertness and helps to induce relaxation, without the crash in energy levels typical with drinking caffeinated drinks. This euphoric sensation of mental alertness and deep relaxation has been compared to the effects of meditation. EGCG has been shown in some studies to inhibit disease progression and reduce the risk of inflammation in OA and RA. Green tea also includes EGCG, but less than matcha, and steeping tea leaves has a lower polyphenol content than that made from the powdered form (matcha is ground young green tea leaves in their purest form). Matcha can be purchased from a number of brands, but unfortunately, low cost equals low quality. Aside from price, the colour is an indication of its quality: higher grade ceremonial matcha will have a bright green-blueish hue , whereas lower grade matcha will appear a dull yellow-brown.
Probiotics, genistein	Miso paste is a fermented food made from soybeans and is full of probiotics. Probiotics are emerging positively in research, especially relating to chronic disease and health, and although their efficacy is hard to pin down due to variants such as diet, age, BMI, stress and gut microbiome, it seems that they hold potential in clinical therapy as anti-inflammatory agents. Probiotics could be useful in assisting with the use of DMARDs for RA – in one recent study a specific probiotic bacterium has been proven to improve methotrexate treatment efficacy by lowering inflammation.
Kaempferol	Moringa contains a number of vitamins, minerals, amino and fatty acids, as well as various types of antioxidant compounds such as flavonoids and carotenoids. An acquired, grass-like and earthy taste, it's better suited to boosting curries, soups and smoothies, to not overwhelm a recipe.
Quercetin, carotenoids, vitamin C and rutin	Mulberries, or their extracts, exhibit excellent anti-inflammatory effects and are often used therapeutically to combat different acute and chronic diseases, but more research is needed.
Dietary fibre, proteins, vitamins, essential nutrients, β-glucan, flavonoids, lectins, phenolics, classed also as a prebiotic	Many studies suggest that mushrooms and their extract/concentrate can be considered as a functional food which can control inflammation. They are rich in anti-inflammatory components, such as phytonutrients, fatty acids, carotenoids, vitamins and more. Recent reports indicate that edible mushroom extracts and compounds exhibit favourable therapeutic and health-promoting benefits, particularly in relation to diseases associated with inflammation. Mushrooms act as a prebiotic to stimulate the growth of gut microbiota, conferring health benefits to the host. Shiitake mushrooms are especially healthful, and in one study, consuming them daily was shown to improve immunity, with a reduction in CRP (C-reactive protein) – a marker for inflammation. Despite many studies citing them as both antioxidant and anti-inflammatory, more studies are required – and benefits are dependent upon the type of mushroom.

Mustard seeds	Vegan Chickpea Curry (page 169), Goan Prawn and Cod Curry (page 176), Chilli Apricot Chutney (page 237)	Herbs and Spices
Oats	Indulgent Chocolate Porridge (page 96), Cinnamon Toast Overnight Oats (page 100), Bakewell Tart Overnight Oats (page 101), Carrot Cake Overnight Oats (page 101), Apricot and Almond Baked Oats (page 104), Date, Cacao and Banana Chia Pot (page 109), Apple and Berry Bake (page 182), No-Bake Ginger and 'Caramel' Slices (page 188), Vegan Chocolate Tiffin (page 189), Apricot Chia Seed Bites (page 202)	Grains and Proteins
Olives	Roasted Vegetables with Tuscan White Bean Dip (page 130), One-Tray Roast Chicken with Vegetables (page 150), Katy's Quinoa-Base Pizza (page 166)	Fruit
Onions	Most recipes, excluding Desserts and Drinks, Juices and Smoothies	Vegetable
Pak choi/ Bok choi	Mushroom Noodle Soup (page 136)	Vegetable
Paprika	Sweet Potato 'Hash brown' Patties and Perfect Poached Eggs (page 95), Salmon Fishcakes and Cashew Parsley Sauce (page 116), Bang Bang Cauliflower Salad (page 126), One-Pot Chicken and Prawn Jambalaya (page 140), One-Pot Harissa Tempeh Stew (page 143), Pulled Smoky Jackfruit Salad (page 147), Vegan Chilli (page 156), Spicy and Warming Dahl (page 158), 'Fakeaway' Katsu Curry, or Katsu Curry Salad (page 160), Honey Mustard Chicken or Tofu Salad (page 170), Butternut Squash and Leek Risotto (page 175), Plain Hummus (page 206), Smoky Paprika Crispy Kale (page 211)	Herbs and Spices
Parsley	Salmon Fishcakes and Cashew Parsley Sauce (page 116), One-Pot Harissa Tempeh Stew (page 143), Salmon and Puy Lentils with Orange Dressing (page 148), One-Tray Roast Chicken with Vegetables (page 150), Vegetable-Packed Shepherd's Pie (page 164), Creamy Caesar Salad (page 172), Cashew Parsley Sauce (page 236)	Herbs and Spices

Kaempferol, quercetin, polyunsaturated fatty acids (PUFAs – omega-3)	Omega-3 fatty acids are involved in regulating inflammatory processes in the body and may help to decrease inflammation. Omega-3 may also help to reduce pain in arthritic conditions like RA. However, more research is needed to determine how using mustard oil may affect inflammation in humans. Mustard oil contains allyl isothiocyanate, a chemical compound that has been well studied for its effect on pain receptors in the body, and despite minimal human research, one animal study found that administering mustard oil to drinking water desensitised certain pain receptors and helped treat widespread pain.
Zinc, magnesium, polyphenols, PUFAs	Oats provide a slow release of energy and are known to be good for the heart mainly due to their high β-glucan (beta-glucan) content. They also contain more than 20 unique polyphenols, such as avenanthramides, which have shown strong antioxidant and anti-inflammatory activity. Alongside polyphenols, they also contain proteins, peptides, amino acids, β-glucans, resistant starch, dietary fibres, polyunsaturated fatty acids, vitamins, and minerals such as zinc and magnesium.
Hydroxytyrosol, monounsaturated fatty acids (MUFAs), oleocanthal, vitamins A and E, iron, calcium	Black olives (as with black beans, the darker the better) have a better nutritional profile than green olives.
Kaempferol, quercetin, vitamin C	Onions contain over 25 different varieties of flavonoids or antioxidants, and red onions are the most healthful. Onions are a brilliant source of fibre and prebiotics too, which are necessary for optimal gut (and immune) health. One of the most remarkable properties of quercetin is its ability to modulate inflammation. Quercetin has been shown in some studies to be effective against chronic diseases, including arthritis and psoriasis, and has been shown to reduce inflammatory markers.
Sulforaphane	Sulforaphane has been shown to have anti-inflammatory and anti-arthritic effects in studies, including RA, and promising anti-inflammatory properties for osteoarthritis treatment, but more research is needed.
Vitamin A, capsaicin, carotenoids	Carotenoids and polyphenols play a key role in preventing certain diseases, while vitamin A, capsaicin and carotenoids may help prevent inflammation. Topically applied capsaicin is useful in alleviating pain associated with arthritis, and other chronic musculoskeletal pain.
Polyphenols (apigenin, quercetin, luteolin and kaempferol), carotenoids, vitamin K, vitamin C	Vitamin K is alleged to play an important role in bone health. In one study, participants with low levels of vitamin K were 56 per cent more likely to develop knee OA. Vitamin K has been associated with osteoarthritis and rheumatoid arthritis in a number of studies.

Pecans	Breakfast Granola Bowl (page 108), Apple and Berry Bake (page 182), Pick N Mix Chocolate Fruit Yoghurt (page 194), Sweet Cinnamon Mixed Nuts (page 210)	Nuts and Seeds
Pineapple	Green Dream Juice (page 222)	Fruit
Pistachios	Matcha and Berry Compote with Pistachio Crumb and Chocolate Sauce (page 184), Pick N Mix Chocolate Fruit Yoghurt (page 194)	Nuts and Seeds
Pomegranate seeds	Aubergine Dip Topped with Pomegranate Seeds (page 198)	Fruit
Pumpkin seeds	Breakfast Granola Bowl (page 108), Apricot Chia Seed Bites (page 202)	Nuts and Seeds
Quinoa	Moroccan Salmon with Fresh Mint Quinoa Salad (page 122), Sea Bass with Infused Quinoa (page 139), Katy's Quinoa-Base Pizza (page 166), Honey Mustard Chicken or Tofu Salad (page 170), Creamy Caesar Salad (page 172)	Grains and Proteins
Raspberries	Raspberry Jam (page 234), Pick N Mix Chocolate Fruit Yoghurt (page 194)	Fruit

Zinc, magnesium, polyunsaturated fatty acids (omega-3)	Omega-3 fats are known for easing inflammation, plus, the magnesium and zinc in pecans give the nuts anti-inflammatory properties. Pecans also provide folate*. Pecans have been characterised as having a high concentration of flavonoids and also containing EGCG, a powerful antioxidant, see Green tea (page 71) for more information. *Folate is a general term used to describe the many different forms of vitamin B9, which includes folic acid.
Bromelain	Bromelain is considered a high-value compound as it appears to be an effective treatment for inflammation, osteoarthritis, dental plaque, and more. It exhibits anti-inflammatory properties and one study suggests that it is a possible natural remedy for easing arthritis symptoms, including joint pain and stiffness, but human trials are required to test its efficacy.
Resveratrol, potassium, vitamins A and E, lutein, monounsaturated fatty acids (MUFAs)	Pistachios also contain alpha-linoleic acid (ALA), a beneficial type of omega-3 fatty acid that can be converted to DHA and EPA, the two other forms of omega-3s which are only found in animal sources, helpful for vegans and vegetarians. The polyphenols present in pistachios possess antioxidant and anti-inflammatory properties and have been shown in some studies to significantly reduce inflammation in the body with a positive impact on improving cardiovascular health.
Vitamin C, Vitamin A, folic acid, fibre, potassium, polyphenols	A cup of pomegranate seeds provides 10–20 per cent of the RDA of vitamin C. Pomegranate is also rich in anthocyanins, which have antioxidant and anti-inflammatory capabilities.Some studies have shown that pomegranate extract can block enzymes known to damage joints in people with osteoarthritis, plus it may prevent the onset of OA too. Pomegranate may also have the potential to help reduce inflammation in inflammatory conditions such as rheumatoid arthritis. Although pomegranate fruit extract has been shown to inhibit cartilage degradation in OA, and suppress inflammation and joint damage in rheumatoid arthritis, human evidence remains inconsistent.
Zinc, magnesium, calcium, iron, polyunsaturated fatty acids (PUFAs)	Health-promoting benefits of pumpkin seeds range from reducing inflammation to boosting immunity and alleviating depression. Roasted pumpkin seeds have a higher total concentration of phytonutrients with greater antioxidant properties than raw seeds. Tip: don't throw away pumpkin or butternut squash seeds, season and then roast them.
Quercetin, kaempferol, magnesium	Quinoa is high in protein but gluten-free, and contains PUFAs, carbohydrates, vitamins, minerals and fibre. It contains all nine essential amino acids, is anti-inflammatory with high antioxidant activity, and acts as a prebiotic supplying the fuel for beneficial gut bacteria, which is important for our immune health.
Anthocyanin (flavonoid), vitamin C, quercetin	Emerging preclinical studies (lab-based studies before human studies) provide evidence on the role of whole berries and berry polyphenols in reversing the pathological changes in arthritis, including OA. In one preclinical study raspberry extract was shown to improve the clinical symptoms of arthritis. One study suggests that red raspberry polyphenols may prevent cartilage protection and/ or modulate the onset and severity of arthritis. In an animal study, red raspberry extract decreased depression-like behaviour by modulating neuroinflammation and oxidative stress. Anti-inflammatory compounds, such as anthocyanins, appear to show that raspberries may reduce the symptoms of arthritis. These studies also show a lower risk of developing arthritis as well as less damage to the joints in those that developed the condition. However, more research and human trials are needed to confirm these effects.

Rooibos	Orange and Cinnamon Warmer (page 216)	Herbs and Spices
Sesame seeds (oil, seeds, tahini)	Ready-To-Go Jar Noodle Pot (page 119), Moroccan Salmon with Fresh Mint Quinoa Salad (page 122), Spicy Tahini Prawn 'Submarines' (page 125), Bang Bang Cauliflower Salad (page 126), Brown Rice 'Sushi' Nori Bites (page 128), Mushroom Noodle Soup (page 136), Plant-Packed Chow Mein (page 138), Grandad Speight's Nasi Goreng (page 144), Sticky and Sweet Mixed Veg Stir-Fry with Cashew Nuts (page 152), 'Fakeaway' Katsu Curry, or Katsu Curry Salad (page 160), Butternut Squash and Leek Risotto (page 175), Aubergine Dip Topped with Pomegranate Seeds (page 198), Smashed Cucumber Sesame Seed Salad (page 204), Plain, Hummus (page 206), Roasted Beetroot Hummus (page 207), Sweet Roasted Pepper Hummus (page 207)	Nuts and Seeds
Soy (tofu, tempeh, tamari, edamame)	Ready-To-Go Jar Noodle Pot (page 119), Creamy Mushroom Butter Beans with Asparagus (page 120), Spicy Tahini Prawn 'Submarines' (page 125), Bang Bang Cauliflower Salad (page 126), Brown Rice 'Sushi' Nori Bites (page 128), Mushroom Noodle Soup (page 136), Plant-Packed Chow Mein (page 138), One-Pot Harissa Tempeh Stew (page 143), Grandad Speight's Nasi Goreng (page 144), Sticky and Sweet Mixed Veg Stir-Fry with Cashew Nuts (page 152), Vegetable-Packed Shepherd's Pie (page 164), 'Fakeaway' Katsu Curry, or Katsu Curry Salad (page 160), Honey Mustard Chicken or Tofu Salad (page 170), Creamy Caesar Salad (page 172), Matcha and Berry Compote with Pistachio Crumb and Chocolate Sauce (page 184), Smashed Cucumber Sesame Seed Salad (page 204)	Grains and Proteins
Spinach	Breakfast Savoury Muffins (page 92), Easy Frittata (page 115), Moroccan Salmon with Fresh Mint Quinoa Salad (page 122), One-Pot Harissa Tempeh Stew (page 143), Spicy and Warming Dahl (page 158), Katy's Quinoa-Base Pizza (page 166), Vegan Chickpea Curry (page 169), Butternut Squash and Leek Risotto (page 175), Goan Prawn and Cod Curry (page 176), Italian-Style Chicken with Sweet Potato Wedges (page 178), Bold Beetroot Juice (page 223), Golden Delicious Green Smoothie (page 218)	Vegetable
Sunflower seeds	Moroccan Salmon with Fresh Mint Quinoa Salad (page 122)	Nuts and Seeds
Sweet potatoes	Sweet Potato 'Hash Brown' Patties and Perfect Poached Eggs (page 95), Spiced Sweet Potato Soup (page 132), One-Tray Roast Chicken with Vegetables (page 150), Hasselback Potatoes with Chilli Apricot Chutney and Cashew Cheese (page 163), Vegetable-Packed Shepherd's Pie (page 164), Italian-Style Chicken with Sweet Potato Wedges (page 178)	Vegetable

Quercetin, luteolin	Rooibos has displayed potent anti-inflammatory and antioxidant potential. The research to date seems to support that rooibos tea consumption is associated with both a reduction in pro-inflammatory cytokine signalling and a heightened secretion of the anti-inflammatory cytokine.
	As rooibos tea is caffeine-free, routine intake may be safe and useful in reducing oxidative stress, and it does not disturb sleep, unless you drink it right before bed, which isn't advised (see page 23).
Monounsaturated fatty acids (MUFAs) and Polyunsaturated fatty acids (PUFAs), vitamin E, fibre, and bioactive lignans	MUFAs, PUFAs, vitamin E, fibre, and bioactive lignans have the potential to produce antioxidant and anti-inflammatory activity. Sesamin, one of the most abundant lignans in sesame, has been found to exhibit beneficial effects on inflammatory markers. It also has anti-inflammatory and antioxidant effects that may protect joint cartilage and reduce pain in OA.
Genistein	Genistein has been found to have anti-inflammatory, immunomodulatory, pain-relieving and joint protection properties. A lab-based study found that genistein suppresses TNF-α-induced inflammation and reduces inflammatory cytokines. In another study, genistein used alongside methotrexate was found to be more effective than methotrexate alone in treating RA.
	Genistein has shown to attenuate the progression of OA and genistein-induced pain relief is even being studied to clarify its potential for neuropathic pain. It may have therapeutic value for arthritis in the future, but more extensive research is warranted.
Vitamin A, beta-carotene, lutein, folate, vitamin K, magnesium, carotenoids, potassium	Lower magnesium intake has been associated with worse pain and function in knee OA, especially among individuals with low fibre intake. Magnesium deficiency (MgD) may cause inflammation in the body. Magnesium has been linked to a number of benefits, from fighting inflammation to improving our sleep and reducing stress, even improving pain, energy and emotional wellbeing. Finally, 30g (1 cup) of raw spinach provides 121% of the recommended daily intake of vitamin K, for more information on vitamin K, see Parsley (page 72).
Vitamin E, zinc, calcium	Vitamin E neutralises free radicals and may help to prevent osteoarthritis and rheumatoid arthritis.
Carotenoids, fibre	Research has shown that phytonutrient carotenoids have the potential to help with inflammatory arthritis.

Tomatoes (fresh and/or sun-dried)	Breakfast Savoury Muffins (page 92), Mexican-Style Salad Bowl (page 112), Easy Frittata (page 115), Moroccan Salmon with Fresh Mint Quinoa Salad (page 122), One-Pot Harissa Tempeh Stew (page 143), Pulled Smoky Jackfruit Salad (page 147), One-Tray Roast Chicken with Vegetables (page 150), Sticky and Sweet Mixed Veg Stir-Fry with Cashew Nuts (page 152), Vegan Chilli (page 156), Spicy and Warming Dahl (page 158), Vegetable-Packed Shepherd's Pie (page 164), 'Fakeaway' Katsu Curry, or Katsu Curry Salad (page 160), Katy's Quinoa-Base Pizza (page 166), Honey Mustard Chicken or Tofu Salad (page 170), Creamy Caesar Salad (page 172), Goan Prawn and Cod Curry (page 176), Italian-Style Chicken with Sweet Potato Wedges (page 178), Chilli Apricot Chutney (page 237)
Turmeric	Spiced Sweet Potato Soup (page 132), Grandad Speight's Nasi Goreng (page 144), Spicy and Warming Dahl (page 158), 'Fakeaway' Katsu Curry, or Katsu Curry Salad (page 160), Vegan Chickpea Curry (page 169), Goan Prawn and Cod Curry (page 176), Sunshine Juice (page 222), Turmeric Kick Juice (page 219)
Turnips	One-Tray Roast Chicken with Vegetables (page 150)
Walnuts	Carrot Cake Overnight Oats (page 101), Salmon Fishcakes and Cashew Parsley Sauce (page 116), Moroccan Salmon with Fresh Mint Quinoa Salad (page 122), Apple and Berry Bake (page 182), Carrot (and Courgette) Loaf Cake (page 187), No-Bake Ginger and 'Caramel' Slices (page 188), Vegan Chocolate Tiffin (page 189), Pick N Mix Chocolate Fruit Yoghurt (page 194), Sweet Cinnamon Mixed Nuts (page 210), Apricot Chia Seed Bites (page 202), Roasted Beetroot Hummus (page 207), Walnut Vegan Pesto (page 239)
Watercress	Salmon and Puy Lentils with Orange Dressing (page 148)

Vitamin C, kaempferol, lycopene	Phytochemical lycopene is anti-inflammatory and consuming tomatoes with olive oil increases the absorption of lycopene. However, nutritionist Victoria Jain adds that tomatoes might be an issue for those with compromised digestive functions (or for some people), so if you do feel you have a reaction to eating tomatoes, then see if you feel better removing them your diet using the Trigger Tracker on page 34. Recent research shows it can depend on how and where tomatoes have been cultivated, and their nutrient content, as with many of the ingredients in this table.
Curcumin	Curcumin has been found to be at least ten times more active as an antioxidant than vitamin E. In one animal study, curcumin significantly suppressed the severity of arthritis, exceeding the anti-arthritic activity of NSAID indomethacin. Despite the lack of significant data from clinical human trials, initial research has shown that curcumin can suppress the expression of inflammatory mediators and modulate immune cells, alleviating the course of RA, and so curcumin's immunomodulatory and anti-inflammatory role seems to have the potential to improve RA patients' lives naturally. Curcumin is the main bioactive found in the turmeric root and many studies have shown that it exerts anti-inflammatory properties and may help to fight inflammation. There is sufficient evidence to say that it may have beneficial effects in various conditions, from arthritis to chronic pain. A very recent study analysed 25 clinical trials with a total of 2,253 participants (called meta-analysis) on the potential effects of supplementing curcumin (or turmeric extract). Those in the study were patients with OA or RA. It looked at the various clinical outcomes relevant to arthritis, such as inflammation biomarkers, or joint stiffness. The overall outcome was that supplementation with turmeric extract, or curcumin, reduced disease severity, inflammatory markers, rheumatoid factor (inflammation biomarker), and most importantly pain levels.
Sulforaphane	Sulforaphane has been shown to have anti-inflammatory and anti-arthritic effects in some studies with RA, and promising anti-inflammatory properties for osteoarthritis treatment, but more research is needed.
Polyunsaturated fatty acids (PUFAs – omega-3), magnesium	Omega-3 has been shown in some studies to reduce arthritic pain and rheumatoid arthritis disease activity, including showing that omega-3 supplements along with DMARDS treatment in patients with newly diagnosed RA can be effective in reducing symptoms. Walnuts are significantly higher in omega-3s than any other nut. There is extensive evidence that omega-3 PUFAs can mediate anti-inflammatory effects. A cup (117g) of chopped walnuts has a 44 per cent of RDA for magnesium, for more detail see Spinach (page 74).
Vitamins A, C and E, quercetin, kaempferol, sulfurophane, carotenoids	Watercress is also a source of folate, calcium and iron. Sulforaphane (1-isothiocyanate-4-methyl sulfonyl butane) is a plant extract obtained from cruciferous vegetables, such as broccoli and cabbage, known to exert anticancer, antioxidant and anti-inflammatory effects.

THE RECIPES

'Cooking demands attention, patience, and,
above all, a respect for the gifts of the earth.
It is a form of worship, a way of giving thanks.'

Judith Jones in *The Tenth Muse*,
American food writer and editor

Now, here are over 85 delicious anti-inflammatory recipes that you can make at home, prep and freeze, as well as share with your family and friends. All of the recipes and the meal planner have been checked and approved by nutritionist VJ Hamilton as well. I have put a rough guide of the timings on the recipes, but please note that we all have our own physical ability and cooking skills, so I did not wish for people to feel disheartened if recipes take them longer than the time allotted to it – we all experience our arthritis and pain differently.

Each recipe also has the following tags:

- Meal Prep
- 10 Ingredients or Less
- Freezable
- Under 30 minutes
- Under 1 hour
- Over 2 hours
- Cooking for Friends and Family
- Fakeaway

Meal Prep means that you can prep all the ingredients beforehand and go straight into the cooking. 10 ingredients or Less means that the recipe uses less than 10 ingredients. Freezable means that you can easily freeze the recipe after making it. Under 30 minutes/under 1 hour/over 2 hours are noted on recipes so you know what you're in for and how much time you'll need to commit to each meal. Cooking for Friends and Family indicate recipes where you can easily double the recipes to make great sharing meals. Finally, Fakeaway is for all those meals that you can create when you fancy some real comfort food.

You'll also spot vegetarian (V), vegan (VEG), dairy-free (DF) and gluten-free (GF) notes on all the recipes.

I've included a super handy meal plan – which stretches across 6 weeks – to get you started!

Enjoy!

Here's a handy key for all the tags - look out for them on the recipes

Meal Prep	Cooking for Friends and Family
Freezable	10 Ingredients or Less
Cook time	Fakeaway

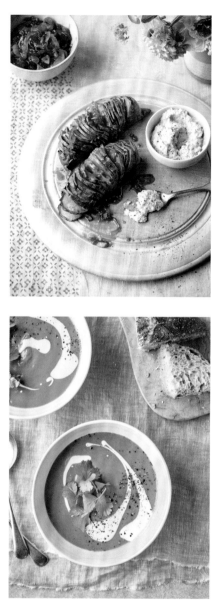
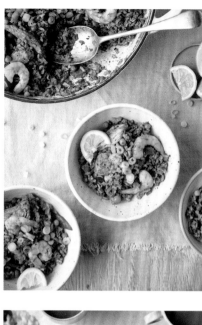
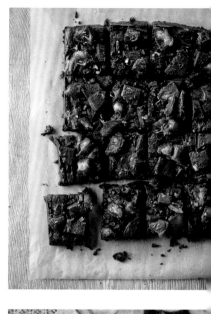
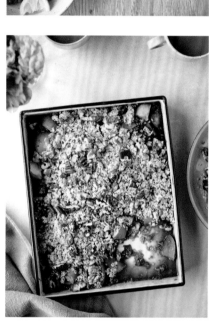
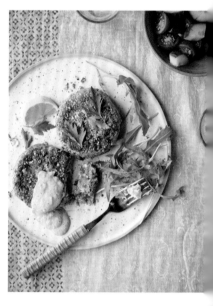
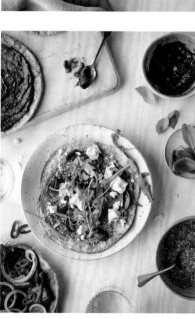
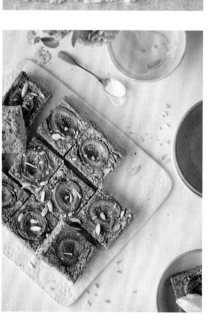
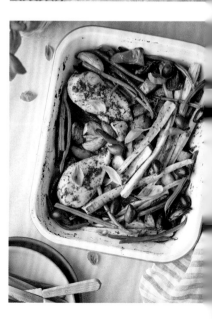

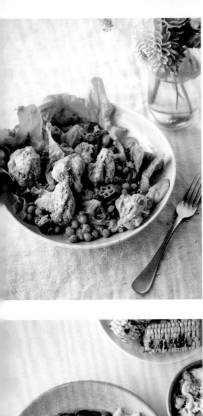
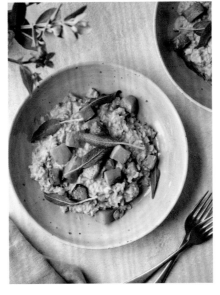
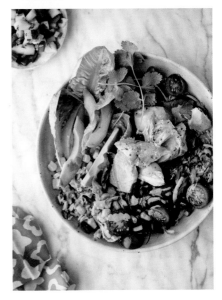
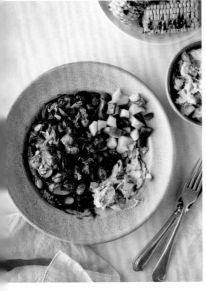
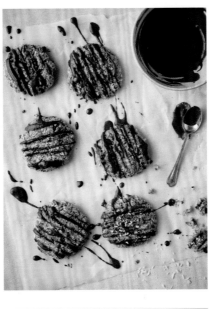
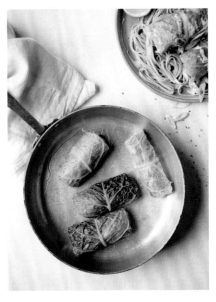
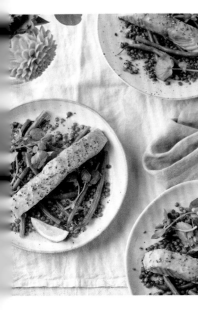
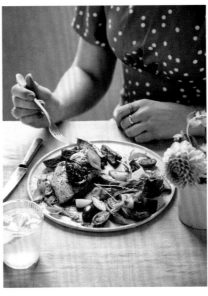
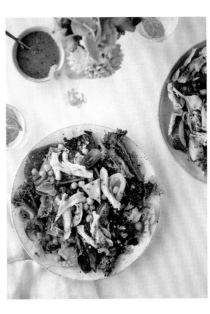

WEEK 1

DAY	BREAKFAST	LUNCHTIME	EVENING MEAL	DESSERTS	SNACKS	DRINKS/NOTES
MONDAY	Cinnamon Toast Overnight Oats (page 100)	Ready-To-Go Probiotic Noodle Jar (page 119)	One-Pot Chicken and Prawn Jambalaya (page 140) [freeze 2 of the 6 portions]			Calm and Energising Matcha (page 226)
TUESDAY	Cinnamon Toast Overnight Oats (page 100)	Ready-To-Go Probiotic Noodle Jar (page 119)	One-Pot Chicken and Prawn Jambalaya (page 140)			Turmeric Kick Juice (page 219) [drink for the next following 2 days]
WEDNESDAY	Cinnamon Toast Overnight Oats (page 100)	Ready-To-Go Probiotic Noodle Jar (page 119)	One-Pot Chicken and Prawn Jambalaya (page 140)			Turmeric Kick Juice (page 219)
THURSDAY	Indulgent Chocolate Porridge (page 96)	Spiced Sweet Potato Soup (page 132) [freeze 2 of the 4 portions]	One-Pot Chicken and Prawn Jambalaya (page 140)			Turmeric Kick Juice (page 219) [freeze any remaining]
FRIDAY	Breakfast Savoury Muffins (page 92) [2 of them, freeze 6 of them]	Spiced Sweet Potato Soup (page 132)	Sea Bass with Infused Quinoa (page 139)	Pick N Mix Chocolate Fruit Yoghurt (page 194)		Calm and Energising Matcha (page 226)
SATURDAY	Breakfast Savoury Muffins (page 92) [2 of them]	Brown Rice 'Sushi' Nori Bites (page 128)	Sea Bass with Infused Quinoa (page 139)	Pick N Mix Chocolate Fruit Yoghurt (page 194)		Calm and Energising Matcha (page 226)
SUNDAY	Breakfast Savoury Muffins (page 92) [2 of them]	Brown Rice 'Sushi' Nori Bites (page 128) [leftovers]	One-Pot Harissa Tempeh Stew (page 143)	Pick N Mix Chocolate Fruit Yoghurt (page 194)		Calm and Energising Matcha (page 226) Make Breakfast Granola for the week

WEEK 2

DAY	BREAKFAST	LUNCHTIME	EVENING MEAL	DESSERTS	SNACKS	DRINKS/NOTES
MONDAY	Breakfast Granola Bowl (page 108)	Creamy Caesar Salad (page 172) [half the recipe]	One-Pot Harissa Tempeh Stew (page 143)			Anti-Inflammatory Power Juice (page 223)
TUESDAY	Breakfast Granola Bowl (page 108)	Creamy Caesar Salad (page 172)	One-Pot Harissa Tempeh Stew (page 143) [freeze the remaining portion]		Coconut Banana 'Cookie' Bites (page 201)	Anti-Inflammatory Power Juice (page 223)
WEDNESDAY	Breakfast Granola Bowl (page 108)	Pulled Smoky Jackfruit Salad (page 147)	Moroccan Salmon with Fresh Mint Quinoa Salad (page 122)		Coconut Banana 'Cookie' Bites (page 201)	Green tea
THURSDAY	Breakfast Granola Bowl (page 108)	Pulled Smoky Jackfruit Salad (page 147)	Moroccan Salmon with Fresh Mint Quinoa Salad (page 122)	Layered Mango and Passion Fruit Dessert (page 192) [freeze 2 of the 4 portions]	Coconut Banana 'Cookie' Bites (page 201)	Calm and Energising Matcha (page 226)
FRIDAY	Breakfast Granola Bowl (page 108)	Defrosted portion of One-Pot Harissa Tempeh Stew (page 143)	Spicy and Warming Dahl (page 158) [freeze one portion]	Layered Mango and Passion Fruit Dessert (page 192)	Coconut Banana 'Cookie' Bites (page 201)	Note: soak the urad beans this evening for dinner tomorrow
SATURDAY	Sweet Potato 'Hash Brown' Patties and Perfect Poached Eggs page 95)	Creamy Mushroom Butter Beans with Asparagus (page 120) [half the recipe]	Spicy and Warming Dahl (page 158)	Apple and Berry Bake (page 182) [make half the recipe, or freeze half in portions for breakfasts]		Orange and Cinnamon Warmer (page 216)
SUNDAY	Sweet Potato 'Hash Brown' Patties and Perfect Poached Eggs (page 95)	Creamy Mushroom Butter Beans with Asparagus (page 120) [half the recipe]	Spicy and Warming Dahl (page 158)	Apple and Berry Bake (page 182)	Sweet Cinnamon Mixed Nuts (page 210) [makes 10+ servings]	Orange and Cinnamon Warmer (page 216)

WEEK 3

DAY	BREAKFAST	LUNCHTIME	EVENING MEAL	DESSERTS	SNACKS	DRINKS/NOTES
MONDAY	Breakfast Granola Bowl (page 108) or Apple and Berry Bake leftovers (page 182)	Easy Frittata and Crunchy Salad (page 115)	Defrosted portion of One-Pot Chicken and Prawn Jambalaya (page 140)			Orange and Cinnamon Warmer (page 216)
TUESDAY	Breakfast Granola Bowl (page 108) or Apple and Berry Bake leftovers (page 182)	Easy Frittata and Crunchy Salad (page 115)	Butternut Squash and Leek Risotto (page 175)			Orange and Cinnamon Warmer (page 216) Make your raspberry jam/ overnight oats
WEDNESDAY	Bakewell Tart Overnight Oats (page 101)	Defrosted Spiced Sweet Potato Soup (page 132)	Butternut Squash and Leek Risotto (page 175)			Green tea
THURSDAY	Bakewell Tart Overnight Oats (page 101)	Salmon Fishcakes and Cashew Parsley Sauce (page 116) [half the recipe]	Butternut Squash and Leek Risotto (page 175)			Green tea
FRIDAY	Bakewell Tart Overnight Oats (page 101)	Salmon Fishcakes and Cashew Parsley Sauce (page 116) [half the recipe]	Defrosted portion of Grandad Speight's Nasi Goreng (page 144)	Matcha and Berry Compote with Pistachio Crumb and Chocolate Sauce (page 184)		Calm and Energising Matcha (page 226)
SATURDAY	Apricot and Almond Baked Oats (page 104) [freeze two portions]	Salmon Fishcakes and Cashew Parsley Sauce (page 116) [half the recipe]	Defrosted portion of Spicy and Warming Dahl (page 158)	Matcha and Berry Compote with Pistachio Crumb and Chocolate Sauce (page 184)		Calm and Energising Matcha (page 226)
SUNDAY	Apricot and Almond Baked Oats (page 104)	Mushroom Noodle Soup (page 136)	Vegan Chilli (page 156) [freeze 1 portion]	Matcha and Berry Compote with Pistachio Crumb and Chocolate Sauce (page 184)		Calm and Energising Matcha (page 226)

WEEK 4

DAY	BREAKFAST	LUNCHTIME	EVENING MEAL	DESSERTS	SNACKS	DRINKS/NOTES
MONDAY	Apricot and Almond Baked Oats (page 104)	Vegan Chilli (page 156)	Grandad Speight's Nasi Goreng (page 144) [freeze 2 portions]		Cacao and Coconut Energy Balls (page 203)	Green tea
TUESDAY	Apricot and Almond Baked Oats (page 104)	Mushroom Noodle Soup (page 136)	Vegan Chilli (page 156)		Cacao and Coconut Energy Balls (page 203)	Green tea
WEDNESDAY	Defrosted Breakfast Savoury Muffins (page 92) [2 of them]	Grandad Speight's Nasi Goreng (page 144)	Defrosted portion of One-Pot Chicken and Prawn Jambalaya (page 140)		Cacao and Coconut Energy Balls (page 203)	Green tea
THURSDAY	Breakfast Granola Bowl (page 108)	Defrosted Spiced Sweet Potato Soup (page 132)	Sticky and Sweet Mixed Veg Stir-Fry with Cashew Nuts (page 152) [make double the amount]		Cacao and Coconut Energy Balls (page 203)	Green tea
FRIDAY	Breakfast Granola Bowl (page 108)	Honey Mustard Chicken or Tofu Salad (page 170) [make half the recipe]	Sticky and Sweet Mixed Veg Stir-Fry with Cashew Nuts (page 152)			Bold Beetroot Juice (page 223)
SATURDAY	Breakfast Granola Bowl (page 108)	Honey Mustard Chicken or Tofu Salad (page 170)	Sticky and Sweet Mixed Veg Stir-Fry with Cashew Nuts (page 152)			Bold Beetroot Juice (page 223)
SUNDAY	My Fair Lady Pancakes (page 98)	Aubergine Dip Topped with Pomegranate Seeds (page 198) [serve with the Crudités and toasted sourdough]		Carrot (and Courgette) Loaf Cake - to share! Have the leftovers for breakfast too (page 187)		Calm and Energising Matcha (page 226)

WEEK 5

DAY	BREAKFAST	LUNCHTIME	EVENING MEAL	DESSERTS	SNACKS	DRINKS/NOTES
MONDAY	My Fair Lady Pancakes (page 98) [leftovers, freeze the remaining 6/2 portions]	Aubergine Dip Topped with Pomegranate Seeds (page 198) [serve with the Crudités and toasted sourdough slices]	Goan Prawn and Cod Curry (page 176)	Carrot (and Courgette) Loaf Cake (page 187)		Green tea
TUESDAY	Carrot (and Courgette) Loaf Cake (page 187) with coconut yoghurt	Aubergine Dip Topped with Pomegranate Seeds (page 198) [serve with the Crudités and toasted sourdough slices]	Goan Prawn and Cod Curry (page 176)		Sweet Cinnamon Mixed Nuts (page 210)	Green tea
WEDNESDAY	Date, Cacao and Banana Chia Pot (page 109)	Moroccan Salmon with Fresh Mint Quinoa Salad (page 122)	Defrosted portion of Vegan Chilli (page 156)		Sweet Cinnamon Mixed Nuts (page 210)	Green tea
THURSDAY	Date, Cacao and Banana Chia Pot (page 109)	Moroccan Salmon with Fresh Mint Quinoa Salad (page 122)	Bang Bang Cauliflower Salad (page 126)		Sweet Cinnamon Mixed Nuts (page 210)	Green tea
FRIDAY	Date, Cacao and Banana Chia Pot (page 109)	Bang Bang Cauliflower Salad (page 126)	Katy's Quinoa-Base Pizza (page 166)	Almond Butter Brownies (page 191) – share with friends!	Sweet Cinnamon Mixed Nuts (page 210)	Calm and Energising Matcha (page 226)
SATURDAY	Carrot Cake Overnight Oats (page 101)	Bang Bang Cauliflower Salad (page 126)	Katy's Quinoa-Base Pizza (page 166)	Almond Butter Brownies (page 191)	Vanilla Date Hemp Seed Smoothie (page 218)	Calm and Energising Matcha (page 226)
SUNDAY	Defrosted My Fair Lady Pancakes (page 98) – buy fresh fruit to go with them [3 of them, 1 portion]	Bang Bang Cauliflower Salad (page 126)	Vegan Chickpea Curry (page 169) [freeze 3 portions]	Almond Butter Brownies (page 191)	Vanilla Date Hemp Seed Smoothie (page 218)	Make the Chilli Apricot Chutney over the weekend Make the cashew cheese (soak the cashews overnight)

WEEK 6

DAY	BREAKFAST	LUNCHTIME	EVENING MEAL	DESSERTS	SNACKS	DRINKS/NOTES
MONDAY	Defrosted My Fair Lady Pancakes (page 98) [3 of them, 1 portion]	Katy's Quinoa-Base Pizza (page 166)	Vegan Chickpea Curry (page 169)			
TUESDAY	Indulgent Chocolate Porridge (page 96)	Hasselback Potatoes with Chilli Apricot Chutney and Cashew Cheese (page 163)	Vegan Chickpea Curry (page 169)		Sweet Cinnamon Mixed Nuts (page 210)	Green tea
WEDNESDAY	Cinnamon Toast Overnight Oats (page 100)	Hasselback Potatoes with Chilli Apricot Chutney and Cashew Cheese (page 163)	Defrosted portion of Butternut Squash and Leek Risotto (page 175)		Sweet Cinnamon Mixed Nuts (page 210)	Calm and Energising Matcha (page 226)
THURSDAY	Cinnamon Toast Overnight Oats (page 100)	Hasselback Potatoes with Chilli Apricot Chutney and Cashew Cheese (page 163) (new batch of sweet potatoes)	Defrosted portion of Goan Prawn and Cod Curry (page 176)		Sweet Cinnamon Mixed Nuts (page 210)	Green tea
FRIDAY	Defrosted Apricot and Almond Baked Oats (page 104)	Hasselback Potatoes with Chilli Apricot Chutney and Cashew Cheese (page 163)	Italian-Style Chicken with Sweet Potato Wedges (page 178) [halve the recipe]	VJ's Black Cherry Ice Cream (page 195)		Golden Delicious Green Smoothie (page 218)
SATURDAY	Lemon and Berry Muffins (page 107)	Hummus Trio Tray (page 206) [make one for lunch, or more to share!]	Italian-Style Chicken with Sweet Potato Wedges (page 178)	VJ's Black Cherry Ice Cream (page 195)		Golden Delicious Green Smoothie (page 218)
SUNDAY	Lemon and Berry Muffins (page 107)	One-Tray Roast Chicken with Vegetables (page 150)	'Fakeaway' Katsu Curry, or Katsu Curry Salad (page 160)	VJ's Black Cherry Ice Cream (page 195)		Calm and Energising Matcha (page 226) Katsu can be used for lunches or dinners later

KITCHEN NOTES AND TIPS

If you're unsure on how to set up your kitchen, the kind of equipment you need, and how to stock up your store cupboard, fridge, and freezer, please turn back to pages 22–27. There are also some brilliant cooking tools, tips and adaptations with occupational therapist Cheryl Crow on pages 40–43.

Sea salt (or pink Himalayan salt, if you can find it) and ground black pepper	Unless otherwise stated, this is to taste; usually a 'twist' or two of the mills will suffice.
Plant milk	Almond, soya, hemp seed, oat, coconut, cashew, brown rice, hazelnut and tigernut. My recommendation would be almond milk, as it is naturally low in sugars, and to try to get the most whole-food one you can, or even make your own using the recipe on page 229.
Oils	All oil used in these recipes is extra virgin olive oil, unless otherwise stated. If using coconut oil, choose cold-pressed and extra virgin. Unrefined nut oils, like sesame oil commonly used in Chinese dishes, should be refrigerated because they are prone to go rancid and lose their flavour.
Eggs, meat, vegetables and fish	All organic, and GMO-free (if you are unable to find/afford organic eggs, then try to buy free-range), and, where possible, wild-caught salmon like Sockeye salmon for instance, as The European Environment Agency states that 'farmed salmon is the most toxic fish'. Quality over quantity when it comes to meat: pasture-raised and organic, could you head to your local farm shop?
Grating	Use the grater setting on your food processor, or ask for help.
Vegan alternative to honey	Use maple syrup, agave or date syrup.
Vegan alternative to eggs	Use a vegan egg recipe (mix 1 tablespoon chia or ground flaxseeds with 2½ tablespoons water and leave to rest for 10 minutes).
Shop-bought products	Tomato purée, mayonnaise, wholegrain mustard, apple cider vinegar (with the mother), balsamic vinegar (traditional or condiment grade), curry or harissa pastes, herb and spices, oils, nut butters, vegetable stocks, or powders like raw cacao powder, try to choose 100 per cent wholefood, unrefined and organic.
Apple cider vinegar	Make sure it is 'with the mother' (this means it's unfiltered and unrefined, with beneficial bacteria, yeast and protein).

Dried fruits	Choose sulphur dioxide-free and organic (for example, apricots will be brown not orange!).
Tinned coconut milk	Chakoah is the best brand I've found, but there are plenty out there.
Flour-based recipes	I mainly use brown rice flour or buckwheat flour, but other GF options include oat (you can actually blend oats to make this at home), almond, chickpea and coconut.
Pasta	In general use GF versions (e.g. red lentil penne pasta, which nutritionist Victoria Jain (VJ) is also a big fan of too, as typically it is made with 100% red lentil flour).
Rice	Red, black or wild rice has additional nutrient value to brown rice, as the presence of phytonutrient and antioxidant anthocyanin makes it nutritionally super-rich and has been cited for its anti-inflammatory properties in a number of studies.
Noodles	The best brand I have found is King Soba organic brown rice and wakame noodles. Nutritionist VJ recommends quinoa noodles with added protein, but white rice vermicelli noodles may be more accessible.
Quinoa	Quinoa is more prone to pesticide residues and contaminants, and according to VJ a pesticide in quinoa can be quite reactive for some people, so it is always best to rinse it thoroughly first and buy organic if possible.
Roasted garlic	Bash cloves once (which releases some of the health benefits), then cook in the oven (unpeeled) at 190–200°C fan (410–425°F) for 10 minutes. Cool and peel.
Bell peppers	Red bell peppers pack the most nutrition because they've been on the vine longest. Green peppers are harvested earlier, before they have a chance to turn yellow, orange, and then red. This is why, red and orange bell peppers are cited as having the most nutritional value, including vitamin C and beta-carotene (for more detail, see page 89).

Note: The potential health effects of these fruits, vegetables, herbs, and spices and more, depend on the nutritional content, which can fluctuate based on factors such as genetic background, cultivation methods, growth season, available light, ripening stage, and postharvest treatments, etc. Health effects also depend on the ingested amount, or serving size.

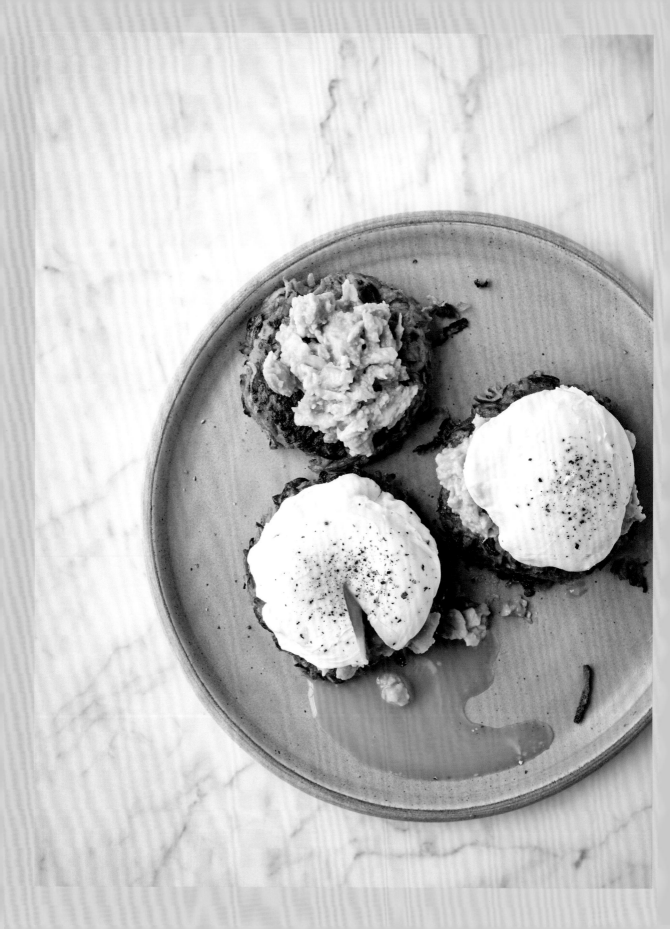

BREAKFAST

BREAKFAST SAVOURY MUFFINS

V, DF, GF

🍴 Meal Prep 👝 10 Ingredients or Less ❄ Freezable 🕐 Under 1 hour

MAKES 12 (SERVES 4-6)

1 red bell pepper
20 baby plum tomatoes
12g (½ cup) basil leaves
115g (2½ cups) baby spinach
Extra virgin olive oil
6 eggs
130ml (½ cup) almond milk
Sea salt and black pepper

Something savoury to whip up and stick in the oven to eat that morning, or keep in the fridge for 3–5 days. Peppers are rich in vitamin C to help with oxidative stress, and eggs are a nutrient-dense food that includes selenium, plus vitamins A and E, which act as antioxidants in the body. You could serve this with the Chipotle Sauce on page 234 and some butter leaf lettuce leaves.

1. Preheat the oven to 180°C fan (400°F).
2. Dice the bell pepper, slice the tomatoes lengthways and then in half, slice the basil, then add everything to a large mixing bowl.
3. Cook the baby spinach with 1 teaspoon of extra virgin olive oil until it wilts (about 1 minute 15 seconds). Drain the excess water by pressing down on the spinach in the pan before adding to the mixing bowl.
4. Whisk the eggs in a jug and stir in the almond milk, adding a pinch of salt and pepper. Add this mixture to the bowl and stir in well.
5. Lightly grease a 12-hole muffin tin with oil, and place in the oven for 3–5 minutes to heat up.
6. Add the chunkier parts of the mixture into the oiled muffin-tin holes using a large spoon, then pour in the liquid on top. (You can add the mixture from the bowl into a jug if that's easier.)
7. Bake for 20–25 minutes until the muffins are fully cooked through (a thin knife inserted into the centre should come out clean).
8. Eat straight away, or cool and store in an airtight container for 3–4 days.

Tip:
If you do not want to eat the muffins for breakfast in the coming days, then chop them up and add to a vegetable stir-fry (see Grandad Speight's Nasi Goreng on page 144).

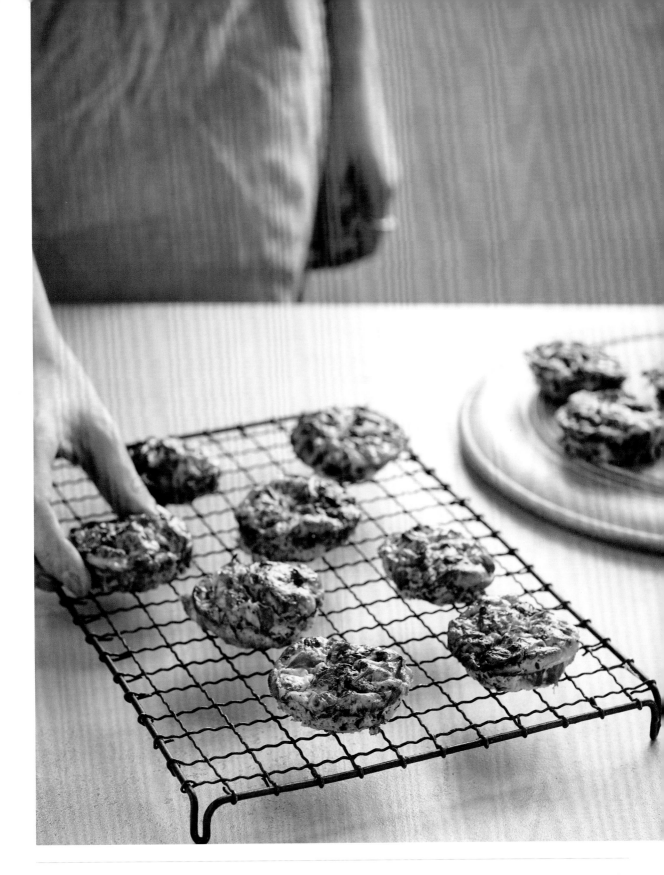

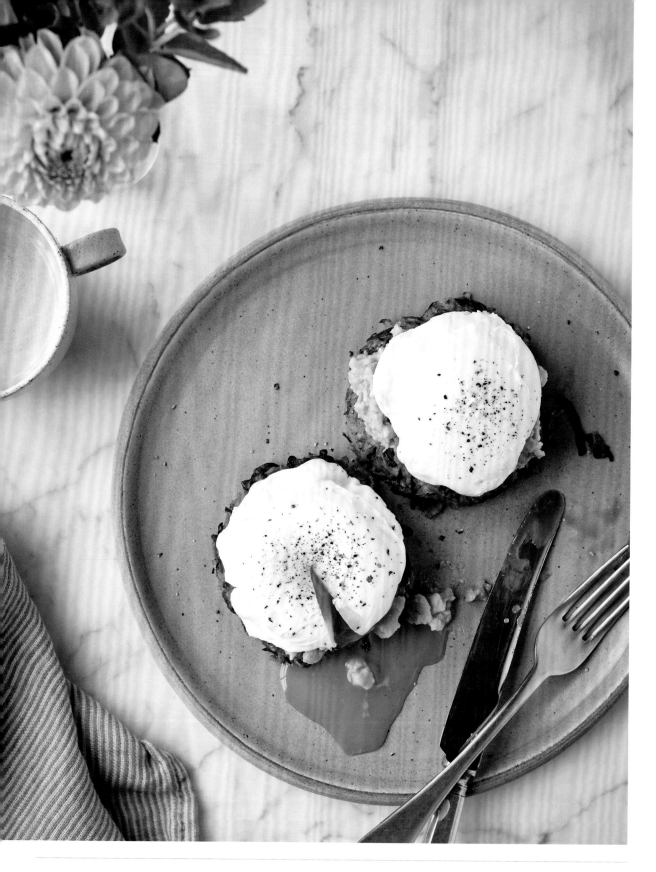

EAT WELL WITH ARTHRITIS

SWEET POTATO 'HASH BROWN' PATTIES AND PERFECT POACHED EGGS

V, DF, GF

✳ Freezable ⊫ Meal Prep 🏷 10 ingredients or Less 🕐 Under 1 hour

SERVES 2 –3/MAKES 6 SMALL OR 6 MEDIUM

2 tbsp chia seeds or ground flaxseeds and 6 tbsp water or 2 small eggs
2 large sweet potatoes (570–590g/18–21oz – peeled weight 520–530g)
1 red onion
1 tsp garlic powder
½ tsp paprika
½ tsp sea salt
½ tsp black pepper
60g (½ cup) chickpea flour (or buckwheat or brown rice flour)
1–2 tbsp extra virgin olive oil

FOR THE TOPPINGS
1 avocado
4 eggs

A quick and easy go-to brunch at home with phytonutrient carotenoids from the sweet potatoes, which have been shown to help with inflammatory arthritis. This can also be made vegan by omitting the eggs and enjoying the fritters with a different topping, such as garlic mushrooms and spinach.

1. Preheat the oven to 190°C fan (410°F) if you want to bake the hash brown pattie.
2. If using vegan eggs, mix the chia seeds and water together in a small bowl and leave to sit for 5 minutes. If using eggs, whisk them in a small bowl and set aside.
3. Peel, then grate the sweet potatoes using the thinnest grating setting on your food processor, then place in sieve over a bowl. With the back of a spoon, press down on the grated sweet potato to release the water into the bowl underneath it.
4. Finely chop the onion into half-moons and add to a separate large mixing bowl. Stir in the grated sweet potato.
5. Mix in all the seasonings, then the flour, then add the vegan egg or beaten eggs.
6. To fry, add 1 tablespoon of oil to a large frying pan and, once hot, scoop the sweet potato mixture into the pan in 6–8 tight mounds. Flatten each one into a hash-brown patty shape with the back of a spatula and cook for 3–5 minutes on each side until they are golden brown.
7. Alternatively, to bake, place the 6–8 fritters on a baking sheet covered with baking parchment and bake in the oven for 20 minutes. Flip and cook for a further 5–10 minutes.
8. When you are halfway through cooking the patties, heat a pan of hot water until it bubbles. Turn the water down to a simmer with tiny rising bubbles visible and plop the eggs in using ramekins or mugs to prevent breaking (if using older eggs, add a splash of vinegar to the water). Time for exactly 3 minutes for perfect poached eggs.
9. Smash or slice the flesh of the avocado in a small bowl.
10. Top your sweet potato fritters with the smashed avocado and poached eggs.

Tip:
You could also serve these with the Chipotle Sauce on page 234.

INDULGENT CHOCOLATE PORRIDGE

V, VEG, DF, GF   Cooking for Friends and Family   10 Ingredients or Less   ✳ Under 30 minutes

SERVES 1

40g (½ cup) whole
    rolled oats
250ml (1 cup) plant milk
150ml (⅔ cup) water
1 tbsp raw cacao powder
2 tsp date syrup

**FOR THE TOPPING
(OPTIONAL)**
strawberries
banana
nut butter of choice (VJ's
    preference is macadamia,
    and my choice would be
    almond butter, but there's
    plenty to choose from!)
cacao nibs

Porridge is perfect as it is, but sometimes we all crave the indulgence of chocolate, and this recipe is one way to get that. With resveratrol from the cacao powder, and plenty of gut-feeding fibre from the oats, this also provides a slow release of energy.

1. Pour the oats into a pan and mix in your plant milk and water.
2. Place on a high heat until it starts to steam and lightly bubble (around 3–5 minutes), then reduce the heat to low–medium, simmer and stir.
3. Lightly whisk in the cacao powder and date syrup. Stir continuously for around 5–8 minutes, or until all the liquid has been absorbed and your porridge has a thick and creamy consistency.
4. Remove from the heat and leave to cool for 1 minute. Serve with the toppings of your choice.

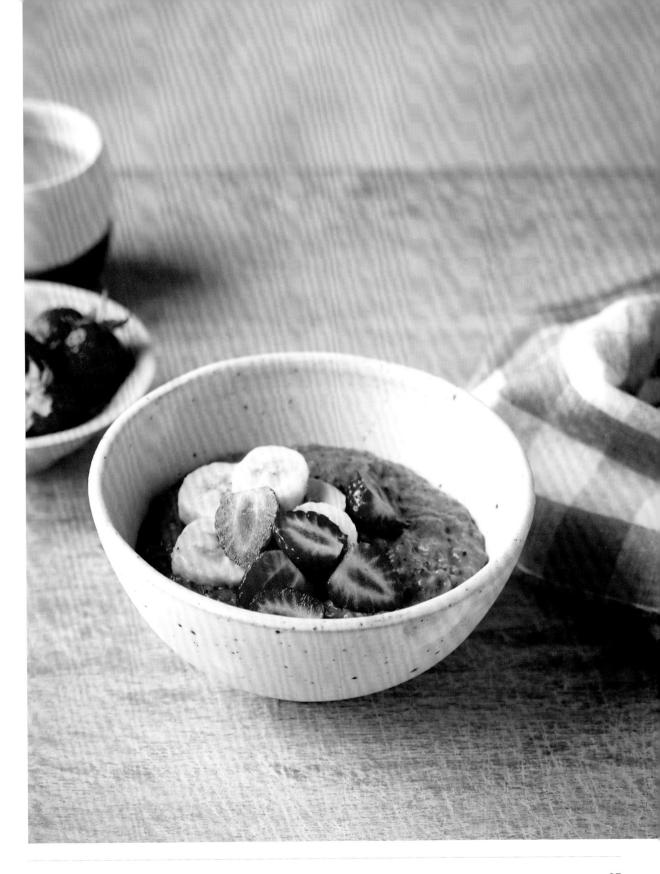

MY FAIR LADY PANCAKES

V, DF, GF

🥄 Cooking for Friends and Family ✳ Freezable 🕐 Under 1 hour

MAKES 12 (SERVES 4–6)

**FOR THE
PANCAKE BATTER**
225g (1½ cups)
  buckwheat flour
¼ tsp ground cinnamon
1 tsp baking powder
260ml (1 cup) plant milk
Juice of 1 large orange
  (55ml or ¼ cup)
Juice of 1 lemon (55ml
  or ¼ cup)
2 eggs, beaten (or vegan
  eggs, see page 88)
2 tsp coconut oil,
  or olive oil, per two
  pancakes for frying

**FOR THE STRAWBERRY
TOPPING**
400g (2½ cups)
  sliced strawberries
80ml (⅓ cup) water
2 tbsp honey (or maple
  syrup, if vegan)

**FOR THE TOPPINGS
(PER PERSON)**
Squeeze of orange juice
2 tbsp coconut yoghurt
Sprinkle of lemon zest
2–3 whole strawberries

Strawberries, oranges, cinnamon and more, these pancakes are named after a cocktail invented by the legendary barman Joe Gilmore, who created it to mark Julie Andrews' first night in the musical *My Fair Lady*, hence the name. It's delicious, but it may spike blood sugar, which could be inflammatory for some people. This recipe is one for the weekend and is not recommended as an everyday dish. If freezing, wrap the pancakes in baking paper two at a time.

1. To make the pancakes, fill a large mixing bowl with all of the dry ingredients and mix well.
2. Slowly add all of the wet ingredients, pouring in the plant milk first, then the fruit juices, then the eggs. Combine well.
3. To make the strawberry topping, place the strawberries in a pan with the water and cook on a low–medium heat for 5 minutes. Add the honey or maple syrup and simmer for another 15-20 minutes until thickened.
4. Meanwhile, heat 2 teaspoons of coconut oil in a large flat frying pan and cook the pancake mixture (2 pancakes at a time, around 1-2 ladles per pancake) for about 1-2 minutes on each side. You can either have two medium ones, or three small ones cooking at the same time. Pile the pancakes onto a plate, as you cook them.
5. Keep stirring the strawberry mixture while you cook the pancakes.
6. Cut the pile of pancakes into quarters like a slice of cake, or have the pancakes individually, and top with your orange juice, coconut yoghurt, lemon zest, strawberry topping and fresh strawberries.

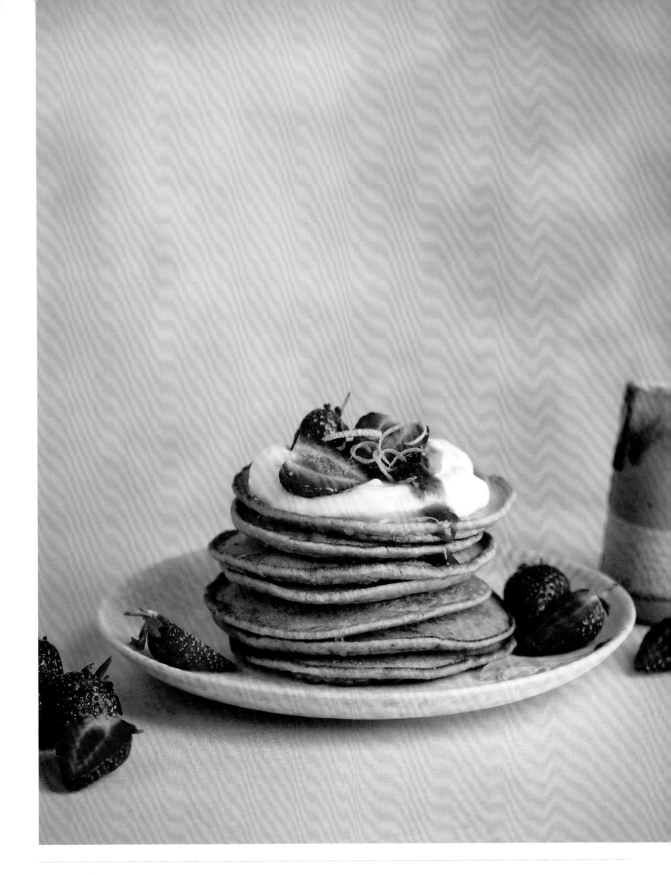

OVERNIGHT OATS, THREE WAYS

V, VEG, DF, GF

🍴 Meal Prep 🥣 Cooking for Friends and Family 🧴 10 Ingredients or Less
🕐 Under 30 minutes

Running out of meal-prep ideas for breakfast? Just multiply the recipe by the number of jars you're making and make more than one at the same time, as they store and keep in the fridge for 3–5 days if in a sealed jar or container. (However, the carrot one will need eating the morning after making it or add the grated carrot fresh in the morning).

Cinnamon Toast Overnight Oats

This recipe reminds me of cinnamon toast. Remember cinnamon is packed with the phytonutrient cinnamaldehyde too. It is always best to start the day with protein to keep your blood sugar balanced if you can, so adding the nut butter here helps with this.

SERVES 1

40g (½ cup) whole rolled oats
1 tbsp chia seeds
2 tsp ground cinnamon
½–1 tsp honey (or a vegan alternative, see page 88)
¼ tsp ground ginger
¼ tsp vanilla extract
⅛ tsp ground cloves
⅛ tsp ground nutmeg
20g (2 tbsp) cashew nuts
200ml (¾ cup) plant milk
45g (½ cup) sultanas
1 tbsp nut butter of your choice (optional)

1. Place the oats in a 500ml (17fl oz) jar or container, then add all of the dry ingredients (apart from the sultanas), followed by the plant milk and honey. Stir well, place the lid on and put in the fridge overnight.
2. Add the sultanas and nut butter (if using) in the morning to serve.

EAT WELL WITH ARTHRITIS

Bakewell Tart Overnight Oats ❷

These are based on the delicious traditional Bakewell Tarts from Bakewell in Derbyshire. As a child my dad would sometimes go there for work, and he would always bring us back a freshly baked one! With my stepdad and stepsisters all from Derby, I thought it was a lovely homage to their home town too.

SERVES 1

40g (½ cup) whole rolled oats
1 tbsp chia seeds
1 tbsp ground almonds
½ tsp honey (or a vegan alternative, see page 88)
1 tsp almond extract
½ tsp grated lemon zest
235ml (¾ cup + 2 tbsp) almond milk (or other plant milk)

FOR THE TOPPINGS
3 tsp homemade Raspberry Jam (see page 234)
2 tbsp flaked almonds
6 fresh raspberries

1. Place all of the ingredients in a jar or container, apart from the toppings.
2. Stir well, or shake if in a jar, and leave in the fridge overnight.
3. In the morning, pour into a bowl and add the raspberry jam, flaked almonds and raspberries.

Carrot Cake Overnight Oats ❸

Carrot cake is my favourite cake, so I wanted to create an indulgent overnight oats recipe. Carrots, walnuts, cinnamon, ginger and nutmeg are the anti-inflammatory stars in this one.

SERVES 1

40g (½ cup) whole rolled oats
½ small carrot, peeled and grated
1 tsp ground flaxseeds
½ tsp ground cinnamon
½ tsp ground ginger
Pinch of ground nutmeg
½–1 tsp honey (or a vegan alternative, see page 88)
½ tsp vanilla extract
200ml (¾ cup) plant milk
3 dates, pitted and chopped
2 tbsp sultanas
20g (¼ cup) walnuts
1 tbsp coconut yoghurt, to serve (optional)

1. Add all of the dry ingredients, except the fruit and walnuts, to a jar or container, then add the honey, vanilla extract and plant milk and stir well. (Leave out the walnuts here if you want them as a topping rather than in the mixture.)
2. Put on the lid and place in the fridge overnight.
3. In the morning, add the fruit and walnuts (if not added previously). Add the coconut yoghurt to serve, if you like.

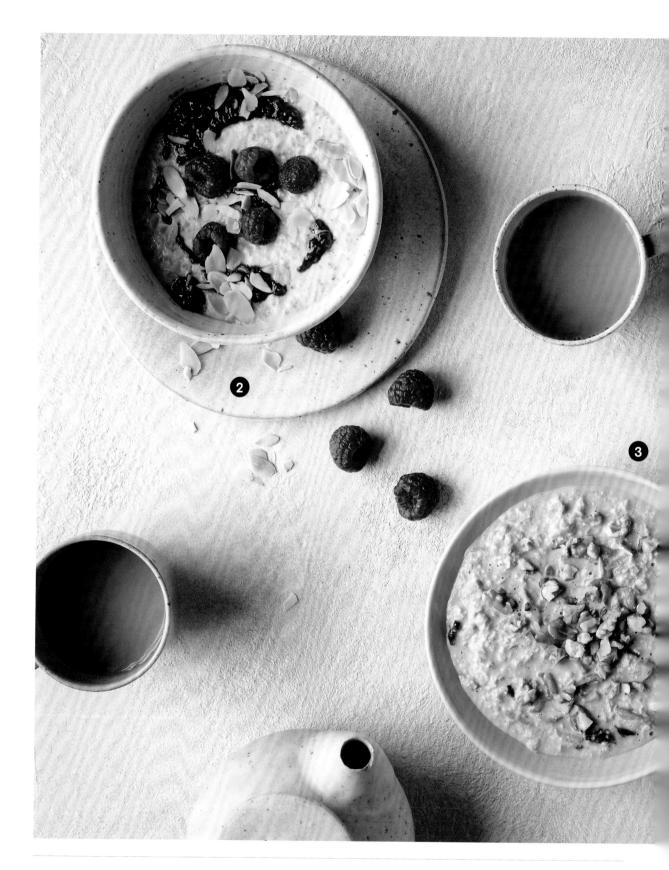

EAT WELL WITH ARTHRITIS

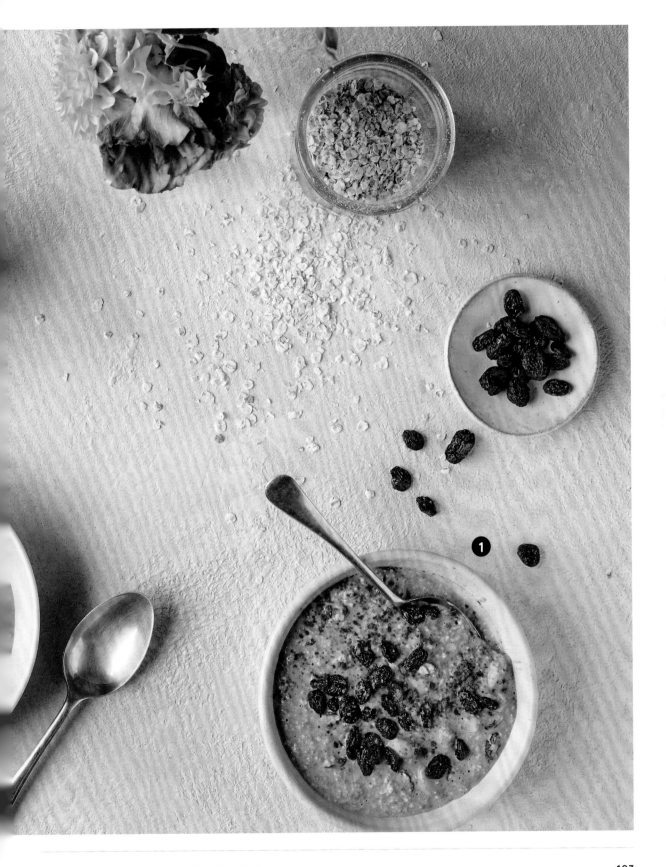

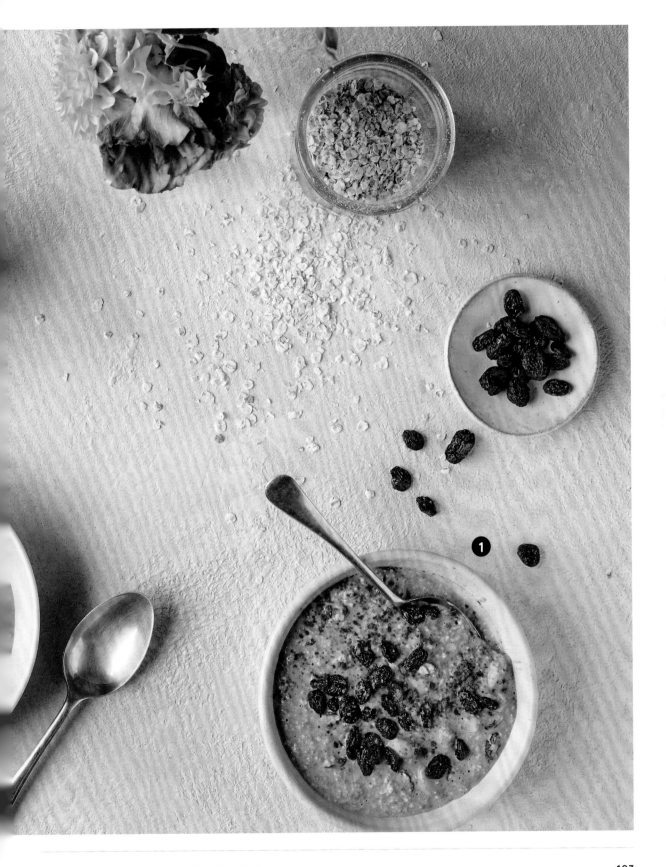

APRICOT AND ALMOND BAKED OATS

V, VEG, DF, GF ✳ Freezable ▯▮ Meal Prep ◗ Cooking for Friends and Family ◷ Under 1 hour

SERVES 6

Coconut oil, for greasing
6 apricots (280g/9½oz,
    I use variety Faralia Spain)
2 eggs (or vegan eggs,
    see page 88)
600ml (2½ cups) plant milk
1 tsp vanilla extract
160g (1½ cups) whole
    rolled oats
1 tbsp chia seeds
50g (½ cup) flaked almonds
1 tsp ground cinnamon
Pinch of nutmeg
1 tsp honey (or maple
    syrup, if vegan)

FOR THE TOPPING
(PER PORTION)
3–4 tbsp coconut yoghurt
1 tbsp flaked almonds
1 tsp Manuka honey (or
    maple syrup, if vegan)

I tried mashed banana baked oats, but they didn't seem to last very long in the fridge. This recipe keeps better, if you don't serve it all at once, and I love the soft, sweet apricots paired with delicate almonds. A warming recipe that can be served on its own or with some coconut yoghurt and Manuka honey for some extra prebiotic goodness.

1. Preheat the oven to 190°C fan (410°F). Smother a 26 x 20cm (10 x 8in) Pyrex baking dish with a thin layer of coconut oil using a pastry brush, or your fingertips.
2. Slice your apricots in half, remove the stones and set aside.
3. Whisk the eggs and plant milk in a jug, then add the vanilla extract.
4. Add the oats, chia seeds, flaked almonds, ground cinnamon and the pinch of nutmeg to the prepared baking dish.
5. Pour the egg mixture over the dry oat mixture and stir thoroughly in the baking dish.
6. Lay the apricot halves, cut side up, evenly across the oat mixture so that you have 12 apricot halves staring up at you.
7. Place in the oven for 20-22 minutes, or until all of the liquid has been absorbed, turning the tray around halfway through.
8. Take out of the oven and leave to cool for 3–5 minutes. Then slice into pieces, 2 apricot pieces per person. Top with coconut yoghurt, flaked almonds and a drizzle of honey or maple syrup to serve.

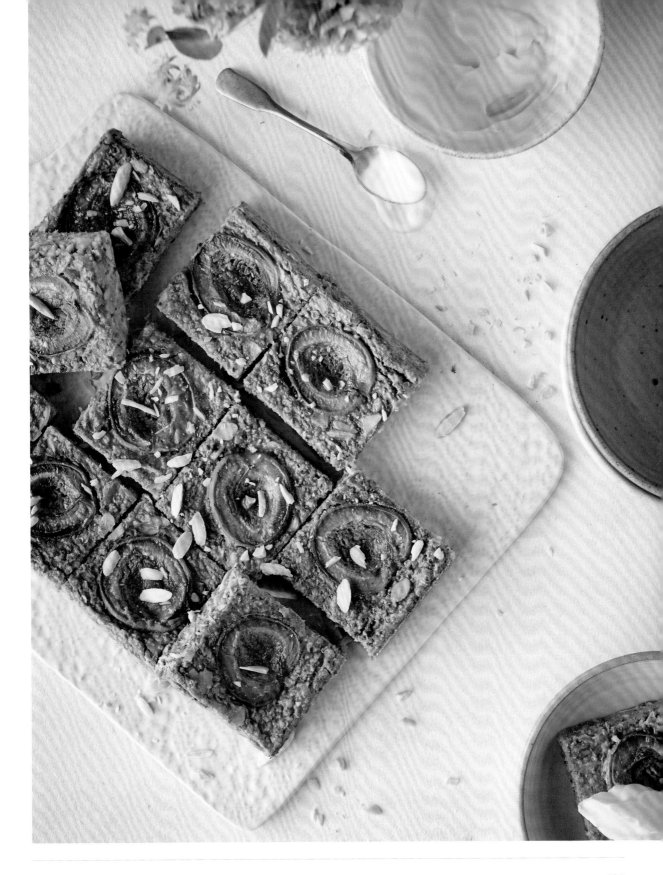

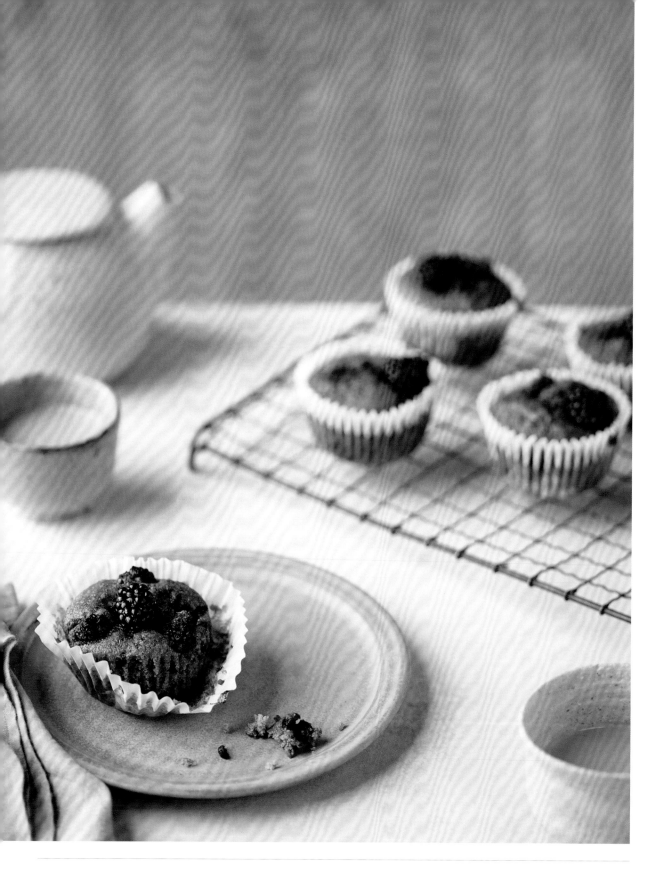

EAT WELL WITH ARTHRITIS

LEMON AND BERRY MUFFINS

V, VEG, DF, GF   ⎮⎮ Meal Prep 🍵 Cooking for Friends and Family 🕐 Under 1 hour

MAKES 12

190g (1⅓ cups) brown
    rice flour
150g (1 cup + 1 tbsp)
    unrefined natural
    caster sugar
2 tsp baking powder
¼ tsp sea salt
Zest of 1 lemon,
    plus juice of ½
1 egg (or vegan egg,
    see page 88)
80ml (⅓ cup) plant milk
85ml (⅓ cup + 2 tbsp)
    coconut oil, melted
1 tsp apple cider vinegar
1 tsp vanilla extract
280g (1½ cups) blackberries
36 white mulberries
    (optional)
Coconut sugar, for sprinkling

Sweet, sharp and lemony, these muffins are packed with berries, which are really good for us. If you can get hold of white mulberries all the better, as they are especially rich in vitamin C, which is great for our immune system and is an antioxidant with anti-inflammatory properties. Nutritionist Victoria Jain suggests trying cassava flour for this recipe, as it may be better for those with autoimmune conditions.

1. Preheat the oven to 200°C fan (425°F) and line a 12-hole muffin tray with paper cases.
2. Whisk together the flour, sugar, baking powder, sea salt and lemon zest in a large bowl.
3. In a measuring jug, mix together the wet ingredients, then combine the two mixtures before folding / mashing in the blackberries.
4. Divide the mixture between the 12 cases – about 2–3 tablespoons in each – and push 3 mulberries (if using) into the centre of each muffin.
5. Sprinkle with coconut sugar, then bake for 20 minutes, turning halfway through.
6. Remove from the oven when the muffins bounce back when pressed – they will be a beautiful purple colour. Leave to cool, then eat straight away, or store in an airtight container and eat within 3–4 days.

BREAKFAST GRANOLA BOWL

V, VEG, DF, GF

🍴 Meal Prep 🥣 Cooking for Friends and Family 🛍 10 Ingredients or Less 🕐 Under 1 hour ❄ Freezable

SERVES 1

FOR HOMEMADE GRANOLA (MAKES 7-8 PORTIONS)

275g (3 cups) whole rolled oats
200g (1¼ cups) mixed nuts and seeds of choice, suggested: 90g (½ cup) unblanched whole almonds, 70g (½ cup) pecan halves, 40g (¼ cup) pumpkin seeds
½ tsp sea salt
2 tsp ground cinnamon
100g (¼ cup + 1 tbsp) honey (or maple syrup, if vegan)
100ml (½ cup) melted coconut oil
2 tsp vanilla extract
80g (1 cup) raisins

TO SERVE
3 tbsp coconut yoghurt
Handful of fresh or dried fruit
1 tsp honey (or a vegan alternative, see page 88)
Sprinkle of ground cinnamon

For this recipe there is the option to make your own granola, or alternatively, choose a ready-made one that is packed with nuts, seeds and dried fruit, with no added refined sugar or preservatives. It's an easy way to get your daily fibre to promote a healthier gut, which is essential to the functioning of your immune system. You can also sprinkle the granola on top of your porridge or add to your smoothie bowls.

1. If making the granola from scratch, make sure to do this the day before, as it will need time to cool before you can use it.
2. Preheat the oven to 160°C fan (350°F) and line a large oven tray with baking parchment. A large oven tray could easily be the grill tray with the rack removed.
3. In a large mixing bowl, combine the oats, nuts and seeds, salt and cinnamon.
4. In a saucepan on a low heat, melt together the honey, oil and vanilla extract. Pour over the dry mixture and stir until it's all coated. Pour the granola on to the prepared tray, making sure it is spread evenly.
5. Bake for around 20 minutes until lightly brown, rotating halfway through.
6. Let the granola cool completely before adding the raisins. It can be stored in an airtight container at room temperature for 1–2 weeks, or in the freezer for up to 3 months.
7. For breakfast, place the granola, coconut yoghurt and your fruit of choice in a bowl, then top with the honey and cinnamon. You could also eat it like you would a bowl of cornflakes with some plant milk and chopped banana.

DATE, CACAO AND BANANA CHIA POT

V, VEG, DF, GF

⏗ Meal Prep 🥣 Cooking for Friends and Family 🛍 10 Ingredients or Less
🕐 Under 30 minutes

SERVES 1

260ml (1 cup + 1 tbsp)
   plant milk
4 tbsp chia seeds
2 tbsp whole rolled oats
2 tsp honey or date syrup
2 tbsp raw cacao powder
½ tsp maca powder
15g (¼ cup) dried
   banana chips
½ banana, sliced (optional)
4 dates, pitted
2 tbsp hazelnuts (or walnuts)
1 tbsp cacao nibs

This is a little more of an indulgent breakfast, but I can promise that it is still good for you – with cacao powder, chia seeds, maca powder and hazelnuts, it tastes good and does good, containing omega-3, gut-nourishing fibre and polyphenols.

1. Place the plant milk, chia seeds, oats, honey or date syrup and cacao and maca powders in a 500ml (17fl oz) jar or container. Stir well, seal and leave in the fridge overnight.
2. In the morning, pour the oat mixture into a bowl and top with the banana chips, fresh chopped banana (if using), dates, hazelnuts and cacao nibs.

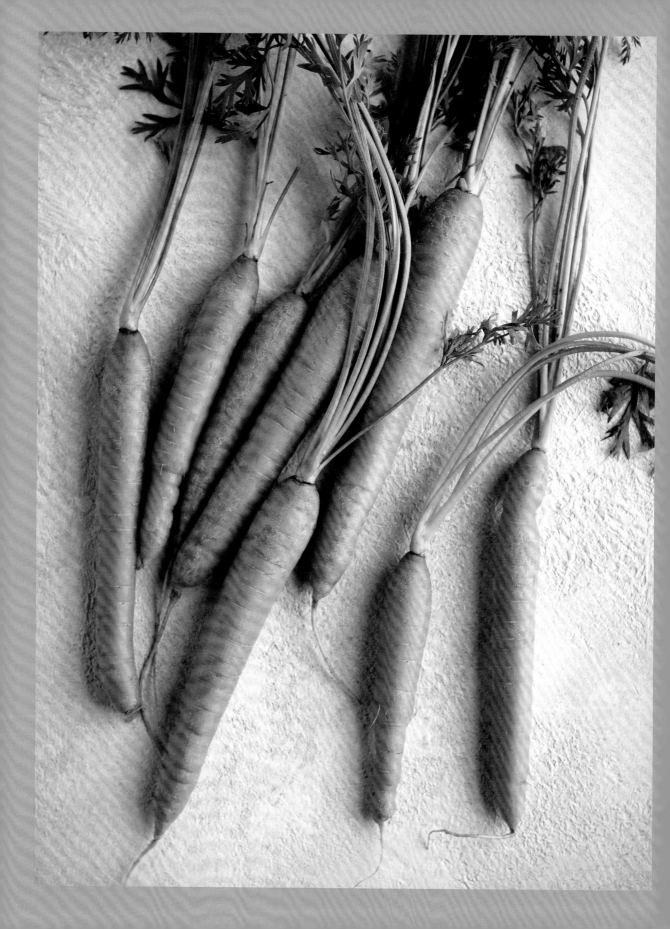

LUNCH AND SMALL PLATES

MEXICAN-STYLE SALAD BOWL

DF, GF   🌿 Cooking for Friends and Family 🕐 Over 1 hour

SERVES 2

2 skinless salmon fillets
    (around 250g/9oz)
1 tbsp extra virgin olive oil
1 avocado
12 cherry tomatoes
1 baby gem lettuce
400g (2½ cups) sweetcorn
    (tinned or frozen
    and cooked)
Sea salt and black pepper

FOR THE FRIED BEANS
1 tsp olive oil
2 fresh red or green chillies,
    deseeded and chopped
1 red onion, sliced
1 red or yellow bell
    pepper, chopped
1 x 350g (12oz) carton
    black beans in water

FOR THE RICE
150g (¾ cup) brown rice
    (or red or wild rice)
7–8g (¼ cup) fresh
    coriander
½ lime

TO SERVE
Chipotle Sauce (see
    page 234)
Mango Salsa (see page 235)

Super nutritious, and if you eat fish, the salmon provides plenty of fatty-fish benefits, like omega-3, although you can still get the delicious healthy fats from the avocado and extra virgin olive oil too. Try swapping the brown rice for red or wild rice, for added nutrient value.

1. Preheat the oven to 190°C fan (410°F).
2. Cook the brown rice according to the packet instructions, or follow my method: Rinse the rice in a sieve under cold running water. Bring 2.5–3 litres (10–12 cups) of water to the boil in a large pot (with an accompanying lid). Add the rice to the water and stir with a sprinkle of salt, then boil uncovered for 28–30 minutes. Drain the rice for about 15 seconds before returning to the pot and covering with the lid for 5–10 minutes of steam time, then fluff through with a fork.
3. Meanwhile, put the salmon on a piece of foil, drizzle with the extra virgin olive oil and season with salt and pepper. Wrap in the foil and bake in the oven for 15–20 minutes.
4. Slice the avocado, tomatoes and lettuce and distribute evenly between 2 bowls. Share out the sweetcorn too.
5. For the beans, heat the olive oil in a pan and cook the chillies and red onion for 3–5 minutes, then add the pepper and then the black beans. Season with salt and pepper.
6. When the rice is cooked, rinse it and stir in the fresh coriander, some salt and pepper, and the lime juice.
7. Divide the black bean mixture, coriander rice and salmon between the 2 bowls. Drizzle with the chipotle sauce and serve with mango salsa.

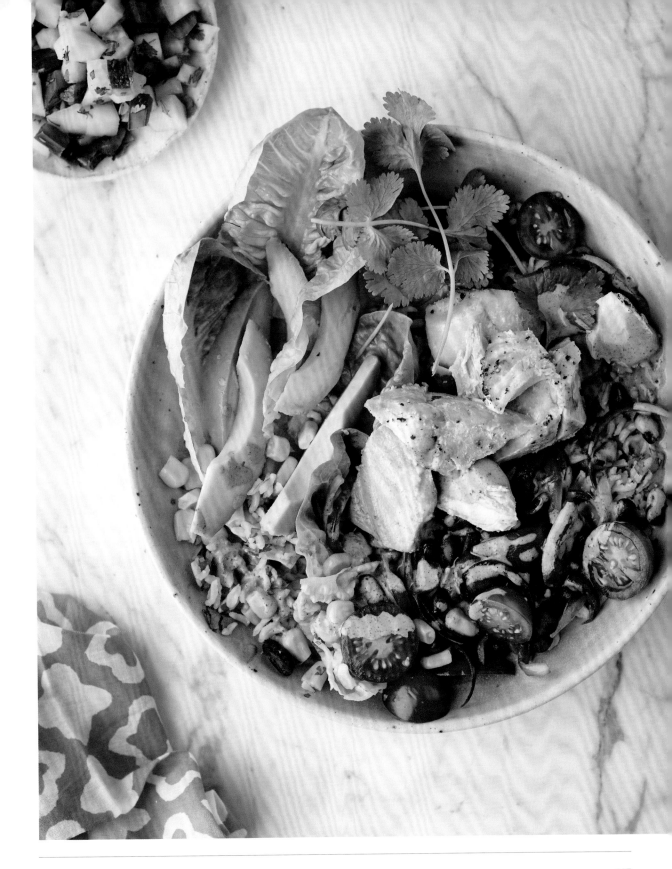

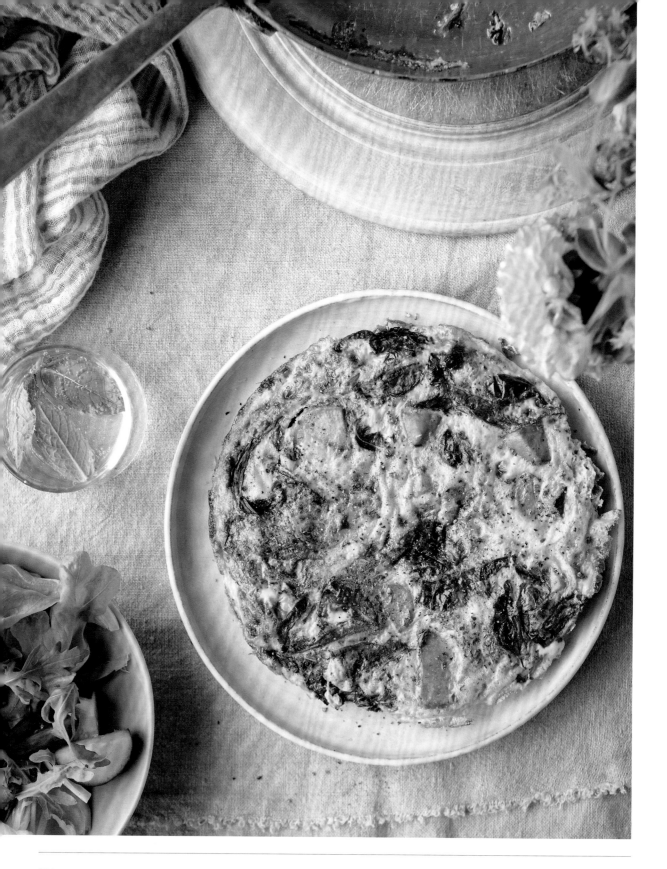

EAT WELL WITH ARTHRITIS

EASY FRITTATA AND CRUNCHY SALAD

V, DF, GF

🍴 Meal Prep   🕐 Under 1 hour

SERVES 2

1 large sweet potato
2 tsp extra virgin olive oil
120ml (⅓ cup + 2 tbsp)
   plant milk
2 large eggs
1 tsp dried oregano
Handful of spinach
Sea salt and black pepper

**FOR THE
CRUNCHY SALAD**
½ cucumber
30g (1oz) rocket leaves
1 baby gem lettuce, sliced
12 plum tomatoes
Classic Salad Dressing
   (see page 236)

Sometimes the simplest recipes are the most comforting. This recipe can be made with pretty much any vegetable you can find in your fridge, and it's a great way to use up leftovers.

—

1. Peel and chop your sweet potato into thin, flat chunks.
2. Add the sweet potato to a large ovenproof frying pan with a little of the oil and cook on a low–medium heat for 5–7 minutes.
3. Whisk the plant milk with the eggs in a jug until fully combined, then add the oregano and sea salt and black pepper to taste.
4. Add the spinach to the frying pan and stir together with the sweet potato for 2–3 minutes until the spinach has wilted.
5. Flatten out the mixture, add a little more oil and then pour in the egg mixture, tilting the pan to even out the mixture.
6. Cook for 4–5 minutes on a low–medium heat, then preheat the grill.
7. Transfer the pan to the grill (leaving the handle outside if it is not oven-proof) and grill for 3–4 minutes until golden on top.
8. Meanwhile, prepare and mix together all the salad ingredients. Mix in the classic salad dressing and serve with the frittata.

SALMON FISHCAKES AND CASHEW PARSLEY SAUCE

DF, GF

🍴 Meal Prep 🕐 Under 1 hour 🌱 Cooking for Friends and Family

MAKES 6

120g (1¼ cups) walnuts
2 skinless salmon fillets
   (around 250g/9oz)
570g (1lb 3oz) sweet
   potatoes (4–5
   depending on size)
1 tsp Dijon mustard
Squeeze of lemon juice
4g curly leaf parsley,
   plus extra to serve
¼ tsp onion granules
¼ tsp paprika
1 large egg
45g (¼ cup) buckwheat flour
Sea salt and black pepper
Extra virgin olive oil,
   for cooking

TO SERVE

1 portion of Cashew Parsley
   Sauce (see page 236)
60g (2¼oz) salad leaves:
   rocket, spinach, kale,
   romaine lettuce leaves
15–20 cherry tomatoes
½ cucumber

OPTIONAL

Tenderstem broccoli
Green beans

In this recipe I have recreated a version of fishcakes with a creamy filling that I had growing up. I have used salmon, but you could also swap it for cod, haddock or pollock, which are also a good source of omega-3. There's also plenty of phytochemical nutrition in the walnuts, extra virgin olive oil, parsley and paprika.

—

1. Preheat the oven to 200°C fan (425°F).
2. Blend the walnuts in a food processor and set aside.
3. Place the salmon on to a piece of foil, drizzle with the olive oil and season with sea salt and pepper. Wrap in the foil, place on a baking tray and cook in the oven for 15–20 minutes.
4. Peel and chop the sweet potatoes into chunks, then boil for 15 minutes until soft. Drain.
5. Mash the cooked sweet potato in a mixing bowl; if you are struggling, pulse it briefly in a food processor on a low setting so that it does not get too smooth.
6. Add the Dijon mustard, lemon juice, chopped parsley, onion granules, paprika, ¼ teaspoon of sea salt and ¼ teaspoon black pepper to the sweet potato, then flake in the salmon in chunks so not to break apart too much.
7. Prepare flat bowls: in one bowl whisk the egg, in another bowl add the buckwheat flour, and in the other bowl add the blended walnuts.
8. Mould the sweet potato salmon mixture into patties the size and shape of fishcakes, each one around 120–130g (4–4½oz).
9. Drizzle some extra virgin olive oil in a pan and fry the fishcakes on a medium–high heat for 3–5 minutes on each side. If you have a large flat pan, then you can cook them all at once, otherwise, place on a tray/plate and cover to keep warm as you cook them.
10. Serve with the cashew parsley sauce, fresh parsley and a side salad of salad leaves, cherry tomatoes and cucumber. Alternatively, serve with steamed tenderstem broccoli and green beans.

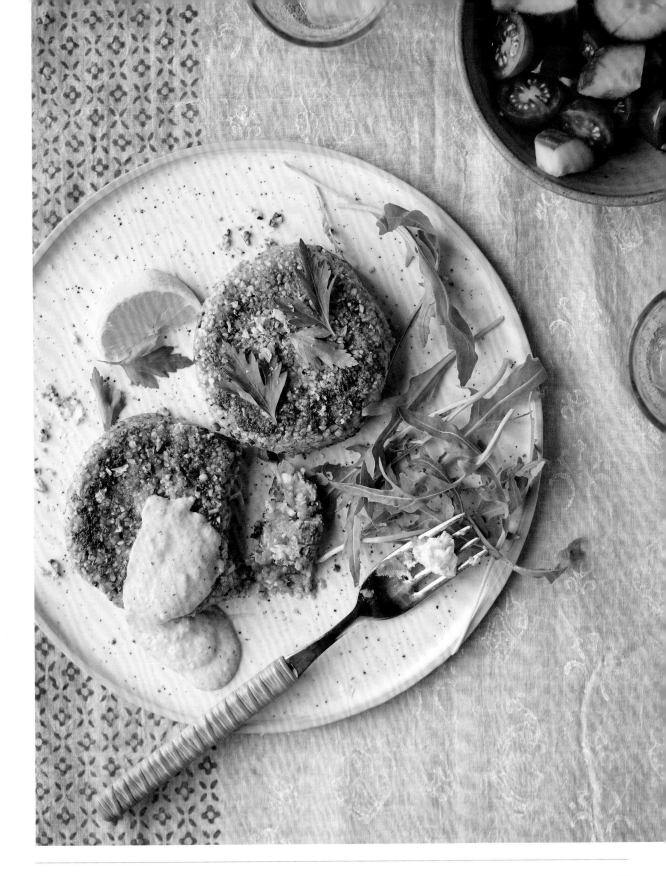

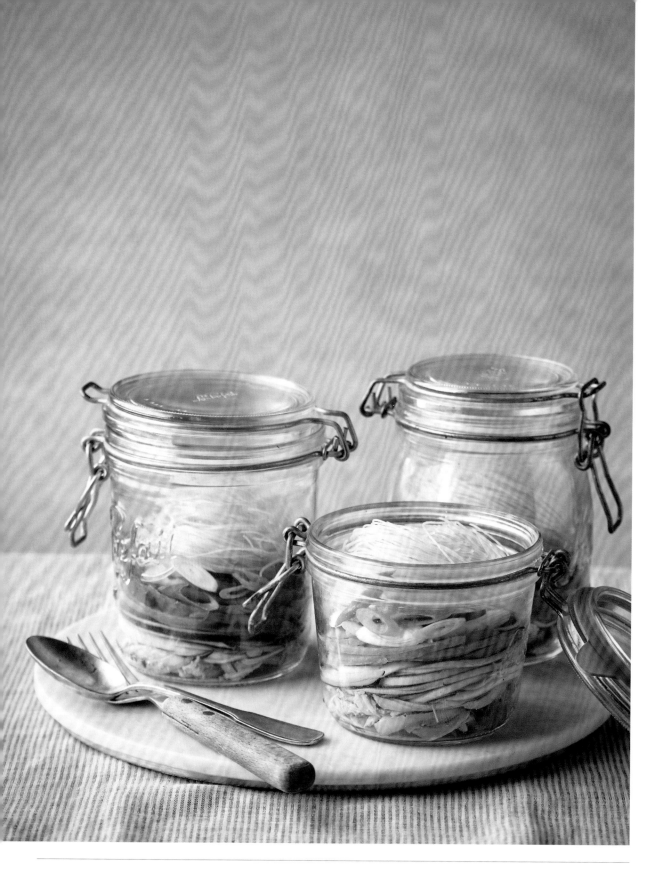

EAT WELL WITH ARTHRITIS

READY-TO-GO PROBIOTIC NOODLE JAR

V, VEG, DF, GF   🍴 Meal Prep ⎮ 'Fakeaway' 🍃 Cooking for Friends and Family 🕐 Over 1 hour

MAKES 3 JARS

2 chicken breasts or
    2 blocks of firm tofu
    or silken tofu

FOR THE SEASONING
1 tsp sesame oil
1 tsp tamari
½ tsp chilli powder
    flakes (optional)
Sprinkle of sea salt
¼ tsp black pepper

FOR THE VEGETABLES
AND NOODLES
1 courgette
2 large carrots (250g/9oz)
2 bell peppers (I use one red
    and one yellow for colour)
6 spring onions
3 (50g/2oz) nests of
    vermicelli rice noodles

FOR THE SPICE MIX
(PER JAR)
½ tsp white miso paste
¼ tsp Chinese five spice
½ tsp sesame oil
¼ tsp garlic granules
1 tsp tamari
1 tsp honey (or a vegan
    alternative, see
    page 88)

TO SERVE (PER JAR)
⅓ sheet of nori, cut
    into strips
1 tsp sesame seeds
Drizzle of chilli oil or 1 tsp
    chilli flakes (optional)

A healthier and more nourishing version of a pot noodle, it is packed with protein, plants and probiotics – if you can find brown rice vermicelli even better! Miso paste is a fermented food made from soya beans and is packed full of probiotics that the gut loves.

—

1. Preheat the oven to 190°C fan (410°F).
2. If you are using chicken, place the seasoning ingredients on a piece of foil and roll the chicken breasts in the mixture. Wrap the chicken in the foil, place on a baking tray and cook for 25–25 minutes, depending on the size of the chicken breasts.
3. If you are using tofu, drain off the excess water, then slice into pieces. You can either heat some olive oil in a pan and lightly fry it until golden brown, or enjoy it raw (silken tastes best raw, firm tastes best cooked).
4. While the chicken is cooking, prepare and chop your vegetables – grate the courgette and carrot separately in a food processor, and place in bowls. Thinly slice the bell peppers and spring onions.
5. Let the chicken rest for 5 minutes, before shredding with a knife and fork.
6. Layer everything into the jars as follows (with the chicken / most moist ingredients at the bottom of the jars):

90g (3oz) shredded chicken or tofu	40g (1½oz) red pepper
80g (2¾oz) shredded courgette	40g (1½oz) yellow pepper
60g (2¼oz) carrot	15g (½oz) spring onion
	1 portion of spice mix
	1 nest of vermicelli noodles

7. On the day of eating, move the jar mixture into a bowl and add 400ml (1⅔ cups) of hot (but not boiling) water (to protect the good probiotics bacteria in the miso) and leave for 5 minutes.
8. Top with the nori strips, sesame seeds and a drizzle of chilli oil or sprinkle of chilli flakes if you like.

CREAMY MUSHROOM BUTTER BEANS WITH ASPARAGUS

V, VEG, DF, GF　　🌿 Cooking for Friends and Family　🕐 Under 1 hour

SERVES 4–6

2 garlic cloves
350g (4½ cups) mushrooms
　of choice (I use 200g/2½
　cups chopped closed cup
　chestnut mushrooms and
　150g/2 cups chopped
　shiitake mushrooms)
1 medium red onion
100g (6 leaves) cavolo
　nero kale
250g (9oz) asparagus
　spears
1 tbsp extra virgin olive oil
1 x 400g (14oz) tin
　butter beans, drained
　and rinsed
250ml (1 cup) plant milk
5 tbsp nutritional yeast flakes
1 tsp ground arrowroot
　(optional, to thicken)
½ tsp dried oregano
1 tsp apple cider vinegar
2 tsp tamari

TO SERVE

4–6 slices of
　sourdough,
　or gluten-free seed-
　based bread (I like
　Seedful), toasted
4–6 tbsp coconut yoghurt
Sprinkle of black pepper
Fresh oregano, chopped
　(optional)

This is so delicious and warming and could even be eaten as a brunch plate on a lazy weekend! You could also have this mixture on seed-based bread for a gluten-free option. Shiitake mushrooms are especially healthy (see page 71).

1. Mince or dice the garlic cloves. Chop the mushrooms and red onion into 1–2cm (½ –¾in) chunks. For the kale, place the leaves on top of one another and slice into strips. Cut the tops off the asparagus and then halve the spears down the middle.

2. Heat the extra virgin olive oil in pan on a medium heat, add the red onion and garlic and fry for 5 minutes. Add the mushrooms and cook for 2–3 minutes, then add the asparagus and cook for 2 minutes. Stir in the kale and butter beans.

3. Add the remaining ingredients, simmer and stir for 20–25 minutes until thickened and all the liquid is absorbed. The mushrooms act like sponges and will absorb all the delicious flavours in the mixture.

4. Place the vegetable mixture on top of your slices of toast, add a dollop of coconut yoghurt to each one, season with black pepper and top with fresh oregano (if using).

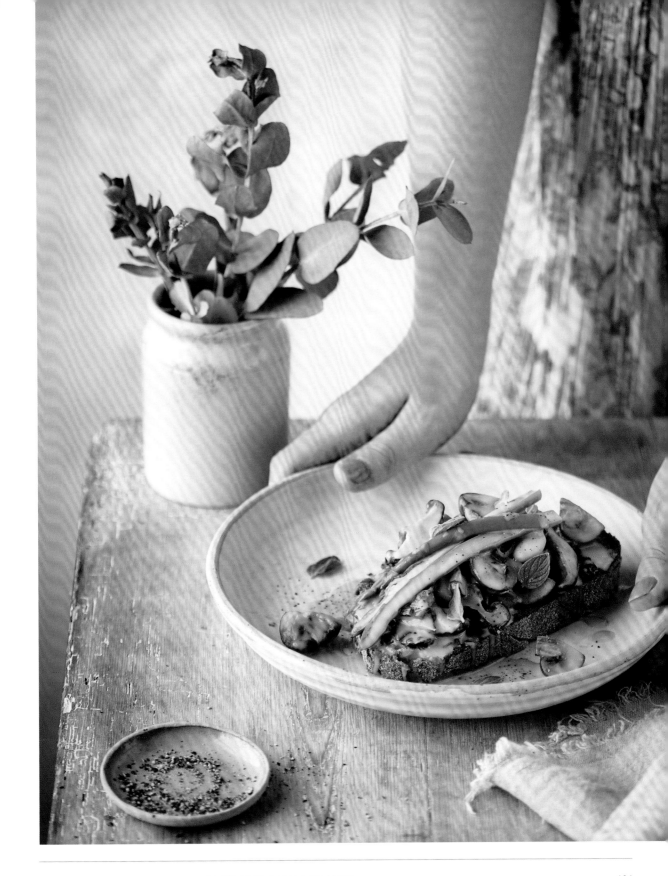

MOROCCAN SALMON WITH FRESH MINT QUINOA SALAD

DF, GF

🍴 Meal Prep 🥣 Cooking for Friends and Family 🕐 Under 1 hour

SERVES 2

100g (½ cup) quinoa
300ml (1¼ cups) water
1 vegetable stock cube
    (I use Kallo)
2 sockeye salmon fillets
2 tsp ras el hanout
1 tsp extra virgin olive oil
½ lemon, sliced into
    6 semicircles
1 avocado, sliced in half,
    then widthways into slices

FOR THE SALAD
½ large red onion
    (or 1 small), chopped
2 tbsp fresh mint leaves
120g (1 cup) Pomodorino
    baby plum tomatoes,
    sliced
2 carrots, peeled and
    grated (120g/4oz)
60g (1½ cups) baby
    spinach leaves
120g (1¼ cups)
    chopped walnuts
85g sulphur dioxide-free
    dried apricots
50g (⅓ cup) sultanas
30g (¼ cup) sunflower seeds

FOR THE DRESSING
Juice of ½ lime
1 tbsp tahini
3 tbsp extra virgin olive oil
Pinch of pink Himalayan salt
1 tbsp water
¼ tsp black pepper
1 tbsp honey
½ tsp balsamic vinegar
¼ tsp ground cinnamon
¼ tsp ground cumin
½ tsp dried oregano

This is so delicious and will definitely impress your family and friends! The salmon, mint, tomatoes, walnuts and spinach are especially powerful anti-inflammatory ingredients. Sunflower seeds are a good source of calcium, balanced with magnesium, they're also an excellent source of vitamin E, which neutralises free radicals and may help to prevent osteoarthritis and rheumatoid arthritis.

1. Preheat the oven to 190°C fan (410°F).
2. Rinse the quinoa, then add it to a saucepan with the 300ml (1¼ cups) water. Cook on a high heat for 5–7 minutes until it reaches a bubbling boil, then stir in the stock cube, turn down the heat and simmer for 12–15 minutes until fluffy and all the water has evaporated. Set aside to cool.
3. Meanwhile, put the salmon on a piece of foil, drizzle with the extra virgin olive oil, scatter 1 teaspoon of ras el hanout on each piece, then top each one with three semicircles of lemon. Wrap in the foil, place on a baking tray and cook in the oven for 10–15 minutes, depending on the size of the salmon.
4. Add all the salad ingredients to a large mixing bowl. Stir in the quinoa.
5. Put all of the dressing ingredients into a jar and stir well.
6. Place the salad onto plates, top with the salmon and avocado, then pour over the dressing.

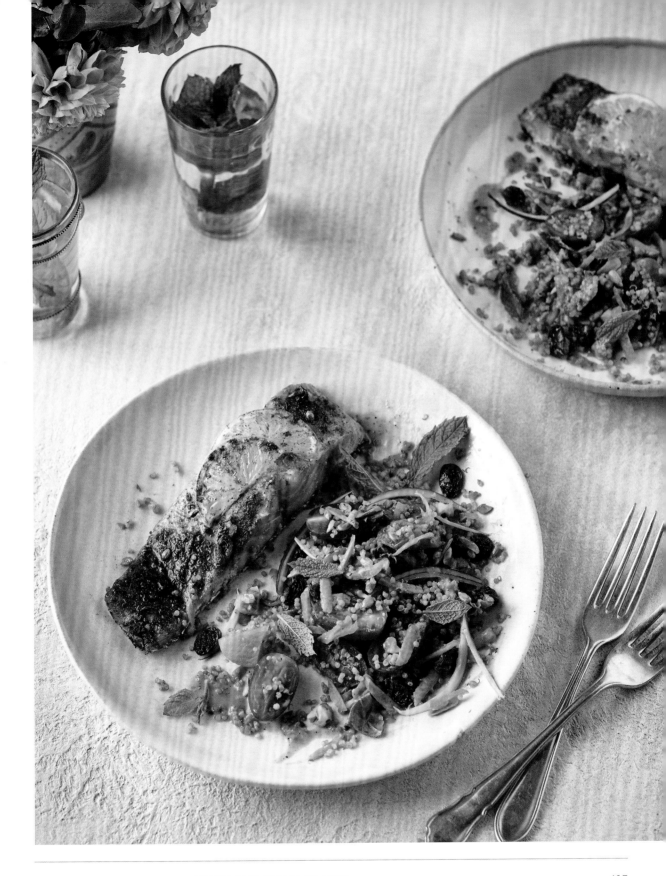

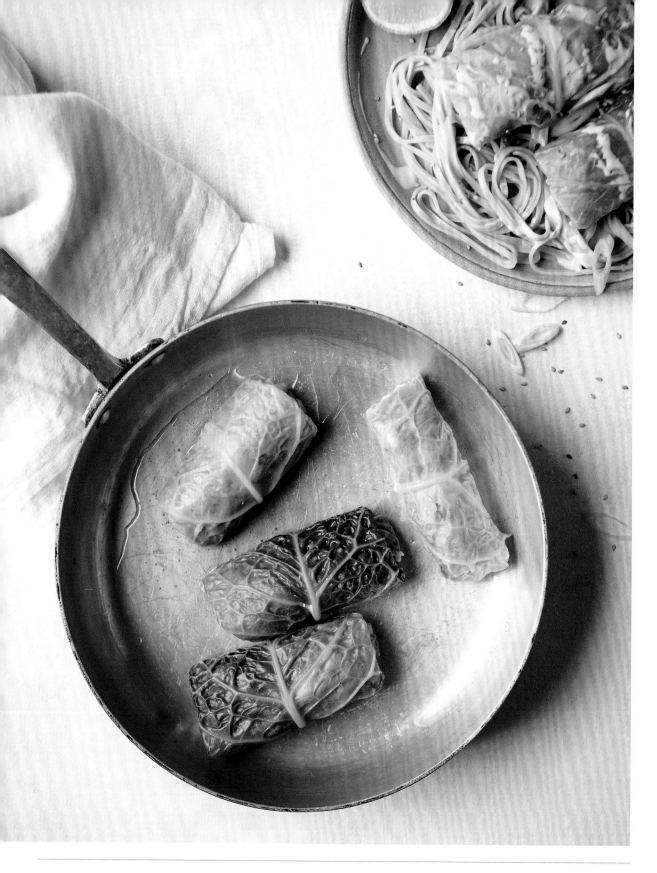

EAT WELL WITH ARTHRITIS

SPICY TAHINI PRAWN 'SUBMARINES' (SUKI ROLLS)

DF, GF

🍴 Meal Prep   🥣 Cooking for Friends and Family   🕐 Over 1 hour

SERVES 4

8 Savoy cabbage leaves
150g (5oz) raw king prawns,
   or extra firm tofu,
   crumbled into chunks
250g (9oz) brown rice
   and wakame noodles (or
   plain brown rice noodles)
3 tsp sesame oil

FOR THE STIR-FRY
VEGETABLES (OPTIONAL)
1 red onion, chopped
1 red chilli, deseeded
   and chopped
1 garlic clove, chopped
1 thumb-sized piece
   fresh ginger, peeled
   and grated
200g (2½ cups) mushrooms
   (shiitake, eryngii and
   oyster if you can), chopped
1 large carrot, peeled
   and grated
150g (1 cup) beansprouts
½ tbsp tamari
½ tsp ground ginger
¼ tsp garlic granules

FOR THE SAUCE
2 heaped tbsp tahini
1½ tbsp tamari
2 tbsp white rice vinegar
2 tbsp water
1 tbsp sesame oil
Pinch of smoked sea salt
   (I use Cornish Sea Salt)
   or pink Himalayan salt
1 tsp chilli flakes
1 tsp honey
¼ tsp garlic granules
¼ tsp ground ginger
Pinch of black pepper

TO SERVE
4 spring onions, chopped
4 tsp sesame seeds
1 lime, quartered

When you're craving something spicy and sweet, which feels like a treat, then this is your dish. This was one of those 'accidental' recipes, using vegetables left in the fridge and a tahini that needing using up, but it's actually something I have made many times since. Thai suki rolls usually have pork in rice paper, but this is harder to roll, and cabbage is thicker and easier for arthritic hands.

1. Separate and soften the cabbage leaves in a large pan of boiling water for 3–5 minutes until soft. Drain, then leave on kitchen paper to absorb the remaining water, dabbing where needed.
2. Mix the sauce ingredients together in a small bowl and set aside.
3. Heat 2 teaspoons of the sesame oil in a frying pan on a medium heat and cook the red onion, chilli, garlic and ginger for 3–5 minutes until browned.
4. Add the chopped mushrooms and soften for 5 minutes. Add the grated carrots, then the beansprouts, tamari, ground ginger and garlic granules. Remove the vegetables and set aside.
5. Gently fry the prawns or tofu in the juices that remain in the pan with another teaspoon of sesame oil.
6. Cook the noodles in a saucepan of boiling water for 5–6 minutes on a medium heat, or according to the pack instructions. Rinse with hot or cold water, depending on your preference, and leave to drain.
7. Take one of the cooked cabbage leaves and place 2–3 tablespoons of vegetable filling 1cm (½in) from the large part of the cabbage leaf vein – you can slice the chunky part of the leaf vein out before assembling the roll if you prefer – then place 2 king prawns or pieces of cooked tofu on top.
8. Fold the left and right side of the cabbage leaf inward, then roll the suki roll upwards from the thick part of the bottom of the leaf. Repeat with the remaining cabbage leaves and filling, until you have 8 rolls.
9. Gently heat a couple of teaspoons of sesame oil in a large shallow frying pan, add the 8 cabbage rolls, cover and cook for 4–5 minutes until slightly crispy underneath.
10. Divide the noodles between 4 plates, top with two suki rolls, drizzle over the sauce and garnish with a sprinkle of spring onions and 1 teaspoon of sesame seeds per plate. Add a wedge of lime to each plate and squeeze over before eating.

Tip:
Use the back of a teaspoon to rub off the skin on fresh ginger.

BANG BANG CAULIFLOWER SALAD

V, VEG, DF, GF   ⫶ Meal Prep ⎮ 'Fakeaway' 🥣 Cooking for Friends and Family

MAKES 2 LARGE PORTIONS FOR DINNER OR 4 SMALLER PORTIONS FOR LUNCH

2 cauliflower heads, broken into florets (850g/1lb 14oz total weight)

FOR THE COATING (WET MIXTURE)
200ml (¾ cup) almond milk
100g (½ cup) brown rice flour
½ tsp smoked sea salt, or Himalayan pink salt
1 tsp black pepper

FOR THE COATING (DRY MIXTURE)
180g (1⅓ cups + 1 tbsp) ground almonds
½ tsp Chinese five spice
½ tsp garlic granules
1 tsp chilli flakes
½ tsp paprika
½ tsp ground ginger
½ tsp ground cloves

FOR THE SPICY VEGETABLE MIX
1 red onion
1 red chilli, deseeded
25g (1oz) fresh ginger, peeled
2 garlic cloves
9 spring onions
175g (1¾ cups) okra
2 red bell peppers
1 tbsp sesame oil
1 x 400g (14oz) tin chickpeas, drained and rinsed
Juice of ½ lime
½ tsp black pepper
3 tsp honey (or a vegan alternative, see page 88)
1 tbsp tamari

Cauliflower contains sulforaphane, which has been shown to have anti-inflammatory and anti-arthritic effects (see page 63). The florets in this salad have a sweet spicy taste and are well accompanied by the dressing (and or dip!). This dish also goes really well with the Smashed Cucumber Sesame Seed Salad on page 204.

1. Preheat the oven to 190°C fan (410°F) and line 2 large baking trays with baking parchment.
2. To make the spicy vegetable mix, finely slice the red onion, chilli, ginger and garlic. Dice the spring onions and okra and cut the bell peppers into strips. Set aside.
3. Cut off the leaves and root of the cauliflower and break into pieces via the natural florets that have formed – there will be a mix of small, medium and larger pieces and that's okay!
4. Combine the wet mixture in one bowl and the dry mixture in another separate bowl. Dip the florets first into the wet mixture, one by one, and then into the dry mixture. Place them on the baking trays, evenly spaced out, with the larger florets in the middle of the trays. Cook in the oven for 15 minutes, turning the florets over and swapping over the trays halfway through.
5. While the cauliflower is roasting, heat the sesame oil and fry the garlic, ginger and chilli for a couple of minutes, then add the red onion and spring onions and cook for 3–5 minutes. Add the okra and allow to soften before adding the peppers. Cook for 5 minutes, then add the chickpeas, lime juice, black pepper, honey and tamari and simmer on a low heat while the cauliflower cooks.
6. To make the sauce, stir all of the ingredients together.
7. Slice the leafy lettuce and divide it between four serving plates, then add the spicy vegetables and cauliflower. Sprinkle over the sesame seeds and fresh coriander, then pour over the sauce (or serve it on the side as a dipping sauce). Only serve the sauce if eating straight away; if not pour it into a jar so it does not make the veg soggy. If you are reheating this dish, use an oven to heat the cauliflower through, as it will go soggy in a microwave, and store the vegetables in a separate container.

FOR THE SAUCE

4 tbsp 100% peanut butter
6 tbsp egg mayonnaise
  (or a vegan alternative)
2 tbsp water
2 tsp sesame oil
2 tsp honey (or a vegan
  alternative, see
  page 88)
1 tsp apple cider vinegar
  or Japanese rice vinegar
½ tsp tamari
½ tsp chilli flakes
½ tsp garlic granules
½ tsp paprika
Juice of ½ lime

FOR THE SALAD

1 curly leaf lettuce
4 tsp sesame seeds
Bunch of fresh coriander

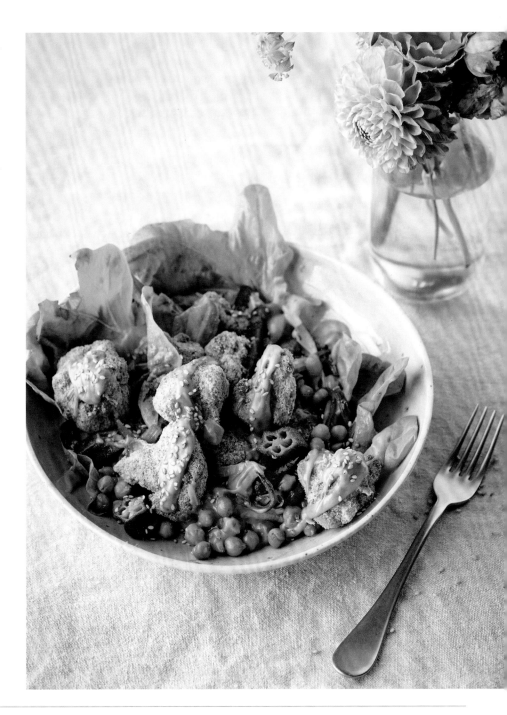

BROWN RICE 'SUSHI' NORI BITES

V, VEG, DF, GF

🍴 Meal Prep ▯ 'Fakeaway' 🥄 Cooking for Friends and Family
🕐 Over 2 hours (including the rice soaking time)

**SERVES 2 AS A MAIN
OR 4 AS A STARTER
(MAKES 4 ROLLS)**

190g (1 cup) short-grain
   brown rice
½ red bell pepper
¼ cucumber
½ avocado
2 spring onions
4 sheets of Sushi Nori
   Seaweed, or 2 packs
   of Clearspring Nori Sea
   Vegetable Thins, or one
   packet of Clearspring Nori
   Sea Vegetable Strips
4 tsp sesame seeds

FOR THE DIPPING SAUCE

2 tbsp soy sauce or tamari
2 tbsp honey (or a
   vegan alternative,
   see page 88)
1 tbsp apple cider vinegar
   or Japanese rice vinegar
1 tsp Shaoxing rice
   wine (optional)
½ tbsp sesame oil
½ tsp ground ginger
¼ tsp chilli flakes (optional)
¼ tsp garlic granules
   (optional, to taste)

These rolls are really easy to make and are great for lunches and/or appetisers with friends. Nori is roasted seaweed (also known as Porphyra tenera) and has been cited in numerous studies as having antioxidative and anti-inflammatory properties, and even improving immune function. If rolling the sushi, you will also need a sushi rolling mat and a bowl of water to wet your fingertips.

1. Cook the short-grain brown rice according to the pack instructions or wash in cold water and drain, then transfer to a saucepan with 600ml (2½ cups) of cold water and leave to soak for 1 hour. Bring to the boil, cover, reduce the heat and simmer for 35–40 minutes or until all of the water has been absorbed Remove from the heat and leave, covered, for 10 minutes. Place the rice on a baking sheet, on top of a tray full of ice cubes, and place in the freezer for around 10 minutes to cool the rice rapidly.
2. Mix together the dipping sauce ingredients in a small bowl. Stir in 1 tablespoon of boiling water, then place in fridge to cool.
3. Deseed and slice the pepper lengthways, cut the cucumber lengthways into strips and cut away the seeded part (as it's too wet to use). Slice the avocado and spring onion thinly lengthways (as thin as you can manage). Place everything on to a plate and set aside.
4. Transfer the cooled brown rice to a bowl.

For sushi rolls

5. Lay a piece of nori shiny side down and textured side up on the sushi rolling mat and wet your fingertips in the bowl of water.
6. Add a thin layer of the brown rice about 5mm (¼in) thick at the very top of the sheet (furthest away from you), leaving about 1cm (½in) empty.
7. About a quarter up from the bottom of the nori sheet, add some fillings – you should be able to fit 3 slices of avocado, 5 strips of spring onion, 2–3 slices of pepper and 3–4 slices of cucumber.
8. Roll the mat away from you over the top of the roll, stopping to tuck it in tightly, pulling the mat at the top at the same time. Roll again and repeat until you are at the end of the mat. Wet the space at the top of the roll with a little bit of water to seal it. Repeat to make 3 more rolls.
9. Place the rolls in the fridge for 10 minutes before slicing into pieces by gently rocking the knife back and forth as you slice downwards. Sprinkle the sesame seeds on top of the rolls, or in the dipping sauce and serve alongside.

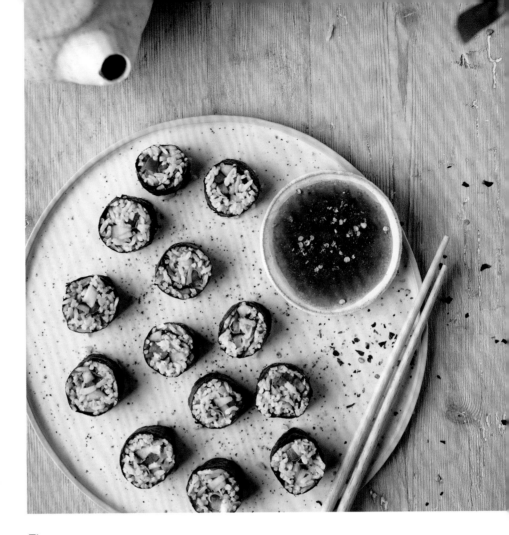

Tip:

If you find that a rolling matt method is too difficult, you can purchase DIY sushi maker kits online that have rice mould shapes. You pack the rice in, then the filling, then another layer of rice, press down and slice.

For nori bites

10. Place the rice in a large bowl, with the strips of vegetables arranged on top, and place the sesame seeds in a separate small bowl.

11. Take a strip of nori and top with 1 tablespoon of rice, then some vegetables, then some sesame seeds. Drizzle with the dipping sauce or dip the loaded nori bite into the sauce with chopsticks or your hands. Definitely good finger food to share with friends! It's best to make the bites then eat straight away, or the nori may get soggy.

Tip:

Other filling ideas: spring onions, salmon and tuna – cooked or smoked, or raw, if raw make sure it is labelled sushi-grade, sashimi grade, or 'for raw consumption', shredded gem lettuce, grated carrots, grated courgettes, cooked tofu, cooked prawns. Also eat it like you would a bowl of cornflakes with some plant milk.

ROASTED VEGETABLES WITH TUSCAN WHITE BEAN DIP

V, VEG, DF, GF

⚄ Meal Prep │ 'Fakeaway' 🍲 Cooking for Friends and Family 🕓 Over 1 hour

SERVES 4

5 parsnips (500g/1lb 2oz)
5 carrots (500g/1lb 2oz)
3 red bell peppers
3 courgettes (500g/1lb 2oz)
40g (1 cup, or
   60 leaves) sage
10g (¼ cup) or handful
   of, fresh thyme
15g (⅓ cup) or handful
   of, fresh rosemary
½ tsp sea salt
1 tsp black pepper
1 Extra virgin olive oil,
   for drizzling
10 big Kalamata olives, pitted
100g (2½ cups) wild rocket
4 large slices of sourdough
   bread, toasted and sliced

FOR THE WHITE BEAN DIP

2 x 400g (14oz) tins
   cannellini beans,
   drained and rinsed
2 roasted garlic cloves
10g (½ cup) fresh
   basil leaves
Zest of 1 lemon
2 tbsp plant milk
8 tbsp extra virgin olive oil
1 tbsp fresh thyme leaves
Squeeze of lemon juice
¼ tsp sea salt
¼ tsp black pepper

This is so delicious on a warm day, one for a BBQ in the back garden, or for lunches. The vegetables are overflowing with phytonutrients. In traditional medicine, sage has been used for the treatment of gout, rheumatism, and inflammation, and rosemary has been used to relieve pain, or for its and anti-inflammatory activity. (For more detail on carnosol, see page 69.)

1. Preheat the oven to 190°C fan (410°F).
2. Peel and cut the parsnips and carrots into strips. Cut the bell peppers in half and deseed them, then cut into chunks. Quarter the courgettes lengthways. Place the peppers on to a baking tray. And the carrots and parsnips to a separate baking tray. Evenly distribute the sprigs of sage, thyme and rosemary across the trays of vegetables, season with the sea salt and black pepper and drizzle with extra virgin olive oil.
3. Place the carrots and parsnips into the oven and cook for 30 minutes, turning halfway through.
4. Roast the pepper chunks for 20–25 minutes, then add the courgettes and cook for 10 minutes until softened and browned.
5. While the vegetables are roasting, blend all of the white bean dip ingredients together. Transfer to a bowl and top with the olives and a drizzle of extra virgin olive oil.
6. Serve the dip with the wild rocket, slices of toasted bread and the roasted vegetables.

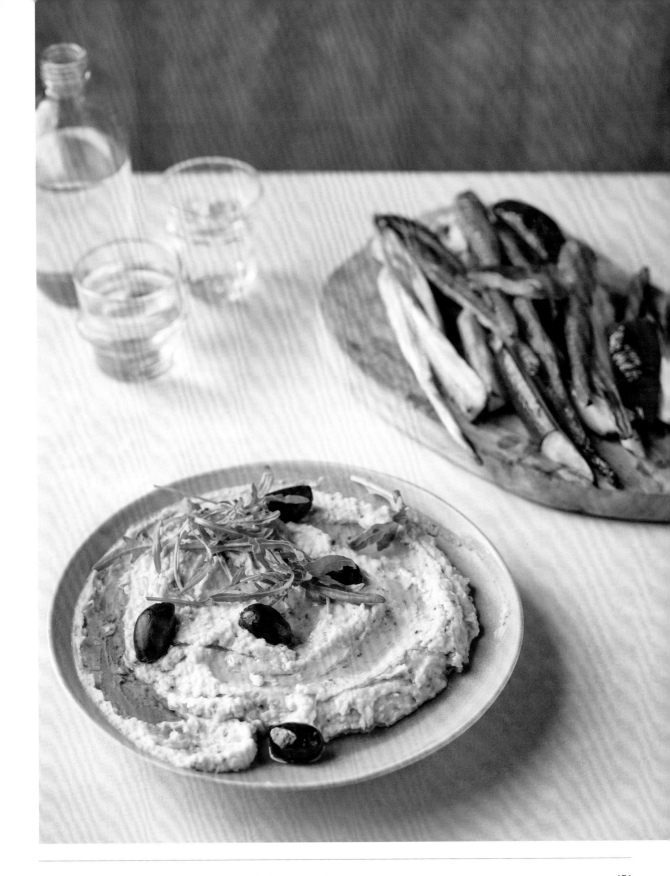

SPICED SWEET POTATO SOUP

V, VEG, DF, GFF   ✳ Freezable ╟ Meal Prep 🥟 Cooking for Friends and Family 🕐 Under 1 hour

**SERVES 4 AS A MAIN OR
6 AS A STARTER**

1 large or 2 small sweet
potatoes (750g/1lb 10oz)
1 tbsp extra virgin olive oil,
plus extra for drizzling
2 red onions
2 garlic cloves
1 vegetable stock cube,
dissolved in 600ml
(2½ cups) hot water
2 tsp creamed coconut
500ml (2 cups) boiled water

FOR THE SEASONING
1 tsp ground turmeric
1 tsp medium curry powder
2 tsp garam masala
½ tsp ground cinnamon
¼ tsp ground ginger
¼ tsp chilli powder
¼ tsp sea salt
¼ tsp black pepper

The 2020 lockdown gave me the chance to get even more inventive with recipes, making use of my spice cupboard and experimenting with flavours. I've since updated this recipe, and it's even more delicious – sweet potatoes are packed with nutrients and gut-loving fibre. And as noted previously, the anti-inflammatory properties of turmeric, especially curcumin, can be especially helpful for those with arthritis.

—

1. Preheat the oven to 200°C fan (425°F). Mix all the seasoning ingredients together in a small bowl.
2. Chop the sweet potato (skin on) into chunks and place in a mixing bowl. Coat with the extra virgin olive oil, then coat with the seasoning.
3. Place the coated sweet potato chunks onto an oven tray and cook for 30 minutes, turning halfway through the cooking time.
4. While the sweet potatoes are cooking, dice the red onions and garlic and set aside.
5. Five minutes before the sweet potatoes are done, heat a drizzle of extra virgin olive oil in a large pan on a medium heat and cook the onions and garlic for 3–4 minutes until softened.
6. Add the roasted sweet potatoes and stir together with the onions and garlic, before adding the vegetable stock and creamed coconut. Stir well.
7. Simmer, covered, for 10 minutes on a low heat, then add the 500ml (2 cups) of hot water and blend using a hand-held blender or add to a food processor and blend.
8. It is delicious as it is, but you could always serve with a dollop of coconut yoghurt and a sprinkle of black pepper on top.

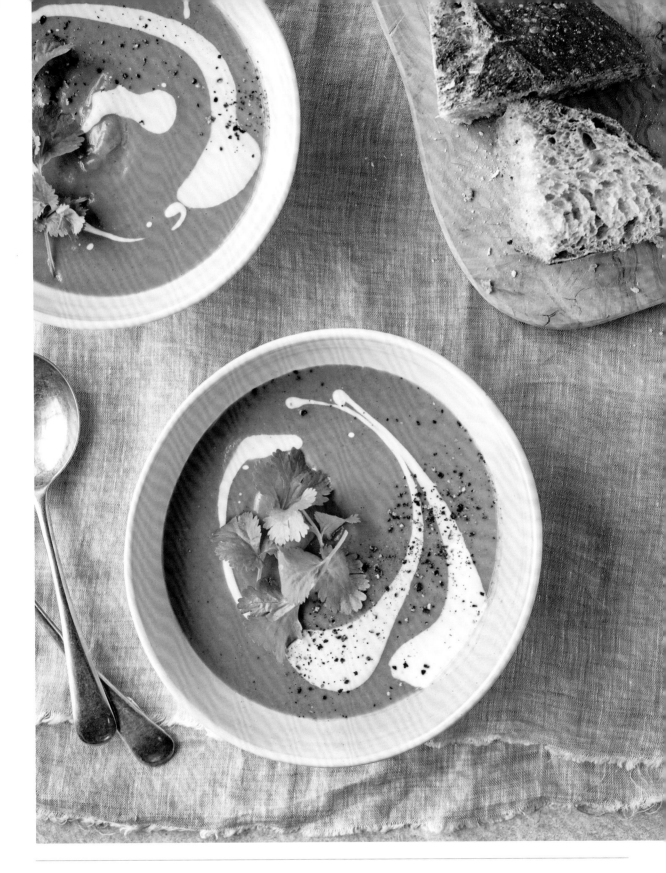

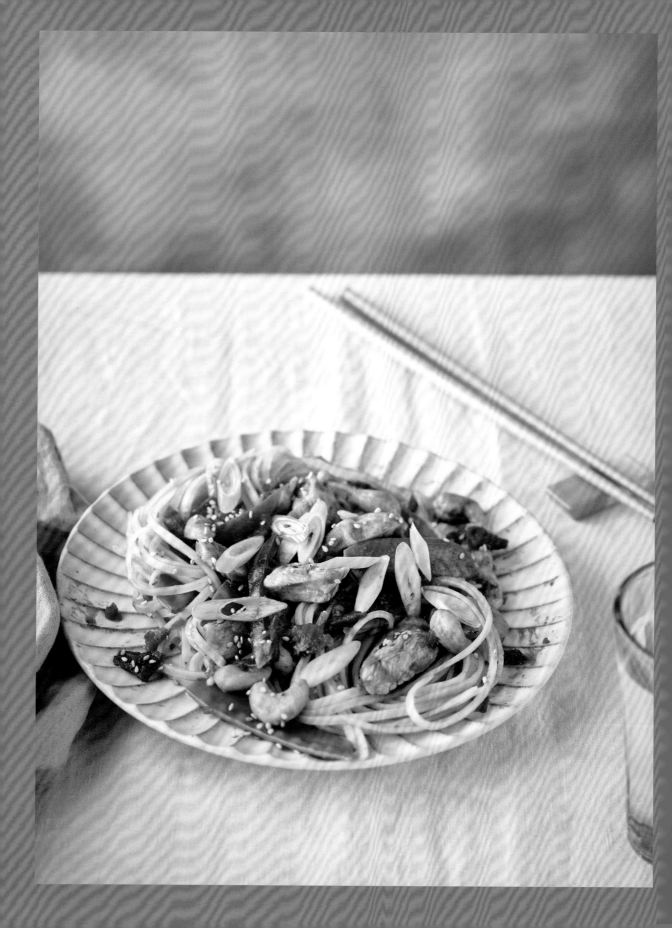

SPEEDY DINNERS

MUSHROOM NOODLE SOUP

V, VEG, DF, GF |'Fakeaway' 🍵 Cooking for Friends and Family 🕐 Under 1 hour

SERVES 2

1 x 300g (10oz) pack
    silken tofu (I like
    Clearspring)
2 large eggs (optional,
    leave out if vegan)
1 tbsp sesame oil
½ red onion, sliced into strips
2 garlic cloves, minced
20g (¾oz) fresh ginger,
    peeled and thinly diced
1 large carrot, grated
150g (1½ cups) closed
    cup chestnut or shiitake
    mushrooms, sliced
2 white cabbage leaves,
    thinly sliced
100g (1 cup) mangetout
1 pak choi, sliced or leaves
    left whole
2 rice noodle nests (brown
    rice if possible)
800ml (3¼ cups) hot
    vegetable stock

TO SERVE (PER PERSON)
1 tbsp tamari
½ tbsp toasted sesame oil
1 tsp chilli oil or chilli
    flakes (optional)
1 spring onion, chopped
1 tsp sesame seeds
4 sprigs of fresh
    chopped coriander
Pinch of black pepper

When you're feeling a little worse for wear, this is such a nourishing and warming bowl that is suitable for everyone, including vegans if you remove the egg. Experiment with the vegetables that you add – the fresh ginger and plenty of vegetables will feel warming and nourishing all at once.

—

1. Drain the silken tofu, cut into 3–4 pieces and set aside.
2. Bring a small pan water to the boil, turn down the heat and gently lower the eggs in. Boil for 6 minutes (for a gooey centre!), remove and place in a bowl of cold water to one side.
3. While the eggs are cooking, heat the sesame oil in a large pan on a medium-high heat, then cook the red onion, garlic and ginger for 2 minutes. Add the carrot and cook for 1 minute, then add the mushrooms and cabbage and cook for a further minute. Finally, add the mangetout and pak choi and cook for 1 minute. Remove from the heat.
4. Peel the eggs and set aside.
5. Put the noodle nests into two large flat soup bowls, then evenly distribute the cooked vegetables on top.
6. Divide the hot vegetable stock evenly between the two bowls. Let the rice noodles soften for 3 minutes, then cut with scissors to make them easier to eat, if preferred.
7. Top each bowl with 2–3 pieces of the silken tofu, followed by the boiled eggs, slicing them while on top of the broth so all the golden runny yolk drizzles into the contents of the bowls nicely. Add the tamari, sesame oil and chilli oil or flakes to taste. Sprinkle over the chopped spring onions, sesame seeds and fresh coriander, and a pinch of black pepper over the egg yolks.

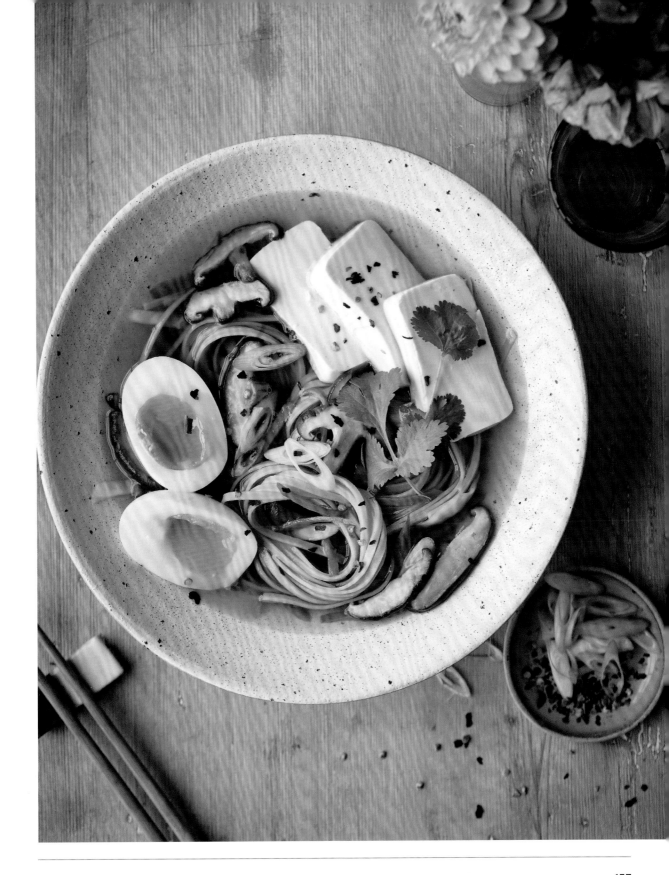

PLANT-PACKED CHOW MEIN

V, VEG, DF, GF ┃ 'Fakeaway' 🍵 Cooking for Friends and Family 🕐 Under 1 hour

SERVES 2–3

200–260g (7–9oz) king
oyster mushrooms

FOR THE MISO MARINADE
3 tsp white miso paste
3 tsp water
2 tsp tahini
2 tsp honey (or maple
  syrup, if vegan)
2 tsp apple cider vinegar
2 tsp sesame oil, plus
  2 tsp for frying
2 tsp tamari
Pinch of sea salt and
  black pepper

FOR THE VEGETABLES
AND NOODLES
1 medium carrot
200g (7oz) closed
  cup chestnut mushrooms
1 bell pepper
4 cabbage leaves
1 green chilli
1 red onion
3 garlic cloves
½ small thumb-sized piece
  fresh ginger (roughly 10g)
1½ tbsp toasted sesame oil
1 tsp onion granules
2 tsp coconut sugar
2 tbsp tamari
2 tbsp dark soy sauce
  (or tamari if gluten-free)
3 tbsp water
1 tsp rice vinegar
1 tsp Shaoxing rice wine
  (or apple cider vinegar)
1 tsp ground arrowroot
2 nests of rice noodles
  of choice

TO TOP
Chopped spring onions
Sesame seeds
Lime wedges
Chopped mint leaves
Chopped coriander leaves

I've packed as many plants as possible into this 'fakeaway' chow mein, combined with miso-soaked king oyster mushrooms for some probiotic and prebiotic goodness too. The miso mushrooms can also be served without the chow mein, on slices of toasted sourdough or brown rice crackers, with the toppings as listed below. To learn more about the anti-inflammatory benefits of miso, see page 70.

—

1. Cut the king oyster mushrooms lengthways into thick 3–4 pieces per mushroom and gently score the back of the mushrooms, diagonally left to right, and right to left.
2. Combine the miso marinade ingredients in a flat bowl and whisk until smooth. Place the mushrooms in the bowl and make sure that they are all well covered with the marinade. Marinate for as long as the other steps take you, or up to 50 minutes, if time allows.
3. Prepare your vegetables: grate the carrot on the grating setting of your food processor, slice the chestnut mushrooms, deseed and slice the pepper lengthways into strips, and roll the cabbage leaves together, then slice along the roll, as if cutting up a cucumber, to create strips of cabbage.
4. Deseed and chop the green chilli, then chop the red onion, ginger and garlic. Place these in the small pestle and mortar setting of your food processor with ½ tablespoon sesame oil and blitz to form a paste.
5. Add the remaining tablespoon of sesame oil to a large frying pan or wok on a medium heat. Add the ginger and garlic paste and cook for 2 minutes, then add the carrot and pepper and cook for 3 minutes.
6. Add the chestnut mushrooms and sweetheart cabbage and cook for 3 minutes, then add all the remaining ingredients, except the noodles and king oyster mushrooms. Turn to a low simmer.
7. In a separate small frying pan, gently heat 2 teaspoons of sesame oil and cook the king oyster mushrooms for 8–10 minutes until golden and crispy on both sides.
8. While the vegetable mix is on a low simmer, soak the rice noodles in boiling water until soft, then drain and add to the pan with the vegetables.
9. Serve in shallow serving bowls, with the miso king oyster mushrooms on top, and sprinkle over the spring onions, sesame seeds, the fresh herbs and some lime juice. If you fancy more spice, sprinkle chilli flakes or chilli oil on top for a real kick!

SEA BASS WITH INFUSED QUINOA

DF, GF

🍲 Cooking for Friends and Family   🕐 Under 1 hour

SERVES 4

160g (1¼ cups) frozen
   garden peas
1 red onion
7–8 mixed baby
   sweet peppers
100g (½ cup) quinoa
4 sea bass fillets
100g (6 leaves) cavolo nero
1 x 400g (14oz) tin red kidney
   beans, drained and rinsed
Handful of fresh basil leaves

FOR THE INFUSED OIL

4 tbsp extra virgin olive oil
1–2 garlic cloves, crushed
½ tsp dried oregano
½ tsp dried thyme
½ tsp onion granules
½ tsp chilli flakes (optional)
Sea salt and black pepper

There are some variations you can try with this recipe; it works well with other white fish such as cod and you can also swap the peas for kale leaves, or spinach. The quinoa is infused using the oil from the roasted sweet baby peppers.

—

1. Preheat the oven to 200°C fan (425°F). Place the frozen peas into a bowl of tepid water and set aside.
2. Peel and chop the red onion into 8 wedges and place in a 26 x 20cm (10 x 8in) Pyrex roasting dish with the baby peppers (leave these whole).
3. For the infused oil, mix all of the ingredients together in a small bowl. Use 3 tablespoons of the mixture to cover the onion and peppers. Roast for 15 minutes in the oven.
4. While the vegetables are roasting, cook the quinoa. Rinse and cook in a pan of salted boiling water on a medium heat for 15–20 minutes, or until tender. Leave to drain in a sieve and set aside.
5. Place the sea bass fillets on a piece of foil, cover with the remaining tablespoon of infused oil, wrap in the foil and place on top of the vegetables. Return to the oven for a further 5 minutes.
6. Chop the cavolo nero into chunks, take the tray out of the oven and roll the chunks through the red onion and peppers. Place the foil sea bass parcel back on top and cook for a final 5 minutes.
7. Remove the tray from the oven and set the sea bass parcel aside. Drain the garden peas, which will now be soft, and add them to the roasting tray.
8. Remove the baby peppers from the tray, open them up with a knife and gently deseed them. Then chop into chunks and return to the roasting tray.
9. Add the red kidney beans and quinoa to the roasting tray and stir everything together. Chop and stir in the basil, plus some more sea salt and black pepper to taste.
10. Divide between 4 plates and top each with a sea bass fillet. Best served straight away.

ONE-POT CHICKEN AND PRAWN JAMBALAYA

DF, GF

✳ Freezable 🍴 Meal Prep ⏐ 'Fakeaway' 🍃 Cooking for Friends and Family
🕐 Under 1 hour

SERVES 6

210g (1½ cups)
   frozen garden peas
2 tbsp extra virgin olive oil
2 garlic cloves, minced
1 red onion, diced
3 chicken breasts, cut
   into strips
1 tbsp tomato purée
2 red bell peppers,
   finely sliced
500g (2½ cups) brown rice
1 x 400g (14oz) tin
   chopped tomatoes
800ml (3¼ cups)
   vegetable stock
700ml (3 cups) water
330g (1½ cups) raw
   peeled king prawns
2 spring onions
1 lemon, cut into 6 wedges

FOR THE SPICES
2 tbsp smoked paprika
2 tsp ground cumin
2 tsp garlic granules
2 tsp paprika
1–2 tsp chilli powder
   (to taste)
2 tsp dried coriander leaf
1 tsp dried rosemary
1 tsp onion granules
1 tsp black pepper
½ tsp Himalayan salt

Plenty of spices and full of flavour, this is a dish that will definitely impress your friends and family. The prawns and chicken can be swapped out for tofu, more beans or tempeh, to get more plants in.

—

1. Place the frozen peas in a bowl of tepid water and set aside.
2. Heat the extra virgin olive oil in a large saucepan and fry the garlic and red onion for 5 minutes before adding in the chicken breast strips. Cook the chicken for 3–5 minutes until it is sealed white on the outside, then add the spices, tomato purée and bell peppers.
3. Add the brown rice, coating it with the spices and herbs, then pour in the tinned tomatoes and veg stock and cook for 20 minutes on a low–medium heat, partially covered. Stir occasionally so that the rice does not stick to the bottom of the pan.
4. Add 300ml (1¼ cups) of water to the saucepan and continue cooking the mixture for 10 minutes before adding another 200ml (¾ cup) of water and cooking for a further 5 minutes. Then add the remaining water and cook for a further 5 minutes.
5. Drain the frozen peas and add them with the king prawns, then cook for 5 minutes, stirring well until the prawns are cooked (but not overcooked).
6. Serve with the spring onions sprinkled on top and lemon wedges to squeeze over before serving.

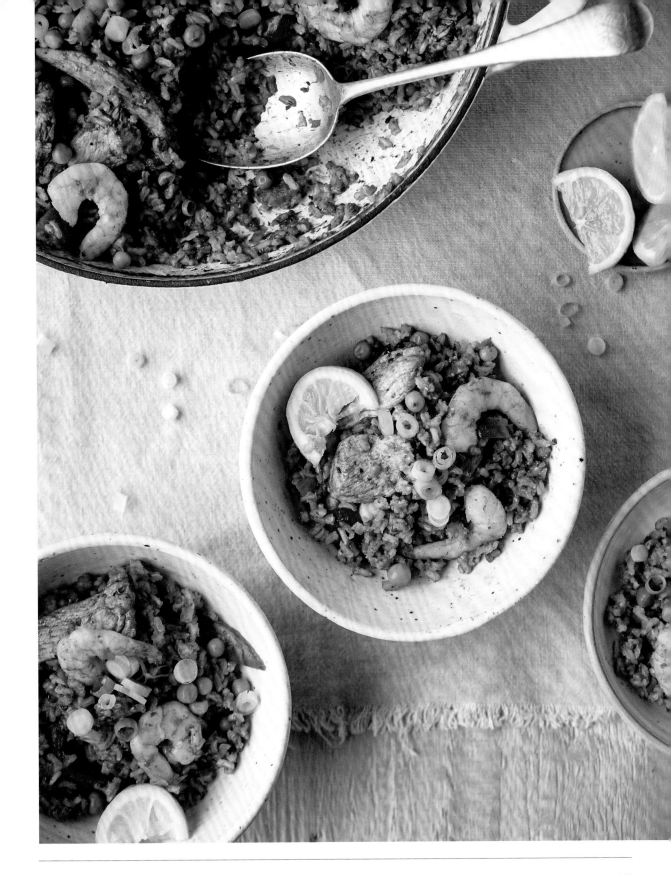

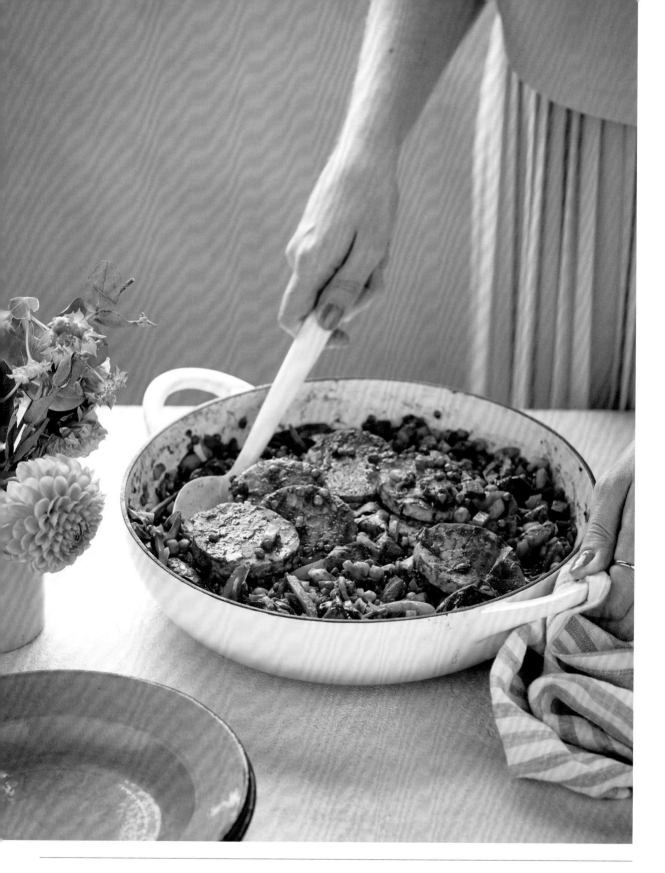

EAT WELL WITH ARTHRITIS

ONE-POT HARISSA TEMPEH STEW

V, VEG, DF, GF   ✳ Freezable 🍴 Meal Prep 🥣 Cooking for Friends and Family 🕐 Under 1 hour

SERVES 4

Extra virgin olive oil
1 red onion, sliced
2 garlic cloves, minced
1 fennel bulb, stalks and root
    removed and finely diced,
    or 1 tsp fennel seeds
1 red bell pepper, sliced
1 yellow bell pepper, sliced
200g (2½ cups)
    mushrooms, sliced
200g (7oz) tempeh,
    cut into slices
5 tsp harissa paste
2 tsp tomato purée
Pinch of saffron threads
½ tsp paprika
½ tsp ground coriander
½ tsp ground cumin
¼ tsp garlic granules
1 x 400g (14oz) tin
    chopped tomatoes
1 tsp maple syrup or honey
200g (1 cup) Puy lentils
1 vegetable stock
    cube, dissolved
    in 600ml (2½
    cups) hot water 1 bay leaf
1 x 400g (14oz) tin
    chickpeas, drained
    and rinsed
100g (2½ cups) spinach
¼ tsp black pepper
Pinch of sea salt

TO SERVE
4 tbsp coconut
    yoghurt (optional)
Handful of fresh flat-leaf
    parsley, stalks and
    leaves separated

I absolutely love this dish: it's easy to make, but feels like a treat. If you have heard of tempeh, but you are not sure where to start with it, or how to cook it, then this is a great recipe to begin with. What is tempeh? Tempeh is made with cooked and fermented soybeans, packed with probiotics for good gut health (important for immune health), phytonutrient and the flavonoid genistein, as well as being rich in calcium and iron, and is a great source of plant-based protein.

—

1. In a large saucepan, gently heat a drizzle of extra virgin olive oil, add the red onion, garlic and fennel and sweat for 5 minutes until softened.
2. Then add the sliced peppers and cook for 3 minutes, before adding the mushrooms with the sliced tempeh and cooking everything for 1 minute.
3. Next, add the harissa paste, tomato purée, saffron threads, paprika, ground coriander, ground cumin and garlic granules. Let it all infuse by stirring for 20 seconds, then stir in the tinned tomatoes and maple syrup (or honey).
4. Add the Puy lentils and coat in the mixture before adding the vegetable stock and bay leaf. Simmer for 35 minutes, covered. Finally, stir in the chickpeas and spinach until the spinach has wilted.
5. Plate up with a dollop of coconut yoghurt and fresh flat-leaf parsley.

GRANDAD SPEIGHT'S NASI GORENG

V, VEG, DF, GF

✱ Freezable ⒕ Meal Prep ║ 'Fakeaway' 🕊 Cooking for Friends and Family
🕐 Under 1 hour

SERVES 4

80g (½ cup) frozen peas
80g (½ cup) frozen
  sweetcorn
3 eggs (optional) with
  30ml (2 tbsp) plant milk
1 red bell pepper
250g (3 cups) mushrooms
2 garlic cloves
1 red onion
½ tsp ground ginger
  (or 1 tbsp fresh)
1 red chilli, deseeded
  (or ½–1 tsp chilli flakes)
350g (1¾ cups) brown rice
1½ tbsp sesame oil
2 chicken breasts, cut
  into strips (optional)
3 tbsp tamari
1 tbsp honey (or
  a vegan alternative,
  see page 88)
½ tsp ground turmeric
¼ tsp sea salt
½ black pepper
4 tbsp cashew nuts

SWAPS AND
REPLACEMENTS
(OPTIONAL)

300g (3 cups) cooked
  king prawns
300g (10oz) firm tofu,
  cut into chunks
2 carrots, grated
1 courgette, grated
½ cabbage, shredded

TOPPINGS (OPTIONAL)

¼ cucumber, thinly sliced
4 spring onions, thinly sliced
4 tsp sesame seeds
1 lime, cut into wedges

My Grandad Speight was famous in his local area for cooking a huge pan of Nasi Goreng for everyone at the pub. Now that Grandad is no longer with us, it's a homage to him. It's packed with plants, and you can use up leftover cooked rice in your fridge, and any vegetables you have to hand.

—

1. Add the frozen peas and sweetcorn to a bowl of tepid water together. In a jug whisk together the plant milk and eggs (if using). Set aside.
2. Prep and slice all of your vegetables – dice the peppers and mushrooms, finely slice the garlic, onion, ginger and chilli (if using fresh) – and set aside (you could do this ahead of time, see the tips on page 49).
3. Cook and drain your brown rice according to the pack instructions.
4. Fifteen minutes before the rice is ready, heat ½ tablespoon of sesame oil in a large pan or wok and cook any optional additions. If using chicken breast, cook for 5–10 minutes to seal, depending on the size of the pieces. Remove from the wok to a plate, cover and set aside.
5. Heat another ½ tablespoon of sesame oil in the same wok, then add the chilli, red onion, garlic and fresh ginger (if using) and cook for 3 minutes, then add the diced peppers and cook for 2 minutes. Add the mushrooms and cook for a further 2 minutes.
6. If using the eggs, gently heat ½ tablespoon of sesame oil in a small frying pan, or in the well of the wok, then pour the beaten egg mixture and cook as though making an omelette. Once firm, gently cut it into strips using a spatula. Add to the wok or stir it in if you have cooked it in the wok. (Cooking it in a small frying pan means the mixture is easier to control.)
7. Drain the peas and sweetcorn, then add to the pan with the vegetables. Add the brown rice, then the tamari, honey, ground ginger (if using), ground turmeric, sea salt and black pepper, plus some more sesame oil, if needed. Add any optional swaps or additions here to heat through thoroughly. Stir and toss for 5 minutes so the rice can soak up the juices nicely.
8. Throw the chicken/prawns/tofu back into the pan, along with the cashews and cook for a couple of minutes.
9. Serve topped with the cucumber, spring onions and sesame seeds, with a wedge of lime alongside. You can always add more tamari here too.

EAT WELL WITH ARTHRITIS

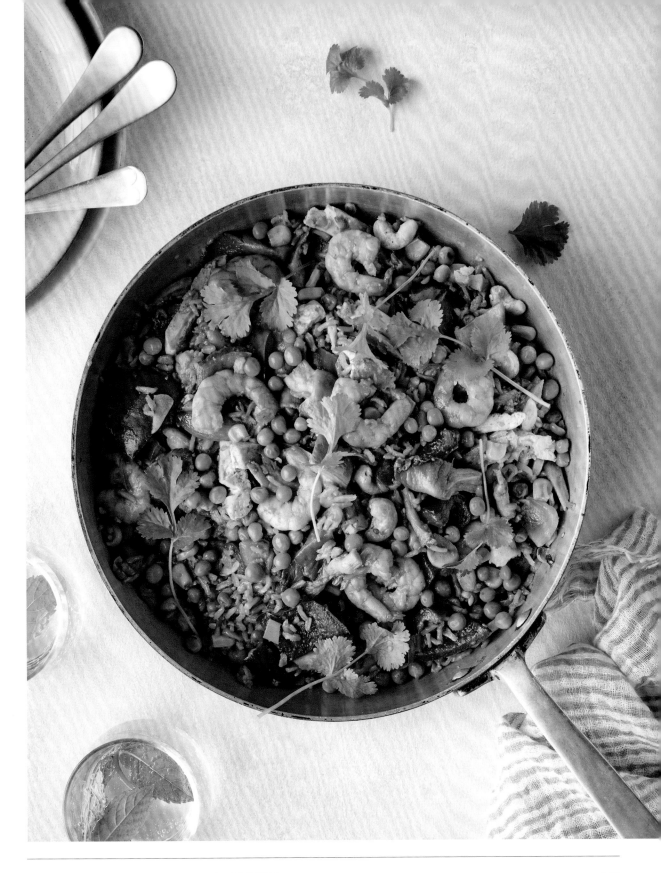

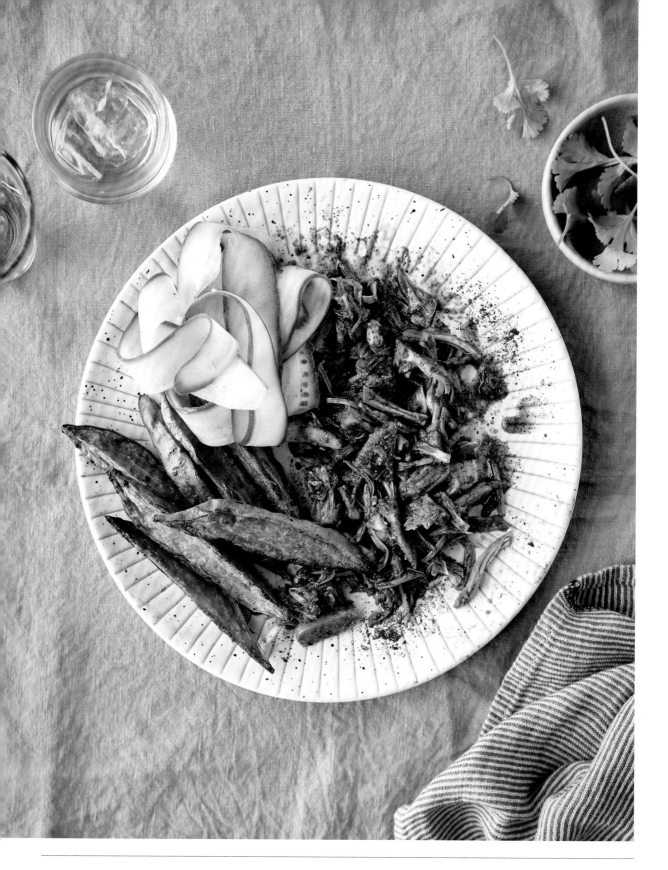

EAT WELL WITH ARTHRITIS

PULLED SMOKY JACKFRUIT SALAD

V, VEG, DF, GF

🍴 Meal Prep ▌'Fakeaway' 🍃 Cooking for Friends and Family 🕐 Under 1 hour

SERVES 2

2 tbsp extra virgin olive oil
2 tsp tomato purée
2 tsp apple cider vinegar
1 tsp garlic granules
    or garlic paste
½ tsp chilli flakes
1 tsp smoked paprika
3 tsp date syrup
½ tsp onion granules
1 tsp ground cumin
⅛ tsp ground ginger
Pinches of sea salt
    and black pepper
1 x 400g (14oz) tin jackfruit
    in water, drained

TO SERVE (OPTIONAL)
Grated carrots
Sliced cucumber
Baby gem lettuce
Tomatoes
Diced peppers
Red onions
Butter beans
Kidney beans
Cooked quinoa
Sweet potato wedges
1 tbsp sunflower seeds
1 tbsp pumpkin seeds

All the smoky flavours of pork . . . without the pork. Delicious served with sweet potato wedges, butter beans or in a sourdough bun (if you're not gluten-free). Jackfruit is packed with healthy antioxidants, including vitamin C, carotenoids and flavanones, which help to protect against oxidative stress and inflammation.

—

1. In a small bowl, mix together all the ingredients apart from the jackfruit to make a marinade.
2. Put the jackfruit in a bowl and mash with the back of a fork so it becomes stringy. Drain and place in a container, then add the marinade and leave in the fridge for a few hours.
3. Prepare your chosen sides – I like to roast some skin-on sweet potato wedges with a drizzle of extra virgin olive oil in the oven at 170°C fan (375°F) for 35–40 minutes.
4. Serve the jackfruit alongside your chosen side(s).

SALMON AND PUY LENTILS WITH ORANGE DRESSING

DF, GF

🍵 Cooking for Friends and Family 🕐 Under 1 hour

SERVES 4

240g (1 cup) Puy lentils
700ml (3 cups) water
1 vegetable stock cube
1 bay leaf
1 tsp dried parsley
½ tsp dried oregano
4 salmon pieces
2 tsp extra virgin olive oil
¼ tsp sea salt
¼ tsp black pepper
280g (2 cups) fine
    green beans
80g (2 cups) watercress

**FOR THE ORANGE
DRESSING (MAKES
175ML, OR ⅔ CUP):**

½ tbsp wholegrain mustard
Zest (1½ tbsp) and juice
    of 1 orange (2½ tbsp)
1 tbsp honey
6 tbsp extra virgin olive oil
2 tbsp water
½ tbsp apple cider vinegar
Pinches of sea salt
    and black pepper

TO SERVE (OPTIONAL)
Fresh parsley
Thin slices of orange
    or lemon

This is a really easy and delicious way to get in your daily omega-3, and you can also swap the salmon for sea bass or cod – they work just as well. For other omega-3 ideas, and why it's important, go to the previous chapter on anti-inflammatory ingredients. Watercress also contains dietary nitrates, which boost blood vessel health by reducing inflammation and decreasing the stiffness and thickness of your blood vessels. Poor circulation can contribute to autoimmune diseases, such as arthritis.

—

1. Preheat the oven to 200°C fan (425°F).
2. Rinse the lentils and then add to a pan with the water, vegetable stock cube and bay leaf. Bring it to a rolling boil, then turn down the heat to low –medium and simmer for 20–25 minutes, uncovered and gently bubbling, until all of the liquid has absorbed. Stir occasionally so that the lentils do not stick to the bottom of the pan.
3. Drizzle the salmon with the extra virgin olive oil, and then sprinkle over the dried herbs and seasoning. Wrap in foil and cook in the oven for 15–20 minutes, depending on the size of your salmon fillets.
4. While the salmon and lentils are cooking, wash and place the fine green beans in a pan of water. Cook for 3–5 minutes on a high heat until crisp, then drain (do this in the last 5–10 minutes of the lentils cooking time, so they're ready at the same time).
5. For the orange dressing, place all of the ingredients into a jug and stir to combine, or add to a jar, seal and shake to combine. You can always add more honey if the dressing is too bitter.
6. On 4 plates, scatter the lentils as the first layer, then add the watercress, green beans and the salmon, and pour over the orange dressing. If you're feeling fancy, you could also top the dish with fresh parsley and slices of orange.

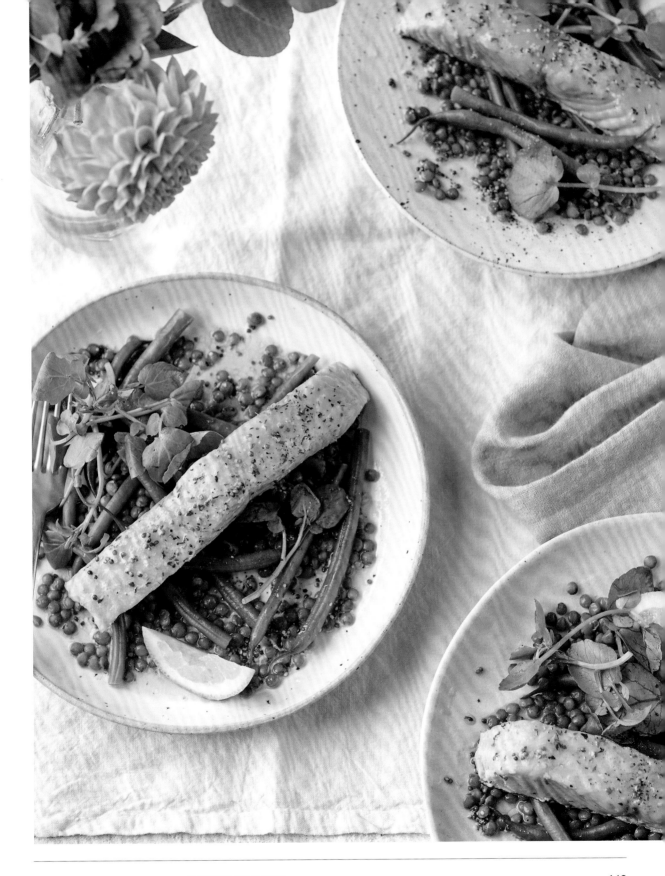

ONE-TRAY ROAST CHICKEN WITH VEGETABLES

DF, GF   🥢 Cooking for Friends and Family 🕐 Over 1 hour

SERVES 4

2 sweet potatoes
3 parsnips
9 long small carrots
3 small–medium red onions
2 bell peppers, 1 red, 1 yellow
2 turnips
220g (8oz) green beans,
   or 1½ cup when chopped
2½ tbsp extra virgin olive oil
4 chicken breasts
Juice of ½ lemon
4 tbsp Kalamata olives

HERBS FOR THE VEGETABLES

2 tbsp fresh thyme leaves
1 tbsp fresh rosemary leaves
½ tbsp dried oregano
½ tsp dried marjoram
1 tsp dried parsley
½ tsp sea salt
½ tsp black pepper

HERBS FOR THE CHICKEN

½ tsp extra virgin olive oil
½ tsp dried rosemary
½ tsp dried marjoram
½ tsp dried thyme
Pinch of sea salt and
   black pepper

FOR THE SAUCE

10 roasted garlic cloves
   (see page 89)
8 tbsp extra virgin olive oil
1 tbsp balsamic vinegar
2 sun-dried tomatoes
Handful of fresh basil leaves,
   plus extra to serve
2 tbsp nutritional yeast flakes
½ tsp maple syrup
Pinch of sea salt
Pinch of black pepper

I have packed as many vegetables as possible into this roast, and the skins are left on to provide extra nutritious fibre. The more organic vegetables that you can use, the better too, as microscopic bugs from the soil that they have grown in will be good for your gut and immune system, and might even boost your mood!

—

1. Preheat the oven to 200°C fan (425°F) and line 2 large flat baking trays with baking parchment (you can use a drizzle of olive oil instead, but the vegetables tend to stick to the trays).
2. Wash and top and tail the sweet potatoes, parsnips and carrots, then slice as follows: sweet potatoes into chunks – circles then into halves, parsnips cut lengthways and then again into strips, carrots lengthways and into strips.
3. Slice the red onions in half, then halve again. De-seed and cut the bell peppers into quarter pieces lengthways. Peel and chop the turnips into chunks. Wash and top and tail the green beans, then leave to drain in a sieve over a bowl.
4. Place all of the vegetables, apart from the green beans, onto the prepared baking trays, add the herbs and 2 tablespoons of the extra virgin olive oil and roast in the oven for 15 minutes.
5. Place the chicken breasts in a bowl with the herbs and the remaining ½ tablespoon of oil and rub them in the seasoned oil.
6. After 15 minutes of cooking, divide the chicken breasts between the trays and cook for another 15 minutes, swapping the trays around in the oven.
7. Swap the trays again, lightly toss the vegetables and scatter the green beans across both trays. Cook for a final 15 minutes.
8. While everything is in its final cooking stage, make the sauce. Blend all of the ingredients together until you have a rich and creamy sauce the colour of gravy. The sauce may separate – but this is normal.
9. Plate up the chicken and vegetables with the Kalamata olives, a squeeze of lemon juice and the garlic 'gravy' sauce. Garnish with a few basil leaves too.

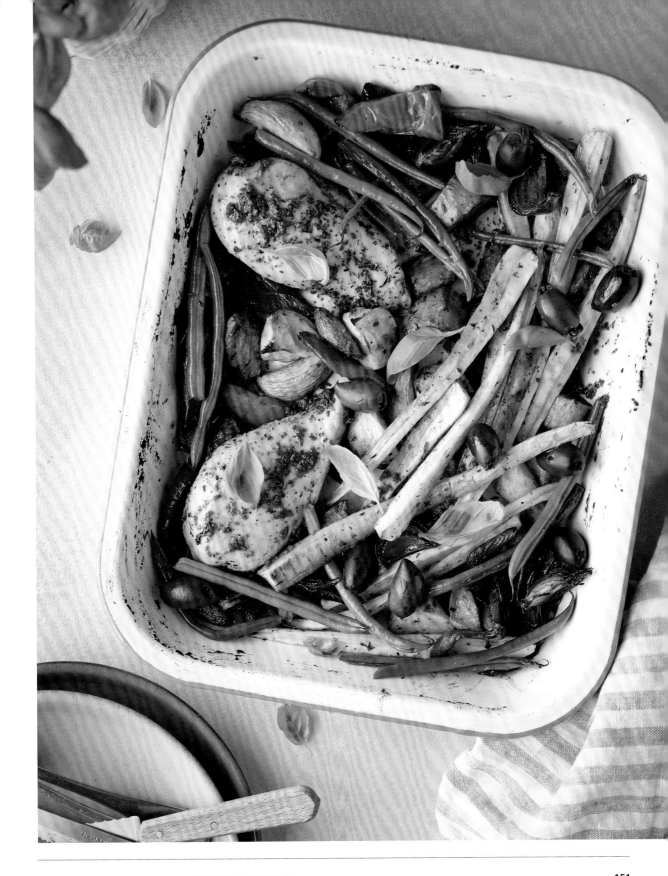

STICKY AND SWEET MIXED VEG STIR-FRY WITH CASHEW NUTS

V, VEG, DF, GF

✳ Freezable ⫴ Meal Prep ❙ 'Fakeaway' 🍃 Cooking for Friends and Family
🕐 Under 1 hour

SERVES 2

2 garlic cloves,
    roughly chopped
1 red chilli, roughly
    chopped (optional)
1 red onion,
    roughly chopped
20–50g (1–2oz) fresh
    ginger, peeled and
    roughly chopped
1 tbsp sesame oil
2 chicken breasts, cut
    into strips (optional)
1 red bell pepper,
    cut into strips
80g (1 cup or a
    handful) mangetout
500g (4 cups) plum
    tomatoes, roughly
    chopped
1 tbsp tomato purée
200ml (¾ cup) water
1 tsp tamari
3 tsp date syrup
½ tsp rice vinegar
    or apple cider vinegar
150g (1 cup) cashew nuts
1 tsp ground arrowroot
    (optional, to thicken)
Sea salt and black pepper

TO SERVE
150g (¾ cup) brown rice,
    or 2 rice noodles nests,
    cooked
2 spring onions, sliced
2 tsp sesame seeds

My grandma is a pescatarian and had almond milk in her fridge even before I was born, and before it was trendy. This is not her recipe, but it is a recipe inspired by her favourite dish – zingy, takeaway-style tomatoes, with the anti-inflammatory power of ginger and nourishing cashew nuts and vegetables, served with brown rice. The chicken is optional, and the dish also works well with tofu or tempeh.

—

1. Blend the garlic, chilli, red onion and ginger in a food processor to form a paste.
2. Gently heat 2 teaspoons of sesame oil in a pan on a medium heat and fry the chicken (if using) with a sprinkle of sea salt and black pepper for 7–10 minutes, depending on the size of the chunks. Remove to a plate, cover to keep warm and set aside.
3. Add another teaspoon of sesame oil to the same pan and gently fry the paste for 2 minutes, then add the pepper strips and mangetout and cook for 5 minutes.
4. Add the tomatoes, tomato purée and the water. Stir well until the tomatoes start to disintegrate and soften, then stir in the tamari, date syrup, vinegar and ground arrowroot (if using). Add the cashew nuts, stirring well, and return the chicken to the pan. Simmer for 3–5 minutes to heat through and thicken.
5. Serve topped with chopped spring onions and sesame seeds, with brown rice or rice noodles alongside.

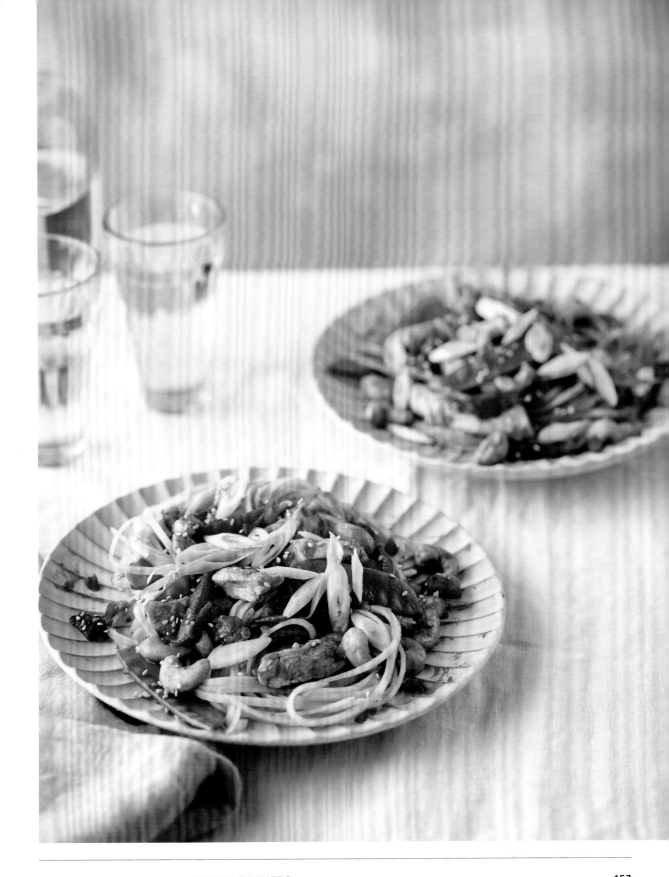

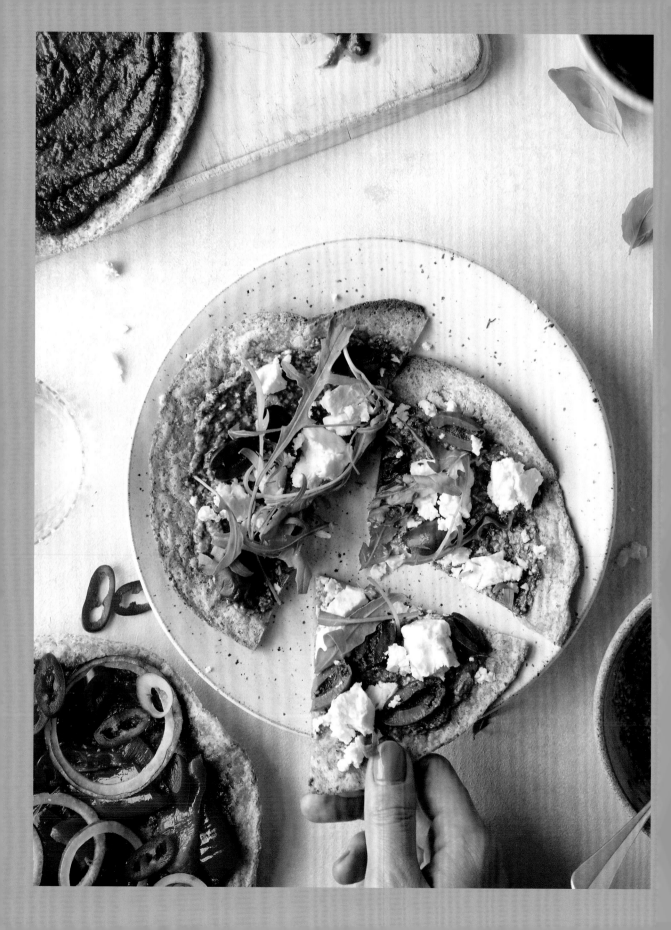

MEAL PREP

VEGAN CHILLI

V, VEG, DF, GF

✳ Freezable ┇ Meal Prep ┃ 'Fakeaway' 🥣 Cooking for Friends and Family 🕐 Over 1 hour

MAKES 4 SMALL OR 6 LARGE PORTIONS

1 tbsp extra virgin olive oil
2 medium red onions,
    thinly sliced
1 red chilli (more to taste
    if you'd like), deseeded
    and finely chopped
2 black garlic cloves (or
    2 normal garlic cloves
    if you're not able to get
    black garlic), thinly sliced
4 carrots, peeled and diced
2 red bell peppers, sliced
    into strips
350g (3½ cups)
    mushrooms, sliced
2 x 400g (14oz) tins
    chopped tomatoes
2 tbsp tomato purée
1 x 400g (14oz) tin red kidney
    beans, drained and rinsed
1 x 400g (14oz) tin cannellini
    beans, drained and rinsed
150ml (⅔ cup) water
Fresh coriander leaves,
    to serve

SPICES 1
2 tsp ground coriander
3 tsp ground cumin
1 tsp smoked paprika
½ tsp dried rosemary
½ tsp dried thyme
½ tsp paprika

SPICES 2
1 heaped tsp raw
    cacao powder
½ tsp garlic granules
½ tsp ground ginger
1 tsp balsamic vinegar
Pinch of chilli flakes
    (optional)

This warming dish is so delicious on a cold winter day, and I've packed in as many key plant phytonutrients as possible, from the ginger and cacao to rosemary, thyme and fresh oregano. Try using wild or shiitake mushrooms for extra nutritional value if you can. It also works in the summer with sweet potato wedges and a side salad. Or swap the red kidney beans for a tin of green lentils and use as a Bolognese-style sauce with brown rice spaghetti. There are two separate spice additions, to get the best flavour from the recipe, but if you do accidently add them all together – that's okay!

1. Add each batch of spices to a separate bowl and set aside.
2. In a large saucepan, heat the extra virgin olive oil and lightly fry the red onions, chilli and garlic for 5 minutes until soft.
3. Add the carrots and cook for 5 minutes.
4. Add the peppers and stir for just under 5 minutes until softened.
5. Add the mushrooms and cook for a couple of minutes before stirring in the first batch of spices. Cook for a minute to infuse, then add the chopped tomatoes, tomato purée, kidney and cannellini beans. Stir in the water and simmer for 15–20 minutes on a low-medium heat, with the lid on.
6. Stir in the second batch of spices for the last 5 minutes of cooking.
7. Serve scattered with fresh coriander and with corn on the cob, smashed avocado or sweet potato wedges alongside.

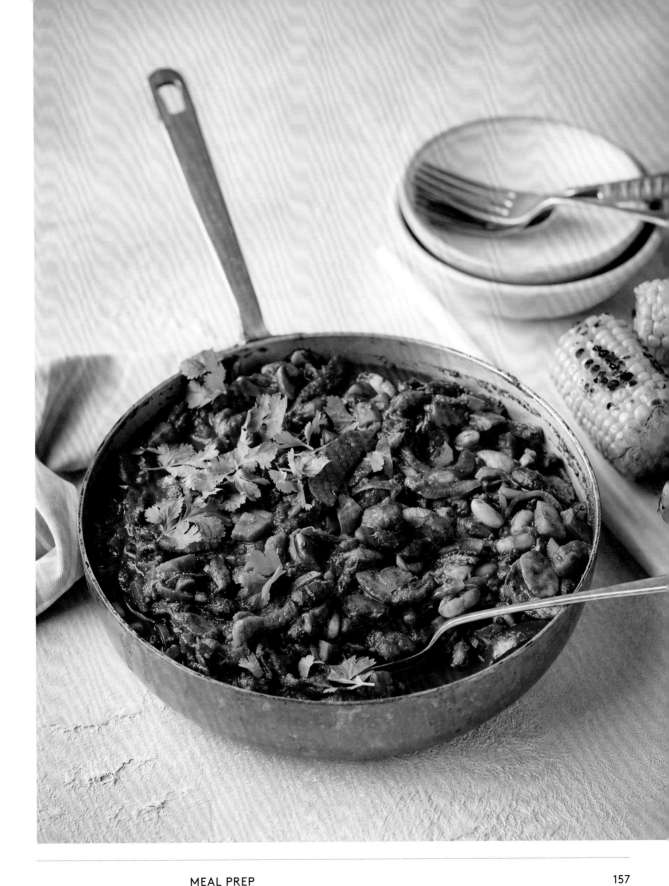

SPICY AND WARMING DAHL

V, VEG, DF, GF

✳ Freezable 🍴 Meal Prep ▌ 'Fakeaway' 🍃 Cooking for Friends and Family
🕐 Over 1 hour (plus 8–9 hours soaking the lentils)

SERVES 4 (WITHOUT RICE) OR 6 (WITH RICE)

270g (1⅓ cups) whole urad dal (whole black gram lentils)
630ml (2⅔ cups) water
3–5 medium tomatoes, chopped, or 1 x 400g (14oz) tin chopped tomatoes
1 red onion, peeled and chopped
40g (1½oz) fresh ginger, peeled and chopped
2 garlic cloves, chopped
1 red chilli, deseeded and chopped
½ tsp ground coriander
1 tsp garam masala
2 tbsp coconut oil
1 bay leaf
1 x 400g (14oz) tin red kidney beans, drained and rinsed
1 x 400ml (14fl oz) tin coconut milk
1 medium dried Kashmiri chilli (optional)
90g (1½–2 cups) spinach

FOR THE SPICES
1 tsp ground turmeric
1 tsp ground fenugreek
1 tsp ground cumin
½ tsp ground cinnamon
½ tsp paprika
½ tsp ground cloves
½ tsp ground cardamom
¼ tsp ground nutmeg or mace (javitri)
¼ tsp sea salt
¼ tsp black pepper

TO SERVE (OPTIONAL)
Fresh coriander
Lime wedges
Brown basmati rice or flatbreads

I know it might seem an affront to the original recipe to make this without dairy, but I really love the creaminess of dahl makhani and wanted to recreate that flavour while keeping it as plant-based as possible. You could also use uncooked red kidney beans, but these require soaking overnight – which is why I find the tinned ones easier. This dahl is packed with powerful spices and has such a warming creamy flavour. Typically, this dish does not have red onion or spinach in it, but I wanted to get in some more vegetables for their phytonutrient content.

—

1. Put the black gram lentils in a large pan or mixing bowl, cover with water and leave to soak for 8–9 hours overnight, or during the day before making the recipe that evening.
2. Drain the lentils well, then rinse a couple of times in water and drain again.
3. Put all of the spices into a small bowl.
4. Transfer the lentils to a large saucepan with the water and set a stopwatch – there's usually one on your phone – so you can track how long they are cooking for. Bring to the boil, this should take around 5–8 minutes, then reduce the heat to a low–medium and cover with a lid.
5. While the black gram lentils are cooking, combine the tomatoes, red onion, ginger, garlic, chilli, coriander and garam masala in a blender until a smooth purée is formed. Add a small amount of water if needed.
6. In a separate frying pan, heat the coconut oil gently on a medium heat (so as not to burn it) and, once hot enough, add the bay leaf and your small bowl of spices and gently cook for a couple of minutes before pouring in the spicy tomato purée mixture from the blender. Stir for about 8–10 minutes on a medium–low heat.
7. By this point, the stopwatch should say 20 minutes, so add the spicy tomato purée mixture to the lentils and stir well.
8. Then add the kidney beans, coconut milk and dried Kashmiri chilli (if using). Simmer for 1 hour, with the lid on, stirring occasionally until nice and thick. Stir in the spinach at the very end (or you can serve it uncooked on top).
9. Remove the bay leaf and dried Kashmiri chilli to serve. Serve the dahl as it is, with fresh coriander and a wedge of lime, or with brown basmati rice or flatbreads to bulk out the portions.

EAT WELL WITH ARTHRITIS

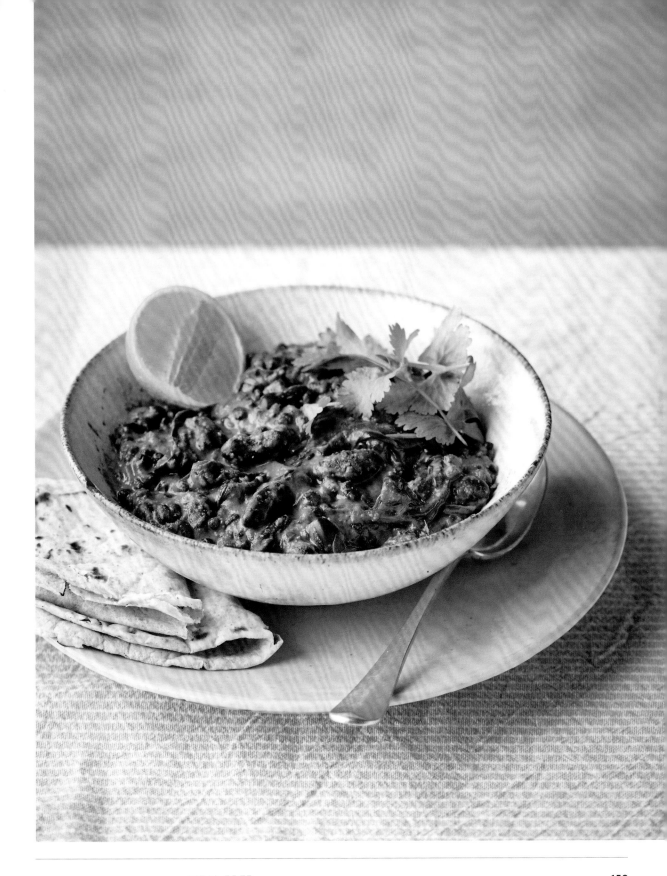

'FAKEAWAY' KATSU CURRY, OR KATSU CURRY SALAD

V, VEG, DF, GF

✳ Freezable 🍴 Meal Prep ▌'Fakeaway' 🥢 Cooking for Friends and Family
🕐 Between 1–2 hours

SERVES 4

350–400g (12–14oz) firm
  tofu, cut into 4 rectangular
  slabs, or 4 chicken breasts
20g (¾oz) fine polenta (tofu)
  or 40g (1½oz) ground
  almonds (chicken)
1 tsp desiccated coconut
1 tsp garam masala
½ tsp ground coriander
½ tsp ground cumin
½ tsp sea salt
½ tsp black pepper
¼ tsp ground turmeric
3–4 tbsp brown rice flour
1 egg, beaten (if
  using chicken)
340g (1⅔ cups) brown rice

FOR THE SAUCE
5 garlic cloves, minced
2 red onions, chopped
  into chunks
½ tbsp coconut oil
2 large carrots, topped
  and tailed and chopped
  into chunks
1 apple, cored and
  chopped into chunks
4 tsp medium curry powder
2 tbsp buckwheat
  or brown rice flour
2 tsp desiccated coconut
2 tsp garam masala
½ tsp paprika
½ tsp ground turmeric
½ tsp ground ginger
½ tsp ground coriander
½ tsp ground cumin
4 tbsp plant milk
2 tbsp honey (or maple
  syrup, if vegan)
3 tbsp tamari
1 vegetable stock cube,
  dissolved in 600ml
  (2½ cups) hot water
2 tbsp sesame oil

This recipe has all the deep flavours of a katsu curry, and if you are craving a classic British chip-shop curry taste, this is a slightly more refined and flavoursome version. It can be made meat-free using tofu too, which I love. Choose between brown rice or salad to enjoy with it.

—

1. If using tofu, mix the polenta with the spices and coat each slab of tofu in the mixture.
2. If using chicken, butterfly each chicken breast and place on a chopping board, cover with a baking sheet and tap with a rolling pin to flatten into two thinner larger pieces. To one side, have a bowl of the flour, a bowl with the beaten egg and a bowl of ground almonds mixed with the spices. Dip the chicken into the flour, then into the egg and then into the ground almond mixture. Set aside.
3. Rinse the brown rice and cook according to the pack instructions or see my method on page 112.
4. To make the sauce, fry the garlic and onions in a large pan with coconut oil for 5 minutes, then add the carrots and apple. After a couple of minutes, add all of the dry ingredients, plus the plant milk, honey and tamari. Let the flavours infuse for a couple of minutes, then add the hot vegetable stock. Stir and simmer for 15–20 minutes until the mixture has thickened.
5. To cook the tofu or chicken, heat the sesame oil in a large shallow pan and cook for 7–9 minutes on each side, taking care not to burn the oil. Use tongs to ensure all pieces are fully cooked and crispy. If cooking the chicken, slice into pieces after cooking. If cooking the tofu, cut each piece into 4 after cooking. Place onto a piece of kitchen paper to drain any excess oil where needed.
6. Blend the sauce using a stick blender or food processor. Return it to the pan if it needs to get thicken.
7. Serve the tofu or chicken with coriander and sesame seeds and the cooked rice alongside. For the salad, simply omit the brown rice, and grate or finely slice the vegetables in a large bowl with lime juice, then add the tofu or chicken. Wait until the sauce has cooled before pouring on top.

Tip:
Freeze the sauce on its own in a flat storage bag, into portions, and take out what you need when you need it'

FOR THE SALAD (OPTIONAL)

½ white cabbage
2 carrots
1 courgette
Handful of cherry tomatoes
1 baby gem lettuce
Juice of ½ lime

TO SERVE

Handful of fresh coriander
    leaves, chopped
4 tsp sesame seeds

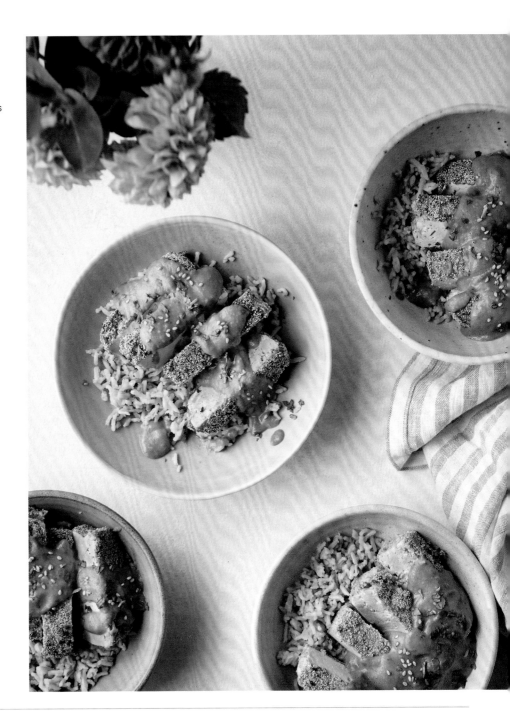

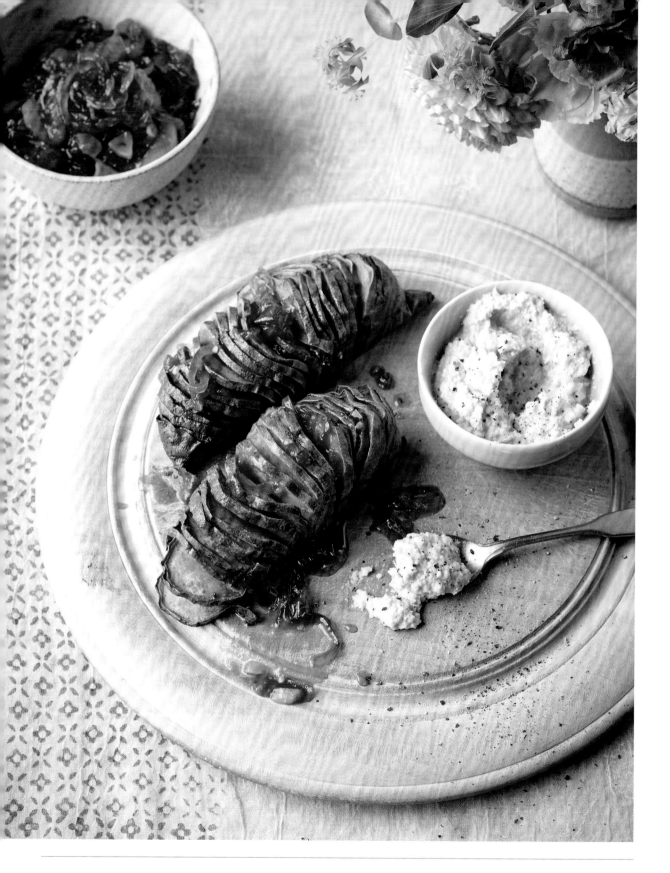

EAT WELL WITH ARTHRITIS

HASSELBACK POTATOES WITH CHILLI APRICOT CHUTNEY AND CASHEW CHEESE

V, VEG, DF, GF

🍃 Cooking for Friends and Family 🕐 Under 1 hour

SERVES 2

2 large sweet potatoes
2 tbsp extra virgin olive oil
Sea salt and black pepper

TO SERVE
Cashew Cheese (see page 237) or cottage cheese
Chilli Apricot Chutney (see page 237)

This is an inventive way to cook and enjoy sweet potatoes, contrasting with creamy cashew cheese and the sharp yet sweet taste of the chutney. For a dairy version, use an organic fermented dairy, such as feta cheese, natural or Greek yoghurt, or cottage cheese, which typically contains probiotics (good for the gut).

—

1. Preheat the oven to 180°C fan (400°F).
2. Hold one sweet potato at one end and gently slice thin sections along it, about two-thirds of the way down into the potato. The easiest way to do this is to place a wooden spoon on either side of the potato to prevent you from slicing all the way to the bottom. Repeat with the other sweet potato.
3. Roll the potatoes on a tray with the oil and some sea salt and black pepper, getting the oil in the gaps. Bake in the oven for 45 minutes.
4. Serve the sweet potatoes topped with the Cashew Cheese, letting it seep into the slices. Add a dollop of chutney too.

VEGETABLE-PACKED SHEPHERD'S PIE

V, VEG, DF, GF   ✻ Freezable ⫚ Meal Prep 🌿 Cooking for Friends and Family 🕐 Over 1 hour

SERVES 4–6

2 large sweet potatoes,
   peeled and chopped
2 tsp extra virgin olive oil
2 garlic cloves, chopped
1 red onion, chopped
2 carrots, peeled
   and chopped
300g (10oz) chestnut
   mushrooms, chopped
3 large tomatoes, chopped
2 x 400g (14oz) tins
   jackfruit, drained
1 tbsp tamari
¼ tsp fennel seeds
½ tsp ground ginger
½ tsp white miso paste
300ml (1¼ cups)
   vegetable stock
1 bay leaf
1 tbsp tomato purée
1 tsp date syrup
150g (1 cup) frozen peas
1 tsp ground arrowroot
   (or brown rice flour)
55ml (¼ cup) plant milk
Sea salt and black pepper

FOR THE SWEET
POTATO TOPPING
2 tbsp nutritional yeast flakes
1 tbsp plant milk
1 tsp extra virgin olive oil
Pinch of sea salt and
   black pepper
Handful of fresh parsley,
   to serve

This is a comforting Sunday dinner, or a great meal to make and store in the fridge or freezer as meal prep for the coming week. Jackfruit flesh has the appearance and texture of meat, so it makes a great meat alternative too. It has a rich source of nutrients, such as vitamin C, and is well known for its inflammatory and antioxidant activities. This recipe contains 95 per cent of your recommended daily intake of vitamin C, key to both preventing inflammatory arthritis and maintaining healthy joints with osteoarthritis.

—

1. Boil the sweet potatoes in a pan of water for 10–15 minutes until soft. Drain and set aside.
2. Heat 1 teaspoon of extra virgin olive oil in a large pan, then cook the garlic and onion with a sprinkle of sea salt and 1 teaspoon of black pepper for 5 minutes. Add the carrots and cook for another 5 minutes.
3. Add the mushrooms and cook for 2–3 minutes until soft, then add the chopped tomatoes and cook for 2 minutes. Add the jackfruit, tamari, fennel seeds, ground ginger and miso paste and stir well.
4. Add the vegetable stock, bay leaf, tomato purée and date syrup. Add the frozen peas, arrowroot and the plant milk.
5. Simmer for 15 minutes; while it simmers, preheat the oven to 200°C fan (425°F).
6. Drain and mash the sweet potatoes for the topping with the nutritional yeast flakes, plant milk, extra virgin olive oil and salt and pepper.
7. Add the vegetables to a 26 x 20cm (10 x 8in) baking dish and top with the mashed sweet potato. Bake in the oven for 20–25 minutes to crisp the top. (You could either remove the bay leaf before doing this or use it as a decoration on top of the sweet potato in the middle of the pie.) Scatter over the fresh parsley before serving.

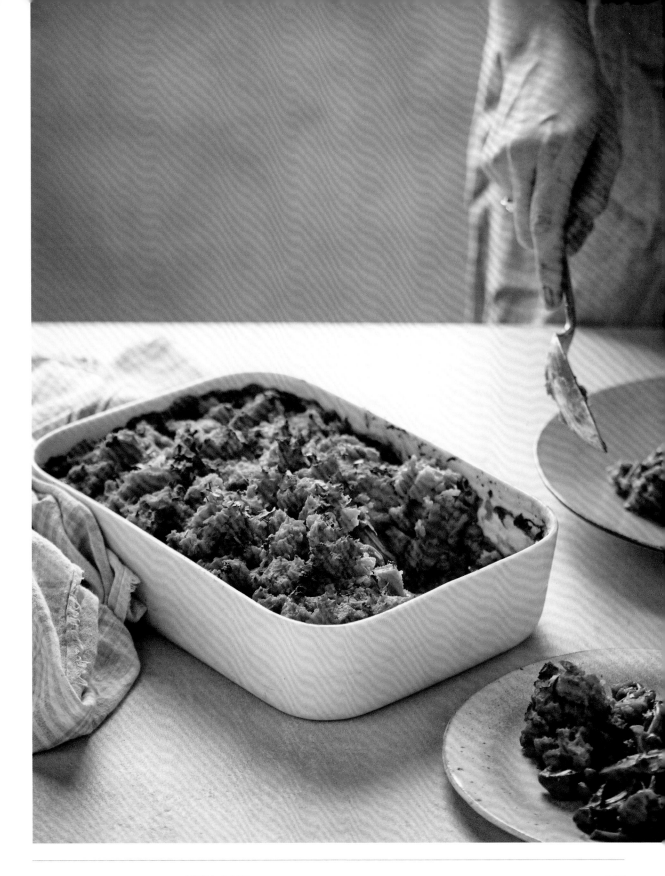

KATY'S QUINOA-BASE PIZZA

V, VEG, DF, GF

✳ Freezable (bases only) ⫴ Meal Prep ▌'Fakeaway'
🥄 Cooking for Friends and Family 🕐 Between 1–2 hours

SERVES 2–4

200g (1 cup +
  ½ tbsp) quinoa
70ml (⅓ cup) water
1 tsp baking powder
1 tsp ground arrowroot
2 tbsp extra virgin olive oil
½ tsp sea salt
½ tsp black pepper
35g (¼ cup) brown rice flour,
  plus extra for dusting
Saucy Vegan Pesto
  (optional, see page 239)
Extra virgin olive oil,
  for drizzling

**FOR THE TOMATO BASE
(OPTIONAL)**
3 tbsp tomato purée
1½ tbsp extra virgin olive oil
2 tsp water
1½ tsp dried oregano
½ tsp black pepper
½ tsp salt

TOPPING IDEAS
Rocket, Kalamata olives and
  Cashew Cheese (page
  237) or feta cheese
Roasted peppers, fresh
  chillies and red onions
Fresh basil leaves,
  shredded sun-dried
  tomatoes and
  baby plum tomatoes
Spinach, mushrooms
  and fresh oregano

A new way to get plant protein and fibre from quinoa, which is widely viewed as a whole grain but is actually a seed. This makes 4 medium pizzas, two each if that's all you're eating, or, one each if you accompany them with a salad and some sweet potato wedges. Choose between tomato or pesto for the base and add whichever toppings you fancy. My sister Katy loves pizza and is a big fan of this recipe (phew)!

1. Preheat the oven to 220°C fan (475°F).
2. Ideally, rinse and cook the quinoa according to the pack instructions in the morning or 1 hour before you make this recipe. Rinse, then leave it to cool and drain for 30 minutes–1 hour before starting the pizzas (don't skip this part).
3. Add the cooked and drained quinoa to a food processor with the water, baking powder, arrowroot, extra virgin olive oil, salt and pepper and mix in intervals for 6–7 minutes until it starts to become smooth. Keep stopping the processor to scrape down the sides, and mix back in to the mixture, so that it all gets processed.
4. Transfer to a large mixing bowl with the brown rice flour and mix together with a spoon or spatula.
5. Line 2 baking trays with baking parchment and sprinkle each one with brown rice flour, dusting your hands too as the dough is sticky, use extra flour where needed..
6. Split the 'dough' into 4 even pieces and place 2 pieces on each lined tray, flattening each one down with the back of a silicone spatula, so that it does not stick to you, so that you have 4 'thin' pizza bases of 5mm (¼in), 2 on each tray. Make sure the bases are not touching.
7. Cook the bases in the oven for 15 minutes.
8. For the tomato base, combine all of the ingredients together in a small bowl.
9. Remove the pizzas from the oven, add your choice of base (tomato or pesto), the toppings of your choice, and return to the oven for 2–3 minutes.
10. Drizzle with oil and serve the pizzas as they are, or with sweet potato wedges and a salad alongside.

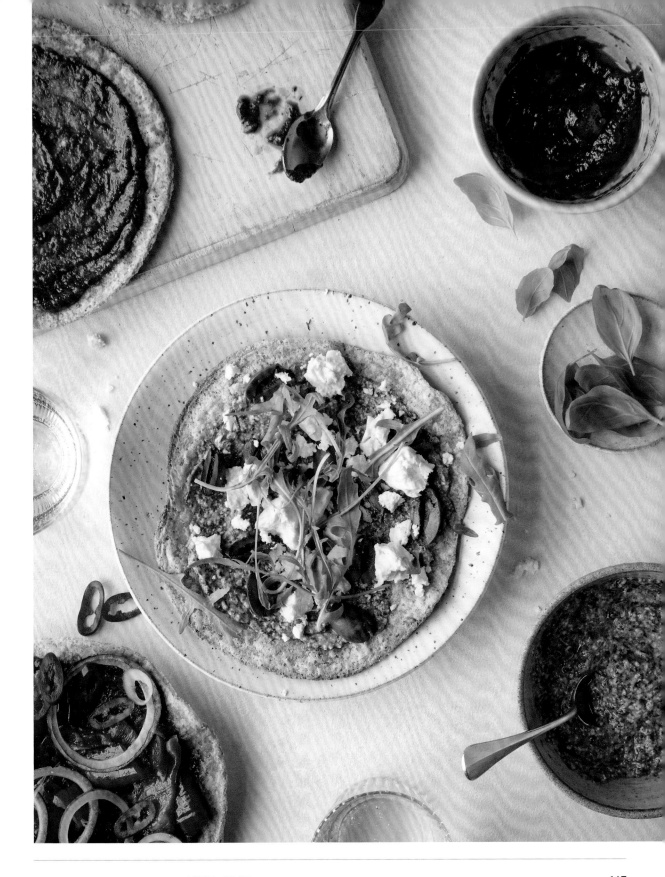

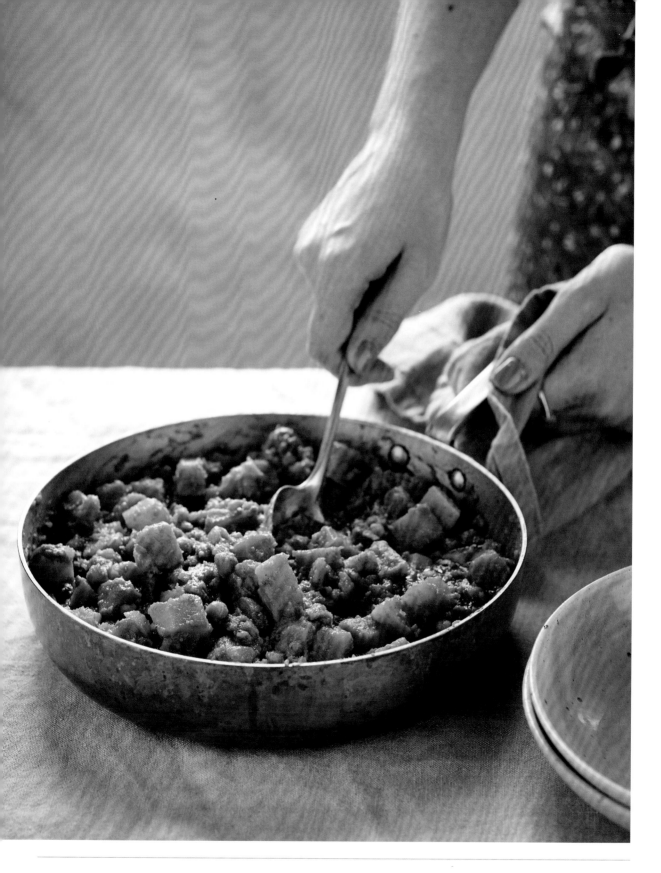

EAT WELL WITH ARTHRITIS

VEGAN CHICKPEA CURRY

V, VEG, DF, GF

✳ Freezable 🍴 Meal Prep ▏'Fakeaway' 🍃 Cooking for Friends and Family
🕐 Under 1 hour

SERVES 4–6

1 tbsp coconut oil
½ tsp black/brown
mustard seeds
1 tsp cumin seeds
(or ground cumin)
1 red onion, finely diced
2 garlic cloves, finely diced
1 green chilli (leave out
if you'd prefer a milder
curry), deseeded and
finely diced
1 tsp ground turmeric
2 tsp medium curry powder
1 tsp ground cumin
½ tsp sea salt
1 tsp black pepper
1 sweet potato,
peeled and cut into
small–medium chunks
1 butternut squash,
peeled and cut into
small–medium chunks
4 carrots, peeled
and cut into small–
medium chunks
1 x 400g (14oz) tin
chickpeas, drained
and rinsed
1 x 400g (14oz) tin
chopped tomatoes
3 tsp tomato purée
1 x 400ml (14fl oz) tin
coconut milk
40g (1 cup) spinach
or kale (optional)

TO SERVE
Brown rice, red rice, wild
rice, black rice or quinoa
Coconut yoghurt
Fresh coriander

Turmeric, namely its bioactive compound curcumin, is one of the most researched anti-inflammatory spices in the world. It has scientifically proven strong anti-inflammatory, antioxidant and immunomodulatory properties. It's not the tastiest spice, with a pungent taste and smell that can be hard to disguise (see page 76). In this recipe, the sweetness of the butternut squash, sweet potatoes, carrots and coconut milk mask the taste of turmeric, which is paired with black pepper (which contains the phytochemical piperine) to support its bioavailability.

—

1. Melt the coconut oil in a large cooking pan on a medium–high heat, then add the mustard and cumin seeds, turn down to medium heat and lightly fry for a couple of minutes (they should sizzle). Add the red onion, garlic and chilli and cook for another 2 minutes.

2. Add the remaining spices, salt and pepper and cook for 30 seconds, then add the sweet potato, butternut squash and carrots with a splash of water. Stir for 2 minutes as the spices become fragrant.

3. Add the chickpeas and stir in for 1 minute, then add the chopped tomatoes and tomato purée and cook for another 2 minutes.

4. Pour in the coconut milk and simmer the curry, with the lid on, for 30–35 minutes until the butternut squash, carrots and sweet potato are tender, but still firm.

5. Stir in the spinach or kale (if using) until it wilts.

6. Serve with rice or quinoa, coconut yoghurt and fresh coriander.

HONEY MUSTARD CHICKEN OR TOFU SALAD

V, VEG, DF, GF ⅏ Meal Prep 🥄 Cooking for Friends and Family 🕐 Under 1 hour

SERVES 4–6

4 chicken breasts
   or 450g (1lb) firm tofu
Extra virgin olive oil
2 sweet pointed peppers
1 yellow bell pepper
260g (1⅓ cups) quinoa
200g (7oz, or 6 pieces)
   tenderstem broccoli
150g (2½ cups) cavolo nero
½ teaspoon paprika
1 sweet gem lettuce
   (155g/5oz)
½ cucumber
200g (1 cup) plum tomatoes
1 x 400g (14oz) tin
   chickpeas, drained
   and rinsed
2 avocados
Sea salt and black pepper

FOR THE DRESSING
150ml (⅔ cup) extra
   virgin olive oil
3 heaped tsp
   wholegrain mustard
1 tbsp apple cider vinegar
2 tsp honey (use maple
   syrup if vegan)
1 tsp balsamic vinegar
½ tsp ground black pepper
Pinch of paprika

When it typing up this recipe I had to ask my sister to remind me how to make it, as she now makes it more than I do! (I gave her the recipe when I first started Arthritis Foodie.) It is so delicious to share or have for lunches.

1. Preheat the oven to 190°C fan (410°F).
2. If using the chicken, place the chicken breasts on a piece of foil, sprinkle with sea salt, ½ teaspoon of black pepper and drizzle over ½ tablespoon of extra virgin olive oil. Wrap it up, place on a baking tray and cook for 35 minutes, turning the tray halfway through.
3. For the vegan version, drain and cut the tofu into chunks. Lightly fry in extra virgin olive oil for 7–10 minutes on each side.
4. Deseed and cut all of the peppers into chunks, place on a separate baking tray and drizzle with 1 teaspoon of extra virgin olive oil. Roast in the oven on the shelf underneath the chicken for 25 minutes, turning the peppers over halfway through.
5. While the chicken and peppers are cooking, cook your quinoa. Rinse the quinoa and place in a pan of salted boiling water on a medium heat for 15–20 minutes, or until tender. Drain and leave to cool. Or to speed up the cooling, rinse in cold water and leave to drain for at least 10–15 minutes.
6. Cut about 1cm (½in) off the ends of the broccoli stems and discard. Bring a pan of water to the boil, add the broccoli, turn down the heat to medium and cook for 5–7 minutes.
7. Cut the cavolo nero into squares and place on a baking tray. Massage with 1 teaspoon of extra virgin olive oil, a pinch of salt, ½ teaspoon of black pepper and the paprika. Cook in the oven for 5–7 minutes at the end of the chicken's cooking time.
8. Take the chicken out of the oven and let it rest for 10–15 minutes.
9. While the chicken is resting, prepare the rest of your salad. Chop the lettuce, cucumber, tomatoes and place in a large salad bowl. Add the drained chickpeas and the quinoa too. To make the dressing, add all of the ingredients to a jug and whisk. If saving some of the salad, store the dressing in a jar separately in the fridge, as it will make the salad go soggy.
10. Chop the avocados and add to the salad at the last minute to stop them discolouring.
11. Shred the chicken with a knife and fork so it has a 'pulled chicken' look. If using tofu, add this to your salad instead. Drizzle the dressing on top and serve.

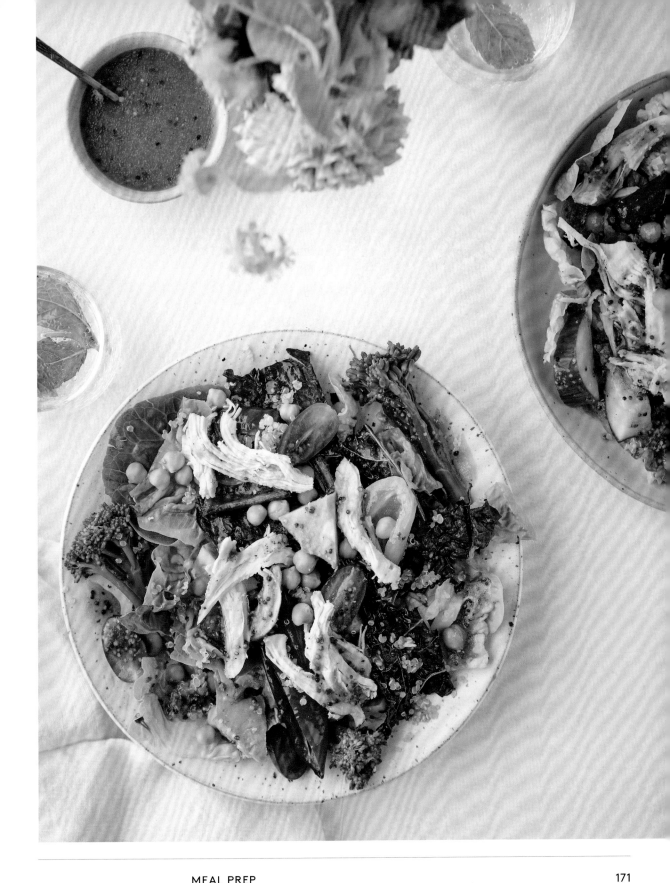

CREAMY CAESAR SALAD

V, VEG, DF, GF　　🍴 Meal Prep ‖ 'Fakeaway' 🥄 Cooking for Friends and Family

SERVES 4

3 chicken breasts or
　280g (9½oz) firm tofu
Extra virgin olive oil
Sea salt and black pepper
1 romaine lettuce
1 red mini Cos lettuce
1 big handful of curly
　leaf kale
1 x 400g (14oz) tin
　chickpeas, drained
　and rinsed
250g (9oz) cherry
　tomatoes on the vine
1 cucumber
2 avocados, sliced
50g (2oz) anchovies
　in extra virgin olive oil

FOR THE SAUCE

2 garlic cloves
80g (½ cup) cashew nuts
½ sheet of nori
3 tsp capers
1 tsp caper juice from the jar
½ tsp white miso paste
1 tsp Dijon mustard
1 tbsp nutritional yeast flakes
125ml (½ cup) almond milk
2 tbsp extra virgin olive oil
1 tsp tamari
1 tsp apple cider vinegar
1 tsp maple syrup
¼ tsp garlic granules
¼ tsp onion granules
⅛ tsp dried oregano
⅛ tsp dried parsley
⅛ tsp ground ginger
Sea salt and black pepper

OPTIONAL SWAPS

1 x 400g (14oz) tin
　of butter beans,
　or cannellini beans
500g (3 cups) cooked quinoa
　(200g/1 cup uncooked)
2 grated carrots
2 sliced red bell peppers

Capers are a superfood and a traditional anti-inflammatory medicine used to relieve the pain and stiffness of rheumatism and arthritis (see page 63). If you aren't vegetarian or vegan, anchovies are a great source of omega-3. These fatty acids have been shown to help to reduce pain and inflammation in both osteoarthritis and rheumatoid arthritis (see page 55).

—

1. Preheat the oven to 190°C fan (410°F).
2. Place the chicken on a piece of foil, sprinkle with sea salt and black pepper and drizzle over some extra virgin olive oil. Wrap it up, place on a baking tray and cook for 30–35 minutes, turning the tray halfway through. Shred while it is still hot, then leave to cool for 10 minutes.
3. For a vegan version, slice the tofu into cubes and gently fry in extra virgin olive oil until golden on the outside and a little crispy. Remove from the pan and leave to cool.
4. Meanwhile, make the Caesar sauce (while the chicken is cooking, or after you have cooked the tofu). Add the garlic cloves to the oven and roast alongside the chicken for 15 minutes. At the same time, soak the cashews in boiling water for 15 minutes, then drain.
5. Peel the roasted garlic cloves and blend with the cashews and the rest of the sauce ingredients until smooth. Add a dash of water or almond milk if you like a thinner sauce.
6. Slice and wash the lettuce and kale leaves, using a salad spinner to spin out the excess water, or dab with kitchen paper.
7. Place the leaves in a large mixing bowl, add the chickpeas, then slice and add the cherry tomatoes. Slice the cucumber lengthways twice and then into slices, adding these to the bowl too.
8. Add the shredded chicken or tofu cubes, then toss the sauce into the mixing bowl, shaking in well, or drizzle the sauce on top of the salad when it's served.
9. Plate up the salad and top with slices of avocado and 2–3 anchovies per person (if using). Season with black pepper.

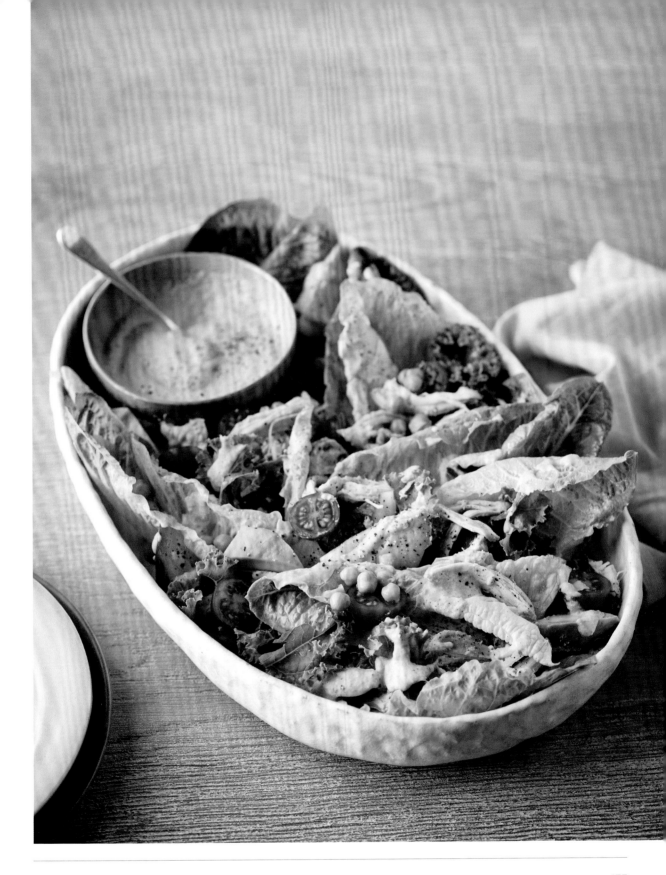

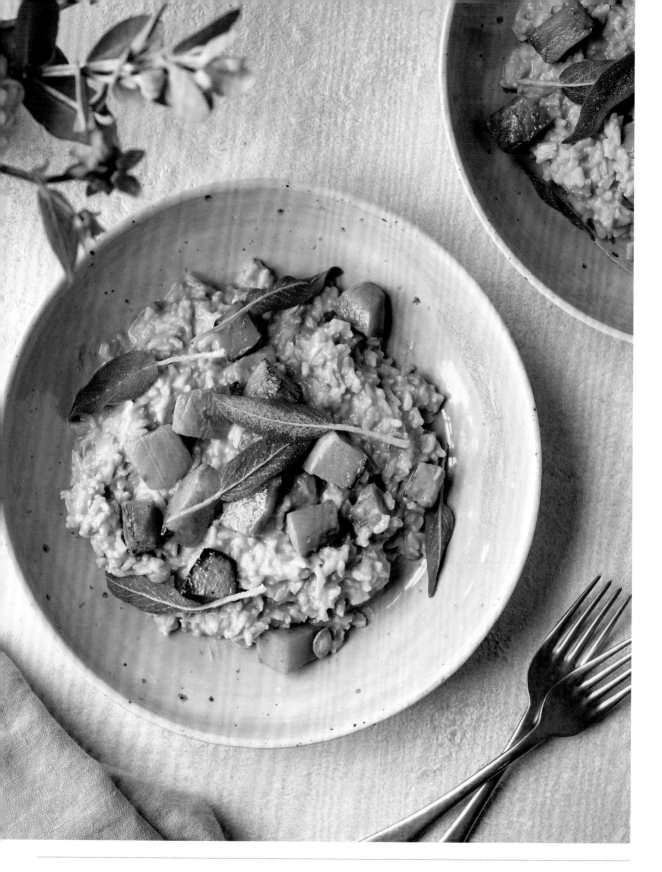

EAT WELL WITH ARTHRITIS

BUTTERNUT SQUASH AND LEEK RISOTTO

V, VEG, DF, GF

✳ Freezable 🍴 Meal Prep 🥄 Cooking for Friends and Family
🕐 Between 1–2 hours

SERVES 4–6

1 butternut squash
Extra virgin olive oil
1 red onion, chopped
2 garlic cloves (I used
    black garlic), chopped
250g leeks, sliced into
    half-moons
300g (1½ cups) brown rice
1 vegetable stock cube,
    dissolved in 800ml
    (3¼ cups) hot water
200ml (¾ cup) plant milk
1 tbsp tahini
1 tbsp nutritional yeast flakes
1 tsp white miso paste
¼ tsp ground nutmeg
¼ tsp paprika
1 tsp apple cider vinegar
200ml (¾ cup) water
300ml (1¼ cups) water
16–24 sage leaves
    (4 leaves per person)
Sea salt and black pepper
2 handfuls of spinach,
    to serve (optional)

Creamy, nutty flavours served with crispy sage makes for a warming and sweet rice dish. Tahini is made with toasted and ground sesame seeds and is rich in selenium, and it's a good source of copper too – a trace mineral essential for iron absorption – which spinach is an excellent source of. Rheumatoid arthritis is often accompanied by low levels of iron. Additionally sage contains carnosol, butternut squash contains carotenoids, and leek is packed with high levels of flavonoids, which are powerful anti-inflammatory compounds.

—

1. Preheat the oven to 200°C fan (425°F).
2. Cut the butternut squash down the middle from the top to the larger bottom end and scoop out the seeds. Lay each side flat down to peel off the skin – it is easier to peel this way. (Or leave the skin on, if you prefer.) Then cut into chunks.
3. Transfer the squash to a roasting tray, sprinkle with sea salt and black pepper and roast for 30 minutes, turning halfway through.
4. Gently heat 1 tablespoon of extra virgin olive oil in a pan, add the onion and garlic and cook for 2 minutes, then add the leeks and soften for 1 minute.
5. Add the brown rice and coat with the oil and juices from the pan and season with a pinch of salt and pepper.
6. Pour in the 800ml (3¼ cups) vegetable stock, then turn the heat to medium–low and gently simmer for 20 minutes, with the lid on.
7. Meanwhile, in a blender, blend 250g (9oz) of the roasted butternut squash (around a third of the yield, or 1½ cups) with the plant milk, tahini, nutritional yeast, white miso paste, nutmeg, paprika, apple cider vinegar and water.
8. After the risotto has simmered for the 20 minutes, add the butternut squash sauce mixture, put the lid back on and cook for 15 minutes with 300ml (1¼ cups) of water, stirring halfway through and 4 minutes before the end.
9. Heat some olive oil in a separate small pan and lightly try the sage leaves until crispy.
10. Stir the rest of the roasted butternut squash into the risotto, or place it on top
11. Serve the risotto topped with the crispy sage leaves and fresh spinach, if liked.

GOAN PRAWN AND COD CURRY

DF, GF

❄ Freezable ❚❚ Meal Prep ❘ 'Fakeaway' 🥄 Cooking for Friends and Family
🕐 Over 1 hour

SERVES 4

1 tbsp coconut oil
2 tsp black mustard seeds
1 red onion, chopped
2 red bell peppers, sliced
1 x 400ml (14fl oz) tin
   coconut milk
3 medium dried
   Kashmiri chillies
485g (17oz) (3-4 fillets) cod
   loin, cut into chunks
165g (2 cups) raw peeled
   king prawns (around 24)
100g (2½ cups)
   baby spinach

FOR THE CURRY PASTE

1 red onion, chopped
30-35g (1-1¼oz) fresh
   ginger, peeled and
   chopped
5 garlic cloves, chopped
2 large tomatoes, chopped
1 red chilli, optional
   deseeded and chopped
2 tbsp desiccated coconut
1 tbsp ground coriander
1 tbsp extra virgin olive oil
3 tsp honey
2 tsp ground turmeric
2 tsp ground cumin
1 tsp ground black pepper
1 tsp tamarind paste
½ tsp ground fenugreek
¼ ground cloves
25-50ml (⅛-¼ cup
   water

TO SERVE

300g (1½ cups) brown rice
Fresh coriander (optional)

The best Goan curry I've tasted is from a restaurant called Chapman's in Canterbury, and ever since then I have been playing with the flavours to get it just as good at home. My version is packed with omega-3 and inflammation-fighting phytochemicals, such as gingerol and curcumin. You could substitute the cod loin for basa, as an economical alternative.

—

1. First, make your curry paste. Put all of the curry paste ingredients into a food processor and blend until smooth.
2. Cook the brown rice according to the pack instructions or use my method on page 112.
3. Gently heat the coconut oil in a large saucepan and, once hot, fry the black mustard seeds with the red onion for around 5 minutes.
4. Add the sliced peppers and cook for 3 minutes, then pour in the curry paste. If you are struggling to get the paste out of the food processor, add another 50ml (¼ cup) of water to loosen it and get all of it into the pan. Fry the curry paste for 2-3 minutes, then add the coconut milk, stir well, and add the Kashmiri chillies. Simmer for 5 minutes, partially covered.
5. Add the cod loin chunks, gently stir on a medium-low heat for 3-4 minutes until they are cooked through (stirring gently so that they hold form and don't flake too much). Add the king prawns and cook for 2-3 minutes until they are pink all the way through.
6. Stir in the spinach to wilt it, then remove the Kashmiri chillies before serving.
7. Serve with the brown rice and top with fresh coriander.

Tip:
Nutritionist Victoria Jain suggests swapping the rice for root vegetables as an alternative to get more fibre for your gut, as she advises her autoimmune clients to try to eat more vegetables with meals rather than grains.

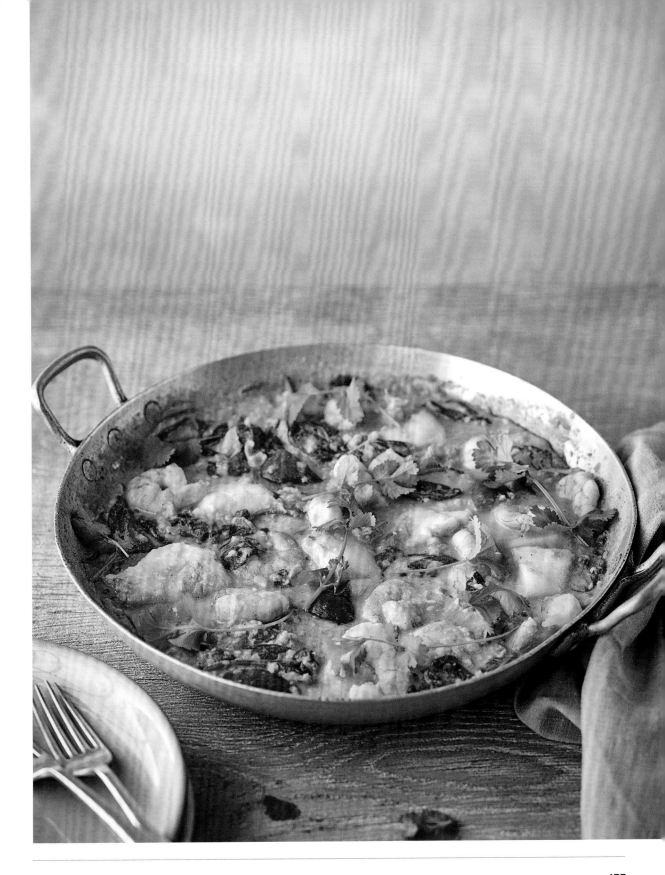

ITALIAN-STYLE CHICKEN WITH SWEET POTATO WEDGES

DF, GF

🍃 Cooking for Friends and Family 🕐 Under 1 hour

SERVES 4

4 chicken breasts,
    cut into chunks
½ tsp balsamic vinegar
½ tsp dried thyme
½ tsp dried oregano
2 tsp roughly chopped
    fresh basil
4 sun-dried tomatoes
2 tsp extra virgin olive oil
Sea salt and black pepper

FOR THE SALAD

320g (11oz) baby
    plum tomatoes, halved
½ cucumber, sliced
    into triangles
125g (4½oz) salad leaves
Classic Salad Dressing
    (see page 236)

FOR THE SAUCE

1 x 400g (14oz) tin
    butter beans, drained
    and rinsed
12 sun-dried tomatoes
2 garlic cloves
2½ tbsp extra virgin olive oil
2 tbsp nutritional yeast flakes
½ tsp apple cider vinegar
1 tsp balsamic vinegar
4 fresh basil leaves
130ml (½ cup) plant milk
3 tsp olive oil (or use
    from the sun-dried
    tomatoes jar)

TO SERVE

3-4 sweet potatoes,
    cut into wedges
2 sweet pointed peppers,
    cut into chunks
3 red bell peppers,
    cut into chunks
2 avocados, sliced
12 sun-dried tomatoes
Handful of basil, chopped

Tomatoes are often misread as being inflammatory, however, there is not enough evidence to prove this. However, nutritionist Victoria Jain adds that tomatoes might be an issue for those with compromised digestive functions, so if you do feel you have a reaction to eating tomatoes, then see if you feel better removing them from your diet. There's also carnosol in the basil, thyme, and oregano in this recipe too. Swap in tofu if you're veggie or vegan!

1. Preheat the oven to 200°C fan (425°F).
2. Prepare your salad, place in a bowl and set side.
3. Put the sweet potatoes on a baking tray, drizzle with extra virgin olive oil and season with pinches of salt and pepper. Cook in the oven for 30–40 minutes, turning halfway through, until soft in the centre and a little crispy on the outside.
4. Place all of the peppers on another baking tray, drizzle with extra virgin olive oil and season with pinches of salt and pepper. Place the chicken in a piece of foil, drizzle with extra virgin olive oil and balsamic vinegar, and scatter over the thyme, oregano and a couple of pinches of salt and pepper. Place the basil and sun-dried tomatoes on top of the chicken breasts, wrap up and place on a baking tray. Roast the chicken and the peppers for 25–30 minutes, turning halfway through.
5. Meanwhile, make the tomato sauce. Add all of the ingredients to a food processor and blend until smooth. Season with salt and pepper, transfer to a bowl and set aside, ready for serving.
6. Plate up! First the chicken, then the roasted peppers, avocado, sweet potato wedges and side salad topped with the dressing. Serve the tomato sauce in a bowl topped with sun-dried tomatoes and fresh basil if you like.

Tip:
Use leftover sauce as dipping sauce for salads, or add to a tofu or roasted vegetable quinoa salad. It will keep in an airtight container in the fridge for 3 days.

EAT WELL WITH ARTHRITIS

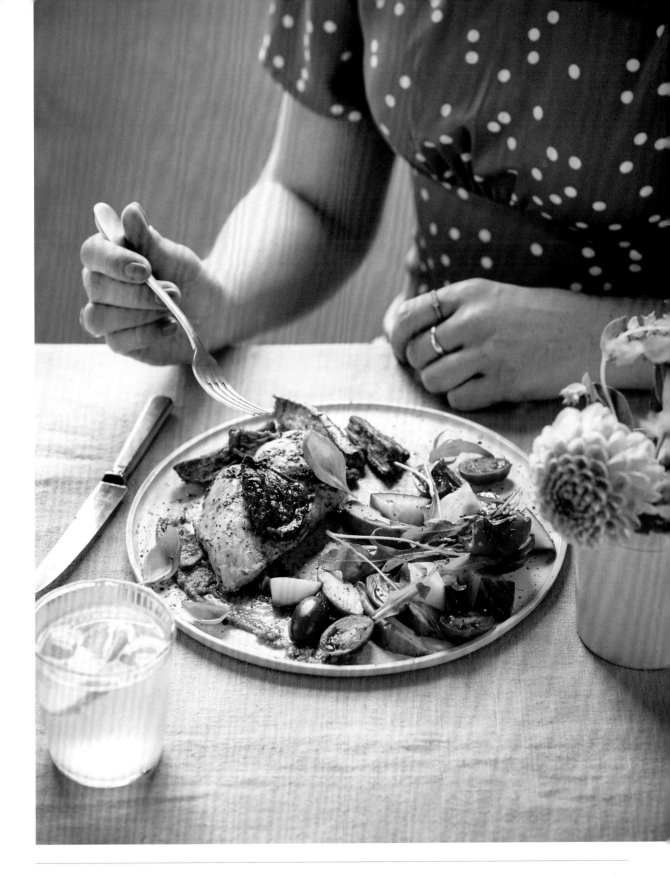

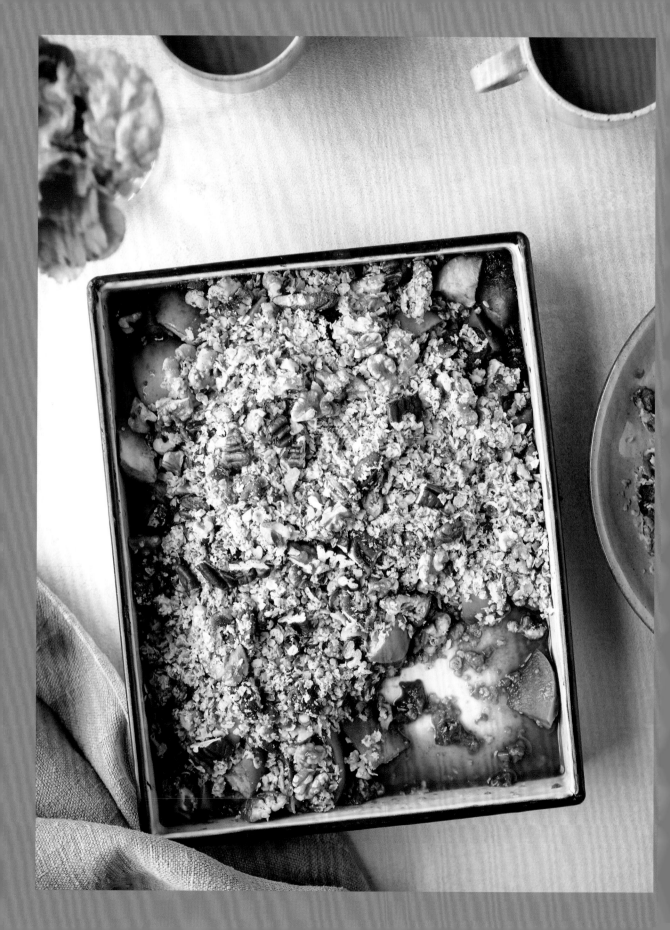

DESSERTS

APPLE AND BERRY BAKE

V, VEG, DF, GF　　　✳ Freezable ▯▯ Meal Prep 🍃 Cooking for Friends and Family 🕐 Under 1 hour

SERVES 8–12

8 Braeburn apples
　(or cooking apples)
200g (1 cup) raspberries
Juice of ½ lemon
2 tbsp melted coconut oil
4 tbsp honey (or a
　vegan alternative,
　see page 88)
½ tsp ground nutmeg
1 tsp ground cinnamon
3½ tbsp coconut sugar
120g (1 cup) roughly
　chopped nuts, I like
　60g (½ cup) pecans
　and 60g (½ cup) walnuts
100g (1 cup) whole rolled
　porridge oats

**TO SERVE WITH (PER
PORTION, IN ORDER)**
2 tbsp coconut yoghurt
1 tsp Manuka honey
　or maple syrup
Sprinkle of ground cinnamon
Extra pecans, nuts, pumpkin
　or sunflower seeds,
　raspberries or sultanas
　(optional)

A modern take on my Nanan's apple pie, you will need a large and deep baking dish for this one, and homegrown cooking apples (if you have them!). It's a really warming dessert, but you could store it in the fridge and have it for breakfast, adding the coconut yoghurt, honey (maple syrup if vegan) and sprinkle of cinnamon when you eat it.

　Keep the skins on the apples if you can as research has shown that peeled apples have less antioxidant activity than apples with their skins on. There are around 300–400 phytochemicals (polyphenols and flavonoids) in apples, depending on the variety, and quercetin (a flavonoid) found in the skin is particularly helpful for modulating inflammation.

—

1.　Preheat the oven to 180°C fan (400°F).
2.　Peel the apples, if you wish, then core and cut into chunks. The skin provides extra fibre, but the apples will be softer when peeled. Add the apple chunks and raspberries to 26 x 20cm (10 x 8in) Pyrex baking dish and coat with the lemon juice, melted coconut oil and 2 tablespoons of the honey.
3.　Add the nutmeg, cinnamon and 3 tablespoons of the coconut sugar to the apples and coat them well. Flatten the apple mixture.
4.　Mix the nuts, 50g (½ cup) of the oats and the remaining ½ tablespoon of coconut sugar in a mixing bowl, then scatter over the apple mixture. Bake in the oven for 20 minutes, then turn and roll the topping in with the filling, gently tossing and turning so they become one mixture.
5.　Before placing back in the oven, top with the remaining 2 tablespoons of honey, flatten the mixture, then sprinkle over the remaining 50g (½ cup) oats. Bake for a further 15 minutes.
6.　Serve with coconut yoghurt, Manuka honey, a sprinkle of cinnamon and any other nuts, seeds or sultanas you'd like. Eat hot, or store in the fridge to eat cold or warm up. It will keep in the fridge for about 5 days.

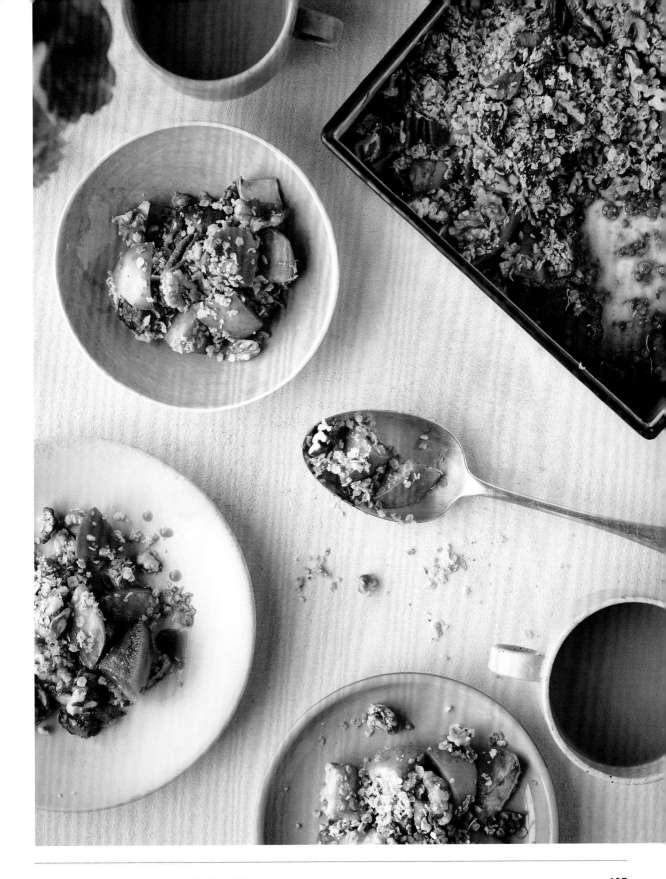

MATCHA AND BERRY COMPOTE WITH PISTACHIO CRUMB AND CHOCOLATE SAUCE

V, VEG, DF, GF

❄ Freezable 🍴 Meal Prep 🍃 Cooking for Friends and Family
🕐 Under 1 hour (or under 30 minutes if you've already made the jam)

MAKES 6

FOR THE FILLING
75g (½ cup) cashew nuts
500g (2 cups) silken tofu
(I like The Tofoo Co for this recipe)
½ heaped tsp ceremonial grade matcha
25g (generous ¼ cup) desiccated coconut
3 tbsp honey (or a vegan alternative, see page 88)
1 tsp lemon juice
¼ tsp almond extract
6 tbsp Raspberry Jam (see page 234 for homemade)

FOR THE TOPPING
3–6 tsp Chocolate Sauce (see page 235)
40g (¼ cup) pistachio kernels, roughly crushed/chopped

I love matcha green tea, and if drinking it isn't quite to your taste yet (it takes time to get accustomed to), then perhaps you could start by trying this dessert with friends and family first. You can read about how to make and enjoy matcha drink, and why it's so healthful, on page 226. Additionally, pistachios are high in potassium and antioxidants, including vitamins A and E and lutein.

1. Add the cashew nuts to a bowl, cover with boiling water and leave to soak for 15 minutes. Drain.
2. Add the soaked cashew nuts and the rest of the filling ingredients, except the raspberry jam, to a blender and blend until smooth. Divide the filling mixture between 6 glass ramekins, add 1 tablespoon of raspberry jam to the centre of each one and place in the freezer, on a tray for ease, for 10 minutes.
3. Pour ½–1 teaspoon of chocolate sauce on top of each ramekin and sprinkle the pistachio crumbs on top. Place back into the freezer and freeze overnight.
4. Take the ramekins out individually and place them in the fridge on the day you wish to eat them. I often take one out in the morning, to have after as a snack in the afternoon, or for dinner that evening. This is great for enjoying with family and friends, and a good way to introduce them to matcha too.

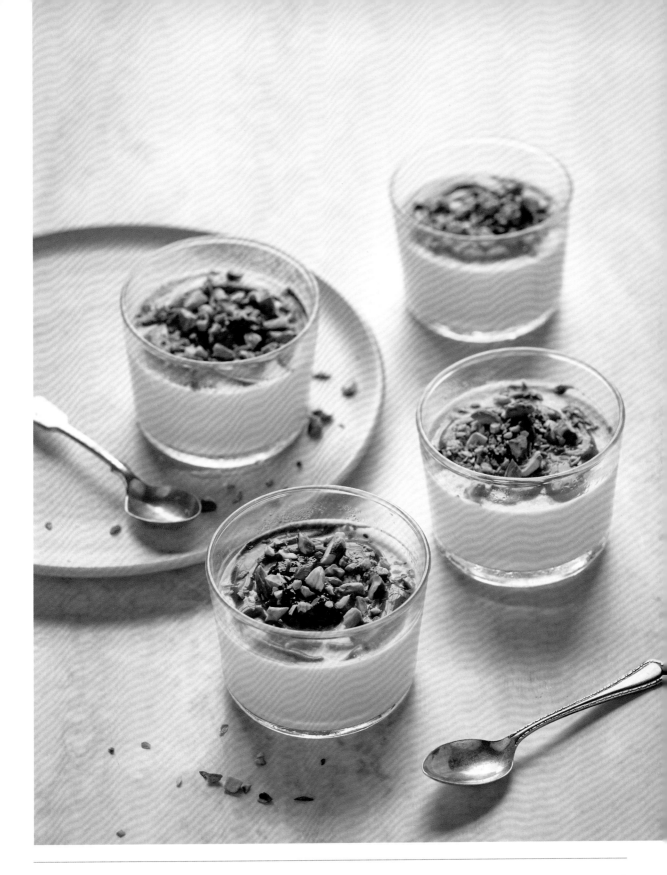

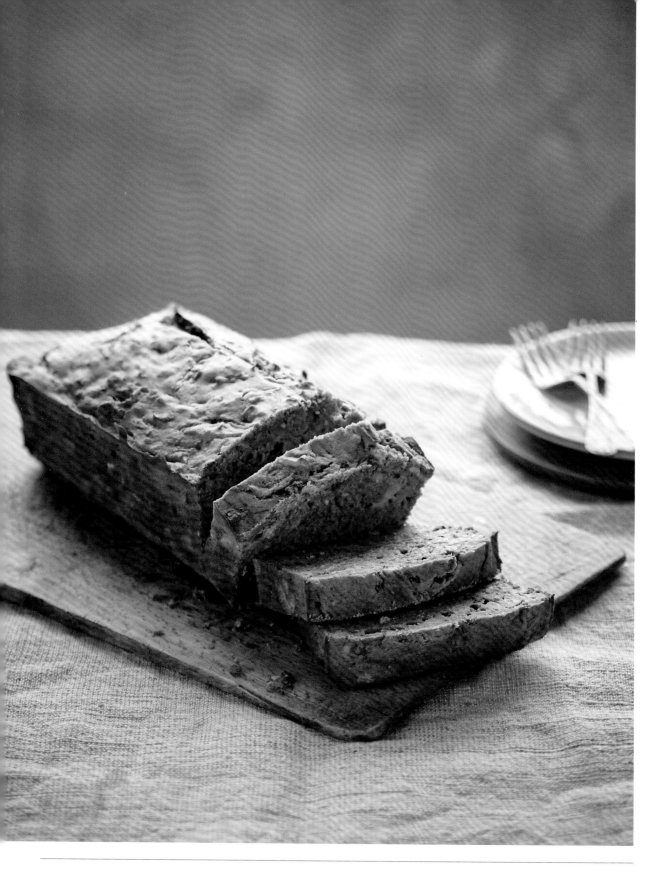

EAT WELL WITH ARTHRITIS

CARROT (AND COURGETTE) LOAF CAKE

V, DF, GF   🍴 Meal Prep   🌱 Cooking for Friends and Family   🕐 Under 1 hour

SERVES 8–12

FOR THE WET INGREDIENTS
150ml (⅔ cup) plant milk
2 large eggs, beaten
1 banana, mashed
1 courgette, grated
2 carrots, grated
5 tbsp honey
4 tbsp coconut oil,
   plus extra for greasing
1 tbsp vanilla extract
1 tbsp apple cider vinegar

FOR THE DRY INGREDIENTS
2 tsp ground cinnamon
1 tsp bicarbonate of soda
½ tsp ground ginger
½ tsp ground nutmeg
Pinch of ground allspice
60g (½ cup) walnuts,
   roughly chopped
250g (1½ cups + ⅓ cup)
   buckwheat flour

Walnuts are packed with omega-3, which has been shown in studies to reduce arthritic pain and rheumatoid arthritis disease activity (see page 77). There are another two noteworthy phytochemicals in this loaf cake too: gingerol (from the ginger) and cinnamaldehyde (from the cinnamon). Gingerol has been shown to reduce inflammation in rheumatoid arthritis and osteoarthritis in pre-clinical trials, suggesting that it might prove helpful as a therapeutic treatment in the future.

—

1. Preheat the oven to 180°C fan (400°F) and brush the insides of a 500g (1lb 2oz) loaf tin generously with coconut oil, or line it with baking parchment.
2. Combine all of the wet ingredients in a mixing bowl, then add the dry ingredients, folding in the buckwheat flour last. Pour the mixture evenly into the loaf tin.
3. Bake for 40–45 minutes, then remove from the oven and leave to cool in the tin for 15 minutes. Remove from the tin and place on a wire rack to cool completely.
4. This will keep in the fridge for 3–5 days – you could even toast slices to warm them and add a little honey or coconut yoghurt to serve.

NO-BAKE GINGER AND 'CARAMEL' SLICES

V, VEG, DF, GF

❋ Freezable 🍴 Meal Prep 🌿 Cooking for Friends and Family 🕐 Under 1 hour

MAKES 12 SLICES

FOR THE BASE
250g (2½ cups)
   walnut halves
200g (1 cup) Medjool
   dates, pitted
2 tsp ground ginger
120ml (½ cup) melted
   coconut oil
2 tbsp raw cacao powder
½ tsp ground cinnamon
40g (½ cup) whole
   rolled oats

FOR THE FUDGE LAYER
1 x 400g (14oz) tin
   chickpeas, drained
   and rinsed
275g (1 cup) almond butter
1 tsp vanilla extract
4 tbsp maple syrup
95ml (½ cup) melted
   coconut oil
¼ tsp pink Himalayan salt
115g (½ cup, or 11) Zamli
   dates, pitted (for more
   caramel flavour, but other
   varieties of dates will work)

**FOR THE
CHOCOLATE LAYER**
Juice of 1 orange
2½ heaped tbsp raw
   cacao powder
½ tsp ground ginger
1 tbsp date syrup
75g (⅓ cup) coconut oil
1 tbsp maple syrup

FOR THE TOPPING
50g (⅓ cup) cashew
   nuts, crushed into
   different sized pieces
Zest of 1 orange
1 tbsp cacao nibs

An indulgent treat that is made purely from plants and requires no baking whatsoever – just a food processor. But, more importantly, it contains Omega-3 from the walnuts, resveratrol from the cacao powder, cinnameldahyde from the cinnamon and zinc from chickpeas – even the Medjool dates contain polyphenols, flavonoids, and carotenoids too. And research suggests that the monounsaturated fats from an almond-rich diet lower some markers of inflammation, so enjoy the almond butter here too.

—

1. Line a 26 x 20cm (10 x 8in) Pyrex baking dish with baking parchment.
2. Blend all of the ingredients for the base in a food processor and place in the lined Pyrex dish, spreading evenly. Chill in the fridge.
3. Blend all of the ingredients for the fudge layer in a food processor and add on top of the base layer – the oil may separate slightly but that's okay. Freeze for 15–30 minutes while you make the remaining layers.
4. For the chocolate layer, gently melt all of the ingredients together in a saucepan. Pour over the top of the other two set layers.
5. Sprinkle over the topping ingredients. Slice into pieces in the dish, then place in the freezer to set for at least 2 hours.

Tip:
This recipe also works well with lime zest and juice instead of orange – but you would need 2 limes.

VEGAN CHOCOLATE TIFFIN

V, VEG, DF, GF   ✳ Freezable 🍵 Cooking for Friends and Family 🕑 Under 30 minutes

MAKES 12–18 SLICES

300g (3 cups) whole
   rolled oats
150g (¾ cup) coconut oil,
   plus extra for greasing
3 tbsp maple syrup
3 tbsp coconut sugar
3 tbsp cacao powder
1 tsp ground cinnamon
50g (⅓ cup)
   almonds, crushed
40g (⅓ cup)
   walnuts, crushed
50g (⅓ cup) cashew
   nuts, crushed
80g (⅓ cup) sulphur
   dioxide-free dried
   apricots, chopped
45g (⅓ cup) crimson,
   golden and flame
   jumbo raisins
55g (⅓ cup)
   dried cranberries
2 pinches of ground nutmeg
Zest of 1 orange (optional)
1 tsp vanilla extract
2 pinches of ground cloves
½ tsp ground ginger
Pinch of sea salt
1 tbsp cacao nibs

**FOR THE CHOCOLATE
TOPPING**

50g (¼ cup) coconut oil
2 tbsp cacao powder
2 tbsp date syrup
1 tbsp coconut sugar

For this recipe there is the option to make your own, or alternatively, choose granola that is packed with nuts, seeds and dried fruit, with no added refined sugar or preservatives. An easy way to get in your daily fibre to promote a healthier gut, which is essential to our immune system. For more details, see page 44 of *Beat Arthritis Naturally*.

—

1. Oil a 20cm (8in) square or 23cm (9in) round baking tin with coconut oil and line it with baking parchment.
2. Add the oats to a large mixing bowl.
3. Melt the coconut oil, maple syrup, coconut sugar and cacao powder together in a pan on a low heat. Pour the mixture over the oats, then stir in the remaining ingredients, apart from the cacao nibs.
4. Pour the mixture into the tin and flatten using a silicone spatula or the back of a large spoon.
5. Gently melt the chocolate topping ingredients in a saucepan, then pour over the oat mixture and spread evenly – it will soak through the gaps, which it is meant to. Sprinkle with the cacao nibs.
6. Place in the fridge to set. To cut into pieces, dip a small knife into hot water and it will be a lot easier to slice.
7. It can be stored in an airtight container, or covered in the tin you made it in, for 5–7 days.

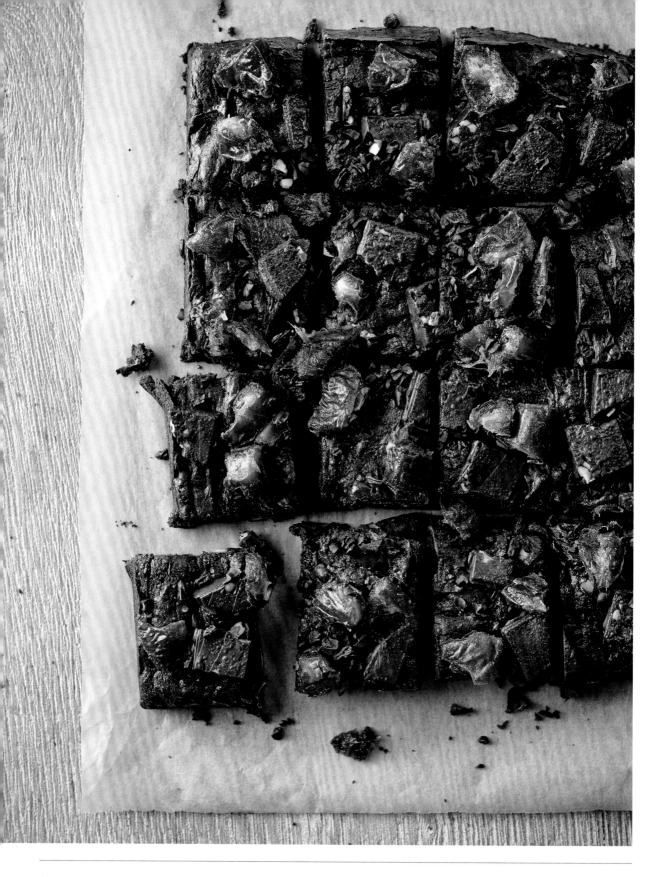

EAT WELL WITH ARTHRITIS

ALMOND BUTTER BROWNIES

V, DF, GF

✳ Freezable ‖ 'Fakeaway' 🍃 Cooking for Friends and Family 🕐 Under 1 hour

MAKES 12 SQUARES

1 ripe avocado
50g (generous ½ cup)
   raw cacao powder
2 large eggs
175g (1 cup) coconut sugar
2 tbsp maple syrup
1 tsp baking powder
¼ sea salt
1 tbsp coconut oil, plus
   extra for greasing
1 tsp vanilla extract
½ tsp almond extract
145g (½ cup) smooth
   100% almond butter
90g (1 cup)
   unblanched almonds
30g (¼ cup) cacao nibs
10 (185g, or 1 cup)
   Deglet Nour or Medjool
   dates, pitted
40g (1½oz or ¼ cup)
   all-natural almond
   and sea salt chocolate

Avocado helps to slow the release of glucose, to help reduce the blood sugar spike which can often trigger inflammation. Avocados and almonds are a great source of monounsaturated fats, as well as antioxidants and there's also resveratrol in the cacao powder too, learn more on page 61.

—

1. Preheat the oven to 170°C fan (375°F). Grease a 26 x 20cm (10 x 8in) Pyrex baking dish or baking tin with coconut oil.
2. Destone and peel the avocado, then add it to a food processor with all of the ingredients apart from the almond butter, almonds, cacao nibs, dates and chocolate.
3. Once combined, mix in the almond butter and almonds, then the cacao nibs. Place in the prepared baking dish and bake in the oven for 20 minutes.
4. Meanwhile, chop the dates and chocolate.
5. Remove the brownie from the oven and scatter over the dates and chocolate, spreading evenly using a spatula. Bake for another 3–5 minutes.
6. Leave the brownie to cool in the baking dish for 1 hour, do not eat or move before this time, as it will fall apart and also taste of avocado!
7. Once cooled, cut into 12 squares, or any shape you prefer – long smaller bites work too. Serve as it is, or with some coconut-based cream or yoghurt.

LAYERED MANGO AND PASSION FRUIT DESSERT

V, VEG, DF, GF

🌿 Cooking for Friends and Family 🛍 10 Ingredients or Less
❄ Freezable ⏱ Under 30 minutes

MAKES 4

1 mango
6 passion fruit
½ tsp vanilla extract
40g (3 tbsp) honey
   (or maple syrup, if vegan)
2 tsp coconut sugar
200g (7oz, or ¾ cup)
   coconut yoghurt
½ tsp chia seeds
Squeeze of lime juice
4 tbsp desiccated coconut

Easily made and stored in the fridge for you and for friends. Mango is rich in polyphenols, carotenoids and vitamin C, and a good source of dietary fibre, which have all exhibited anti-inflammatory properties. Several studies have demonstrated that the prebiotic effects of mango polyphenols and dietary fibre have the potential to lower intestinal inflammation.

—

1. Peel the mango and cut into small chunks. Place in a bowl with the flesh of the passion fruit.
2. Stir in the vanilla extract, honey and coconut sugar. Spoon into 4 glass containers, you should have around 95g (3¼oz) in each one.
3. Chill in the fridge until you are ready to serve.
4. When ready to serve, top each serving with 50g (3½ tbsp) of coconut yoghurt. Sprinkle with chia seeds, lime juice and desiccated coconut.

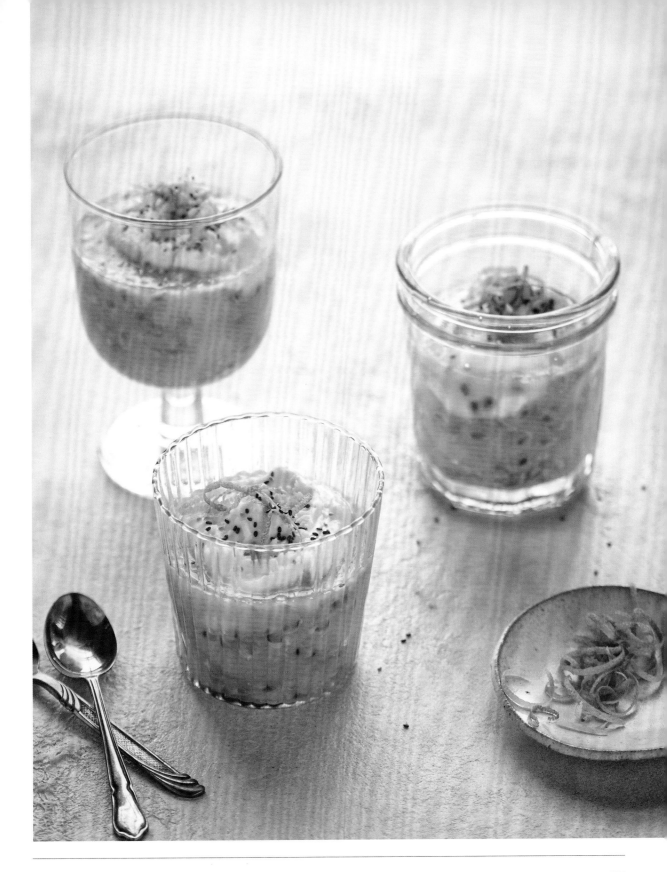

DESSERTS

PICK N MIX CHOCOLATE FRUIT YOGHURT

V, VEG, DF, GF   🍴 Meal Prep 🥄 Cooking for Friends and Family 🛍 10 Ingredients or Less 🕐 Under 30 minutes

SERVES 4

200g (1⅓ cups) fruit and nuts of your choice, such as cherries, raspberries, apples, apricots, mangoes, peaches, blueberries, blackberries, bananas, dates and nuts like almonds, walnuts, cashew nuts, pistachios, pecans and hazelnuts

2 portions of Chocolate Sauce (see page 235)

350g (12oz) coconut yoghurt, or natural yoghurt if eating dairy

4 tbsp cacao nibs

Pack as many anti-inflammatory fruits and nuts into this dish as you can. To recap on the health benefits, such as healthy fats, polyphenols and fibre, go to the anti-inflammatory table on pages 54–77.

—

1. Slice up any fresh fruits that you are using and make the chocolate sauce.
2. In 4 separate 500ml (17fl oz) jars, layer the coconut yoghurt, fruits and nuts and chocolate sauce, then repeat the layers. Sprinkle with the cacao nibs. Eat straight away or place in the freezer for 10 minutes. Enjoy as a dessert, or even for breakfast.

NUTRITIONIST VICTORIA JAIN'S (VJ) BLACK CHERRY ICE CREAM

V, VEG, DF, GF

🍴 Meal Prep 🥄 Cooking for Friends and Family 🛍 10 Ingredients or Less

SERVES 4

72ml/g (¾ cup)
   coconut cream
¼ tsp pink Himalayan salt
4 tbsp lucuma powder
1 tbsp ground arrowroot
2 tbsp water
450g (3 cups) black
   cherries, pitted
2 tbsp collagen powder
1 small banana

FOR THE TOPPING

4 tbsp coconut chips
30g (1oz) vegan
   dark chocolate

As you may be aware, cherries are beneficial for those suffering from gout, a type of arthritis that affects over 3 million people in the US, as they help to lower the amount of uric acid in the body. Cherries have antioxidant and anti-inflammatory properties, so many people with gout may try drinking cherry juice to help treat their symptoms and prevent flare-ups.

—

1. Add the coconut cream, salt and lucuma to a pan on a low heat and stir together until amalgamated.
2. Mix the arrowroot and water together until they form a paste, then add to the pan slowly, stirring constantly. Once the mixture begins to thicken, remove it from the heat and leave to cool.
3. Add the cherries, collagen powder and banana to a blender with the mixture from the pan and blend until smooth. Transfer to a sealable container and freeze for at least 5 hours.
4. Meanwhile, add the coconut chips to a dry pan and toast for 2 minutes until browned.
5. Serve the ice cream topped with toasted coconut chips and grated dark chocolate and enjoy!

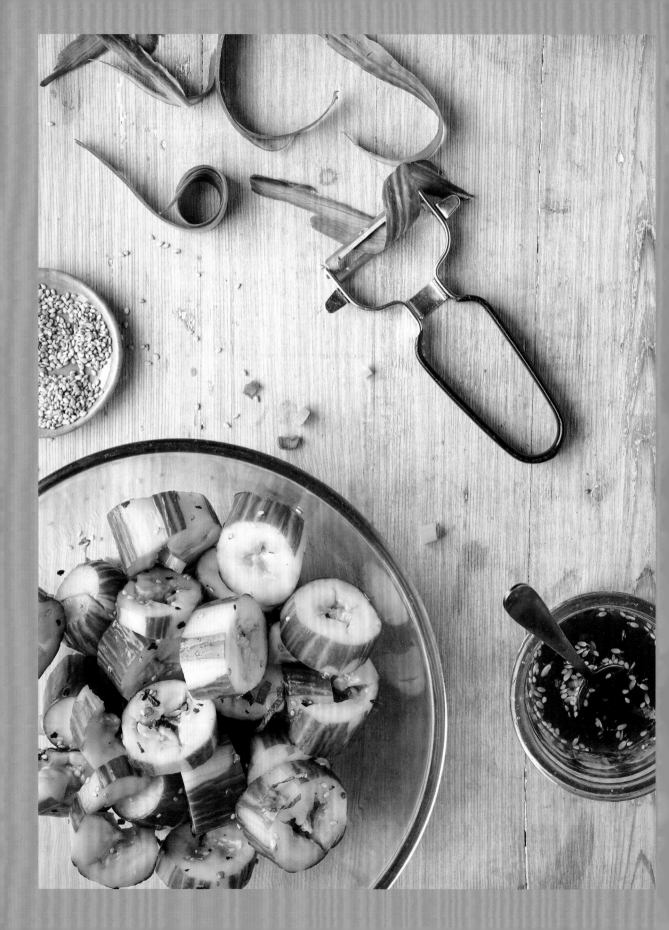

SNACKS
AND SIDES

AUBERGINE DIP TOPPED WITH POMEGRANATE SEEDS

V, VEG, DF, GF

✳ Freezable ⏐⏐ Meal Prep 🥄 Cooking for Friends and Family
🛍 10 Ingredients or Less 🕐 Under 1 hour

SERVES 4

3 aubergines
2 tbsp extra virgin olive oil,
    plus 1 tsp for drizzling
4 garlic cloves
2 tbsp tahini
½ tbsp lemon juice
¼ tsp ground cumin
80g (½ cup)
    pomegranate seeds
Sea salt and black pepper

TO SERVE (OPTIONAL)
Roasted cherry tomatoes
    on the vine
Toasted sourdough slices

Some people believe that the solanine contained in nightshade vegetables (or non-nightshade vegetables like blueberries or artichokes) may make their inflammatory symptoms worse, but there is currently no research to support this, or contradict it. However, you could use the Trigger Tracker to see if it bothers you. The majority of solanine is in the skin and leaves of the vegetables, not typically used in recipes.

—

1. Preheat the oven to 200°C fan (425°F). Line 2 baking trays with baking parchment.
2. Slice the aubergines lengthways and place, flesh-side down, on the baking trays, spread out evenly. Drizzle over 1 teaspoon of extra virgin olive oil and season with salt and pepper. Cook in the oven for 35 minutes, swapping the trays halfway through.
3. Dot the garlic cloves (skin on) onto the top baking tray 10 minutes before the end of the cooking time and roast them for 10 minutes.
4. Once the aubergine has cooked through, remove from the oven and let it cool for 5–10 minutes, before using tongs and a fork to gently peel off the skin – it should come off in one go.
5. Add the aubergine flesh to a mixing bowl, then add the 2 tablespoons of extra virgin olive oil, the tahini, lemon juice, ¼ teaspoon of sea salt, ⅛ teaspoon of black pepper and the ground cumin. Peel and chop the roasted garlic cloves and add these in too. Mash and mix well. The food processor is an option if you are struggling but use it on the lowest setting otherwise you will lose the texture of the aubergine.
6. Transfer the dip to a bowl and sprinkle over the pomegranate seeds.
7. Serve with things to dip, such as any of the suggestions above or see the crudités ideas on page 207.

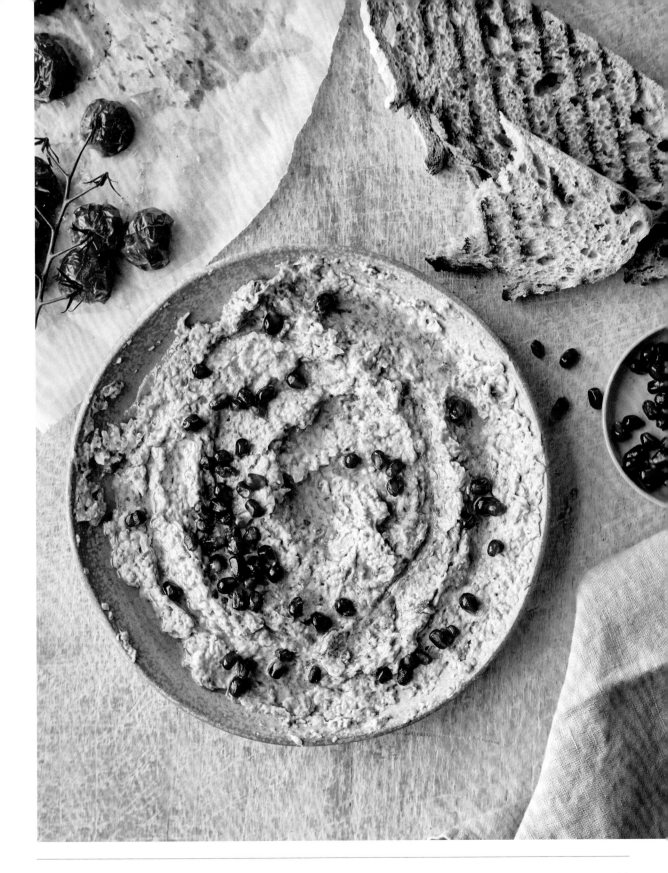

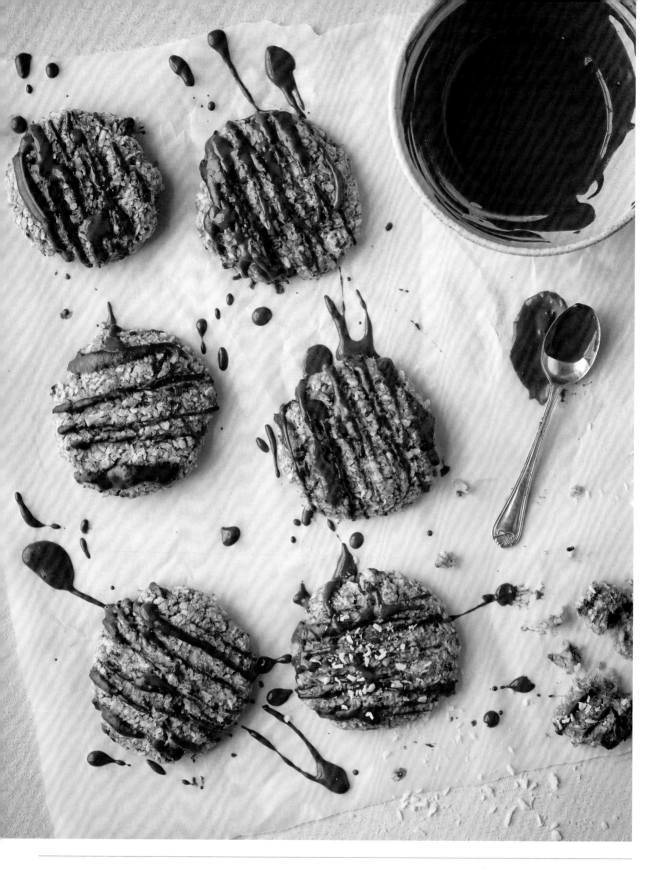

EAT WELL WITH ARTHRITIS

COCONUT BANANA 'COOKIE' BITES

V, VEG, DF, GF 🥣 Cooking for Friends and Family 📦 10 Ingredients or Less ⏱ Under 30 minutes

MAKES 12

3 bananas
2 tsp vanilla extract
2 tsp ground cinnamon
1–3 tsp honey (or
   a vegan alternative,
   see page 88)
270g (3 cups)
   desiccated coconut
Pinch of sea salt

**FOR THE TOPPING
(OPTIONAL)**
Chocolate Sauce (see
   page 235)
3 tsp desiccated coconut

These are really simple bites that you can bake and keep for 3–5 days. Remember to eat as a treat or in moderation though. This recipe provides around 45mcg of selenium, via the desiccated coconut. Selenium is a mineral that helps the body produce enzymes, which enhance the immune system and thyroid function. Desiccated coconut also contains fibre, copper and manganese, and the bananas have plenty of prebiotics and potassium too.

1. Preheat the oven to 180°C fan (400°F). Line a baking tray with a sheet of baking parchment.
2. Mash the bananas in their skins (it is easiest to do this with your hands), then peel them and place the banana flesh into a mixing bowl. Stir in the vanilla extract, cinnamon, honey, desiccated coconut and sea salt.
3. Mould the mixture into 12 cookie-like shapes, placing each one onto the prepared tray, before gently pressing the mixture down with a fork.
4. Bake in the oven for 6–8 minutes until firm, but still moist in the middle.
5. Top with chocolate sauce and ¼ teaspoon of desiccated coconut per 'cookie'. The sauce will set and become fudge-like. Eat straight away, or store in the fridge for 3–5 days to enjoy as snacks.

APRICOT CHIA SEED BITES

V, VEG, DF, GF   🍴 Meal Prep 🥣 Cooking for Friends and Family 🕐 Under 1 hour

MAKES 12

250g (2½ cups) whole
  rolled oats
165g (1 cup) sulphur
  dioxide-free dried apricots
100g (1 cup) pitted dates
1 chia or flax egg (see
  page 88)
100g (1 cup) walnuts
2 tbsp maple syrup or honey
½ tsp vanilla extract
1 tsp ground cinnamon
2 tbsp melted coconut oil
1 tbsp brown rice flour
  (or cassava flour)
30g (¼ cup) pumpkin seeds

These nourishing and fruity bites have a similar texture to flapjacks. They
are packed with fibre from the dried fruit, which helps keep our gut happy.

—

1. Line a baking tray with baking parchment.
2. Combine all of the ingredients, apart from the pumpkin seeds,
   in a food processor.
3. Separate into 12 pieces and mould into cookie shapes on the prepared
   tray. Squish gently down with a spatula, top each 'bite' with pumpkin seeds,
   and press them down again.
4. Refrigerate for 4 hours. Remove from the fridge and cut around the baking
   parchment so that each 'bite' sits on a square of the baking parchment.
   Place in a storage container and keep in the fridge for up to a week.
5. Take out and eat as a sweet treat alternative to a biscuit or a chocolate bar.
   If you want to make it indulgent, you could dip each one in the Chocolate
   Sauce on page 235 and place back into the fridge to set.

CACAO AND COCONUT ENERGY BALLS

V, VEG, DF, GF

✱ Freezable 🍴 Meal Prep 🍲 Cooking for Friends and Family
🔒 10 Ingredients or Less 🕯 Under 1 hour

MAKES 18

100g (1 cup) desiccated
  coconut, plus 30g (⅓ cup)
  for coating
200g (7oz, or 15) Medjool
  dates, pitted
50g (¼ cup) almond butter
  (or macadamia butter)
85g (½ cup + ½ tbsp)
  cashew nuts
40g (⅓ cup) cacao powder
3 tbsp melted coconut oil
2½ tbsp date syrup
Pinch of sea salt

Almond butter, or in particular macadamia butter if you can find it, is high in healthy fats, vitamins, and minerals. And research suggests that the monounsaturated fats from an almond-rich diet lower some markers of inflammation.

—

1. Line a baking tray with baking parchment.
2. Combine all of the ingredients in a food processor (apart from the 30g/⅓cup of desiccated coconut for coating).
3. Mould the mixture into 18 small-medium-sized balls, weighing 25–30g (1oz) each.
4. Place the desiccated coconut in a flat bowl for coating and roll the balls in the coconut to completely coat the outsides. Place them on the prepared tray and put in the fridge for 30 minutes to set.
5. Once set, place them in a container and store in the fridge for 2–3 days. Enjoy as a dessert with the Chocolate Sauce on page 235, or as a snack.

SMASHED CUCUMBER SESAME SEED SALAD

V, VEG, DF, GF 🌿 Cooking for Friends and Family 🕐 Under 30 minutes

SERVES 4

2 cucumbers
2 tsp coconut sugar
  (or honey)
2 spring onions, finely sliced
2 garlic cloves, minced
½ tsp ground ginger
1½ tbsp apple cider vinegar
  or Japanese rice vinegar
1½ tbsp tamari or light
  soy sauce
1 tsp chilli flakes (or
  1 fresh chilli, deseeded
  and thinly sliced)
4 tsp sesame seeds
2 handfuls of fresh mint
  leaves, stems removed
  and finely chopped
½ tsp honey, maple or date
  syrup, or coconut sugar
2 tsp sesame oil

I started making this as a quick go-to summer salad because it tastes pickle-like but feels less acidic. I also added the extra benefits of ground ginger, sesame seeds, sesame oil, and the prebiotic goodness of garlic. For more on the health benefits of garlic in particular, and how to eat it to get the most of its benefits, see page 89.

—

1. Smash the cucumbers using a rolling pin and cut into mishappen chunks. Place in a mixing bowl and add the coconut sugar (or honey). Let the cucumber sit for 15 minutes before draining away the excess water (optional).
2. Add the rest of the ingredients and stir well.
3. Serve immediately, or let it marinate for 10–15 minutes in the fridge. This goes well with the Bang Bang Cauliflower Salad on page 126, and the Nasi Goreng on page 144.

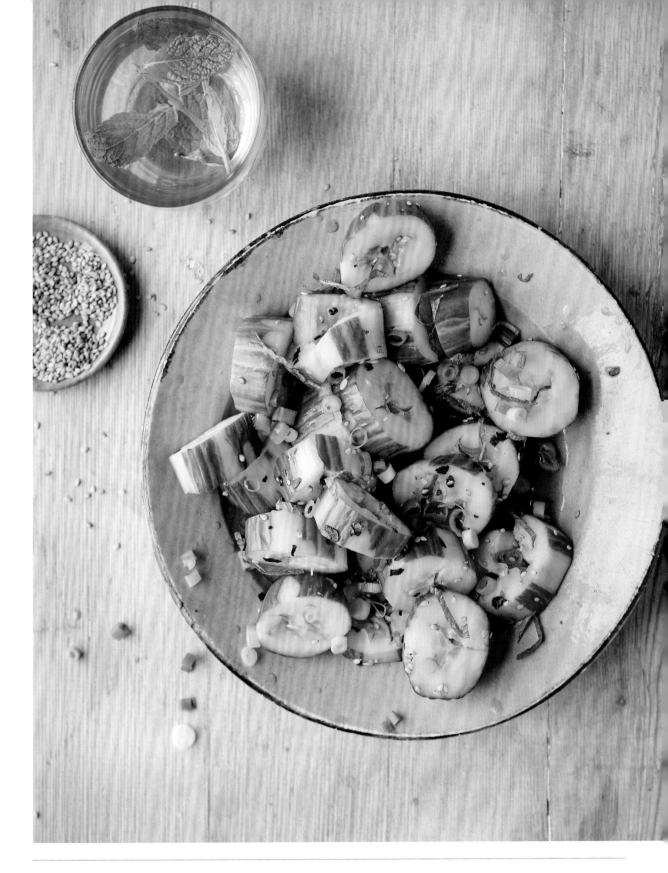

HUMMUS TRIO TRAY

V, VEG, DF, GF   ✳ Freezable 🍴 Meal Prep 🍃 Cooking for Friends and Family
🛍 10 Ingredients or Less 🕐 Under 1 hour

Pulses like chickpeas are full of gut-nourishing fibre and prebiotics and plant protein, as well as being rich in protein, zinc, iron and B vitamins. Hummus is a great way to enjoy them, as well as getting the antioxidant and healthy fats of tahini (from the sesame seeds) too.

Plain Hummus

—

MAKES 2–3 DIPPING BOWLS

2 roasted garlic cloves (see page 89)
2 x 400g (14oz) tins chickpeas,
   drained and rinsed
1 tsp ground cumin
2 tbsp tahini
100ml (¼ cup + 3 tbsp) water
100ml (¼ cup + 3 tbsp) extra virgin olive oil,
   plus extra for drizzling
Squeeze of lemon juice (optional)
Sea salt and black pepper
Pinch of paprika, to serve

1. Mix all of the ingredients in a food processor. Transfer to a bowl, drizzle over some oil and scatter with the paprika. Serve with your choice of crudités and store any leftovers in the fridge for 3–4 days.

Roasted Beetroot Hummus ❷

—

MAKES 4–5 DIPPING BOWLS

4 medium beetroots (520g/1lb 3oz)
100ml (¼ cup + 3 tbsp) extra virgin olive oil,
    plus extra for drizzling
2 x 400g (14oz) tins chickpeas,
    plus the water from one tin
1 tbsp tahini
2 roasted garlic cloves (see page 89)
1 tsp ground cumin
Squeeze of lemon juice (optional)
Sea salt and black pepper
Chopped walnuts, to serve

1. Preheat the oven to 200°C fan (425°F). Line
   a baking dish with foil or baking parchment.
2. Chop the ends off the beetroot and cut into
   slices. Place in the prepared dish, drizzle over
   some oil and season with sea salt and black
   pepper. Roast for 30 minutes.
3. Blitz the roasted beetrool with the rest of the
   ingredients in a food processor. Transfer to a
   bowl, drizzle over some oil and scatter with the
   walnuts. Serve with your choice of crudités and
   store any leftovers in the fridge for 3–4 days.

Roasted Sweet Pepper Hummus ❸

—

MAKES 2–3 DIPPING BOWLS

260g (9oz, or 9) baby sweet peppers
125ml (½ cup) extra virgin olive oil,
    plus extra for drizzling
2 roasted garlic cloves (see page 89)
1 tbsp tahini
1 x 400g (14oz) tin chickpeas, drained and rinsed
Squeeze of lemon juice (optional)
½ tsp ground cumin
Sea salt and black pepper
Pinch of chilli flakes, to serve

1. Preheat the oven to 200°C fan (425°F).
2. Place the peppers on a roasting tray, drizzle
   over some oil and season with sea salt and
   black pepper. Roast for 25 minutes.
3. Slice the caps off the roasted peppers and
   remove the seeds.
4. Blitz the peppers with the rest of the ingredients
   in a food processor. Transfer to a bowl, drizzle
   over some oil and scatter with the chilli flakes.
   Serve with your choice of crudités and store
   any leftovers in the fridge for 3–4 days.

Hummus Accompaniments/Crudités
Serve your choice of hummus with Belgian endive
leaves, sliced bell peppers, celery sticks, cucumber
sticks, carrot sticks, and sugar snap peas. You could
also use slices of toasted sourdough.

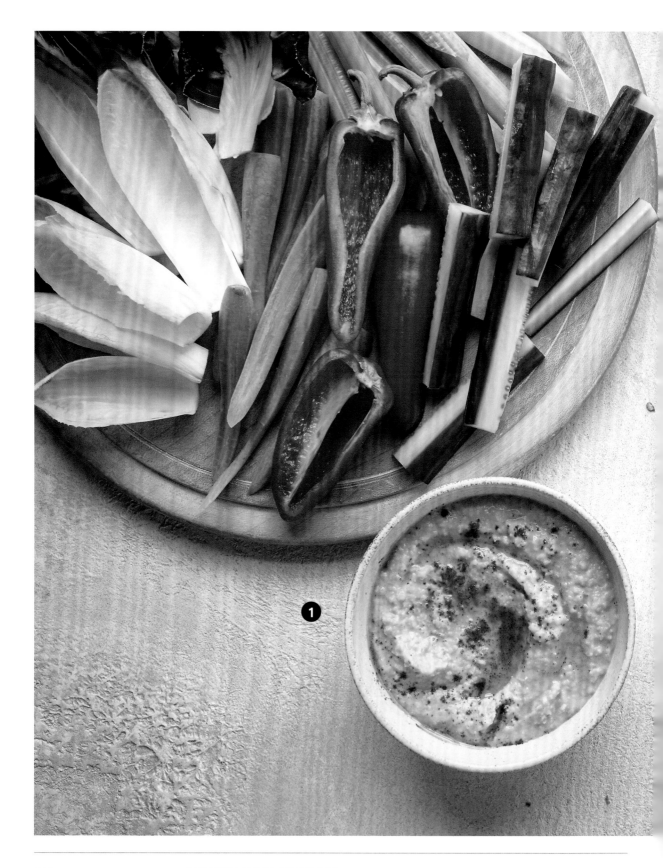

EAT WELL WITH ARTHRITIS

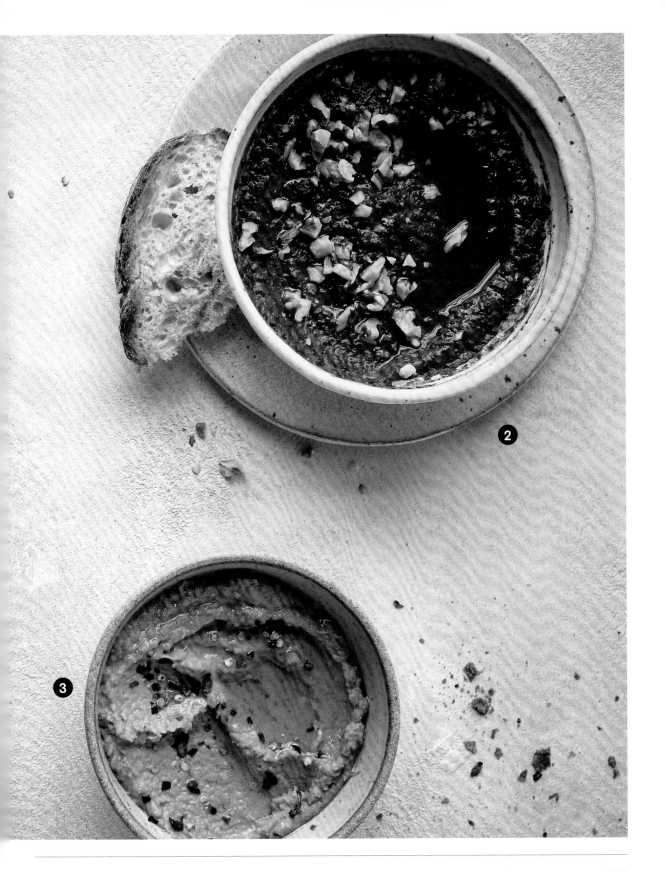

SWEET CINNAMON MIXED NUTS

V, VEG, DF, GF

 Meal Prep Cooking for Friends and Family Under 1 hour

**MAKES ABOUT
10 SERVINGS**

500g (3⅓ cups) assorted
  nuts: cashew nuts,
  almonds, walnut halves,
  pecans, Brazil nuts
1 tbsp coconut oil
3 tbsp maple syrup
1½ tbsp ground cinnamon
¼ tsp pink Himalayan salt
½ tsp vanilla extract
1 tsp ground ginger
½ tsp ground nutmeg
¼ tsp ground cardamom
1 tsp coconut sugar
⅛ tsp (or generous pinch)
  cayenne pepper

In *Beat Arthritis Naturally* I created a savoury, sweet and spicy nut recipe for snacking, but here I wanted to create a sweet-tooth alternative, while still getting in some all-important polyphenols from the spices.

—

1. Preheat the oven to 160°C fan (350°F). Line 2 baking trays with baking parchment.
2. Place the nuts in a large mixing bowl.
3. Heat the coconut oil and maple syrup together in a saucepan on a medium heat until they melted. Pour over the nuts, stirring well and making sure that all of the nuts are coated.
4. Add the remaining ingredients and mix well.
5. Spread onto the lined trays and cook for 15–20 minutes, turning over halfway through.
6. Leave to cool. They may stick together, so use a silicone spatula to separate and store in an airtight container(s) for about a couple of months. I often use jars and take one to work with me each day of the week.

CRISPY KALE, THREE WAYS

V, VEG, DF, GF

🍴 Meal Prep 🥬 Cooking for Friends and Family 🧴 10 Ingredients or Less 🕐 Under 30 minutes

SERVES 4

100g (3 cups) curly leaf
  kale or cavolo nero
1 tsp extra virgin olive oil
¼ tsp sea salt
¼ tsp black pepper

1. CHEESE AND ONION
1 tsp onion granules
¼ tsp garlic granules
¼ tsp dried rosemary
1 tbsp nutritional yeast flakes

2. SALT AND VINEGAR
¾ tsp sea salt (in addition to
  the seasoning from earlier)
2½ tsp balsamic vinegar
½ tsp coconut sugar
¼ tsp nutritional yeast flakes

3. SMOKY PAPRIKA
2 tsp smoked paprika
1½ tsp nutritional yeast flakes
½ tsp garlic granules
¼ tsp onion granules
¼ tsp dried oregano
¼ tsp ground coriander
⅛ tsp ground cumin

Deep-fried white potato salt and vinegar crisps are a treat now because they're definitely on the inflammation scale, so I have come up with an alternative here. I keep these in the fridge and sprinkle on salads or soups, or avocado toast. For more kale crisp ideas see *Beat Arthritis Naturally*. Kale is super nutritious and packed with anti-inflammatory components kaempferol, quercetin, vitamin C, sulforaphane and carotenoids (lutein, beta-carotene).

1. Preheat the oven to 180°C fan (400°F).
2. Place the kale in a large mixing bowl and, with your hands, massage in the extra virgin olive oil, sea salt, black pepper and one of the three seasoning mixes until the kale is fully coated. (Warning: your hands will become paprika red with the smoked paprika seasoning!)
3. Add to a baking tray and bake for 8–12 minutes, turning halfway through. It may need longer or less, depending on the strength of your oven – I have a fan oven and 8 minutes usually does the trick. My advice is to watch the kale and don't leave it alone, as it's quick to burn (I've had plenty of mishaps over the last few years!).
4. These are crispiest when fresh, but you can store them in an airtight container in the fridge for up to 4 days to use as a topping on salads and soups. Make sure they have cooled for 1–2 hours before storing.

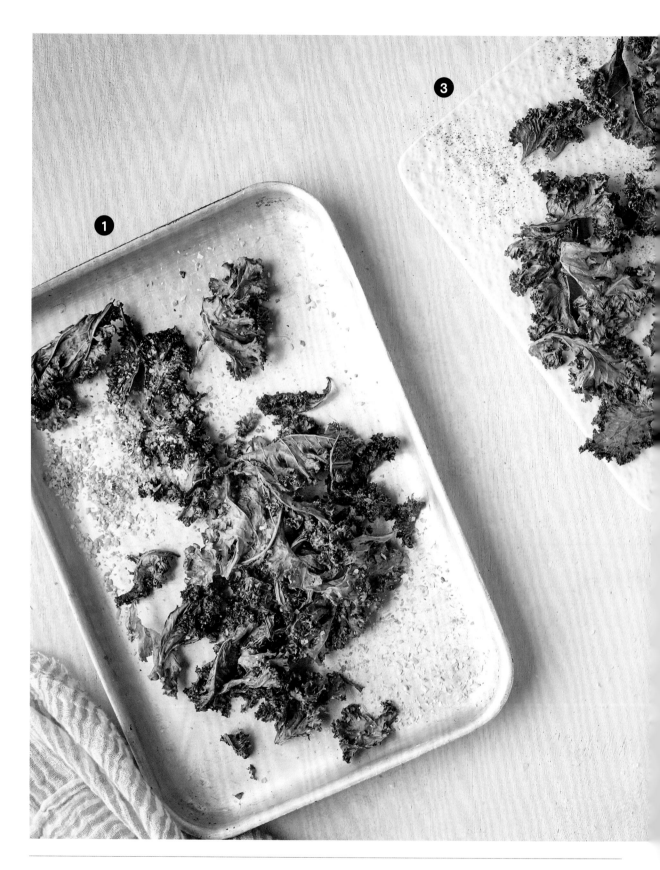

EAT WELL WITH ARTHRITIS

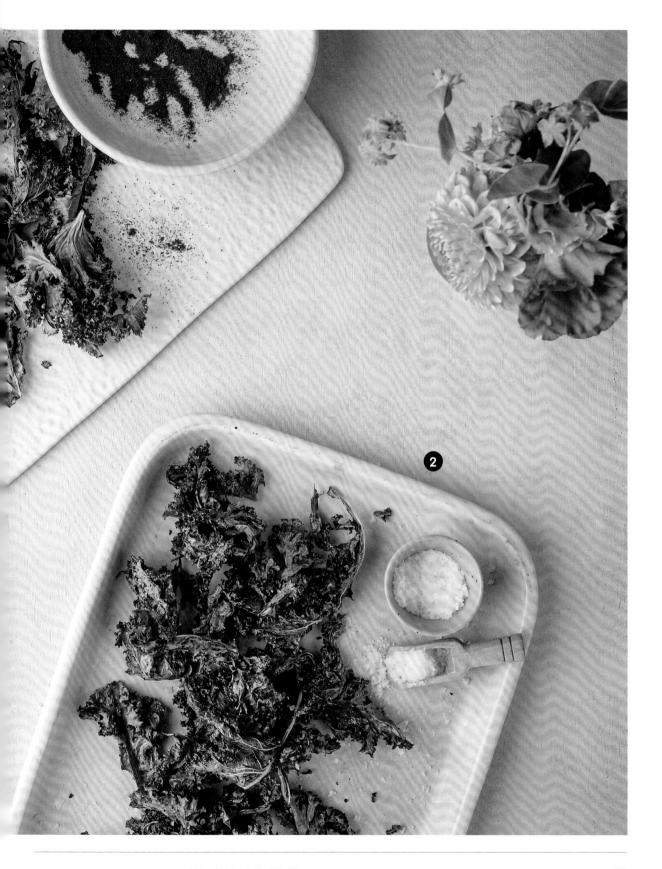

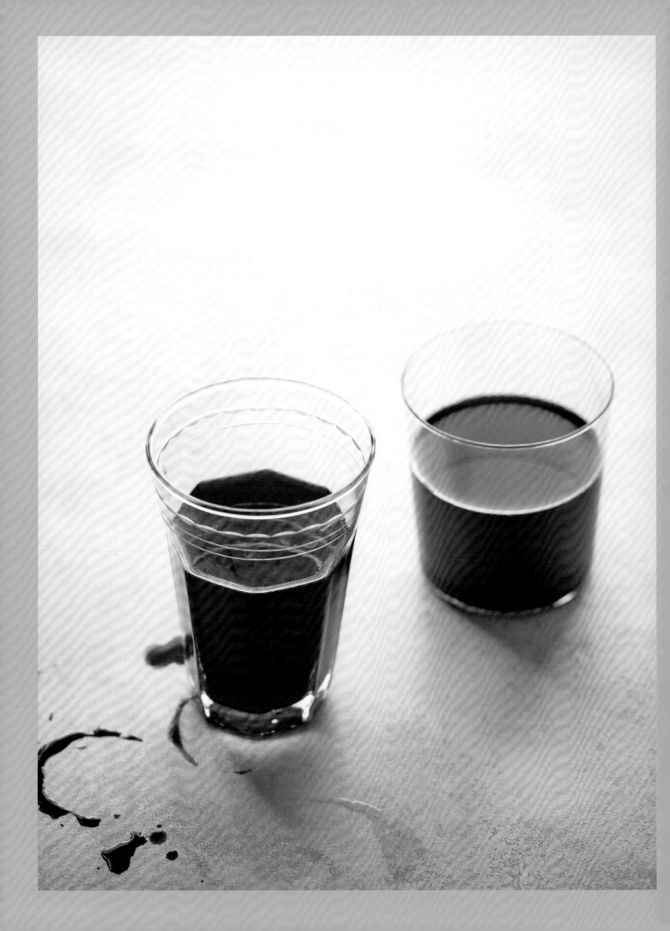

DRINKS, JUICES AND SMOOTHIES

ORANGE AND CINNAMON WARMER

V, VEG, DF, GF

🍴 Meal Prep 🥄 Cooking for Friends and Family 🔒 10 Ingredients or Less
🕐 Under 1 hour

**MAKES 4 SMALL OR
2 LARGE TEA CUPS
OR 4 SMALL GLASSES
COLD WITH ICE**

2 oranges
925ml (4 cups) water
2 rooibos teabags (I like Tick
  Tock) or 2 tsp tea leaves
½ tsp honey (optional)
1 cinnamon stick

TO GARNISH (OPTIONAL)
2–3 sprigs of fresh mint
Lemon wedges

You could have this with breakfast tea leaves if you'd like to, but I keep it caffeine-free. It's refreshing with ice or warm and comforting if it is hot. (Oranges and tangerines are rich in a carotenoid that has been suggested to be protective against rheumatoid arthritis.) Rooibos tea may reduce inflammation, shown in some preliminary studies (see more on page 74). Double the recipe if making for family and friends.

1. Peel and squeeze the oranges, reserving the juice and the peel for the pan. The juice from 2 oranges should yield around 150ml (⅔ cup) of orange juice.
2. Bring the water to the boil in a saucepan on a high heat. When at a rolling boil (this should take 6–7 minutes), turn down the heat and add the tea leaves or teabags, orange peel, honey and cinnamon stick. Stir to combine and let the water simmer for a few minutes on a medium heat.
3. Once the spices and orange flavour are nicely infused in the water, typically 10–15 minutes, depending on how strong you'd like the flavour infusion to be, remove from the heat and add the orange juice. Strain the liquid through a sieve or a straining funnel into a large pot or jug. Remove some of the orange peel from the sieve to place in the cups or glasses as a garnish.
4. Cool then place in the fridge if having cold, or drink straight away, with the mint leaves and lemon, if desired.

Tip:
When freezing liquids, freeze in ice-cube trays or in ziplock bags, flattening to store in the freezer.

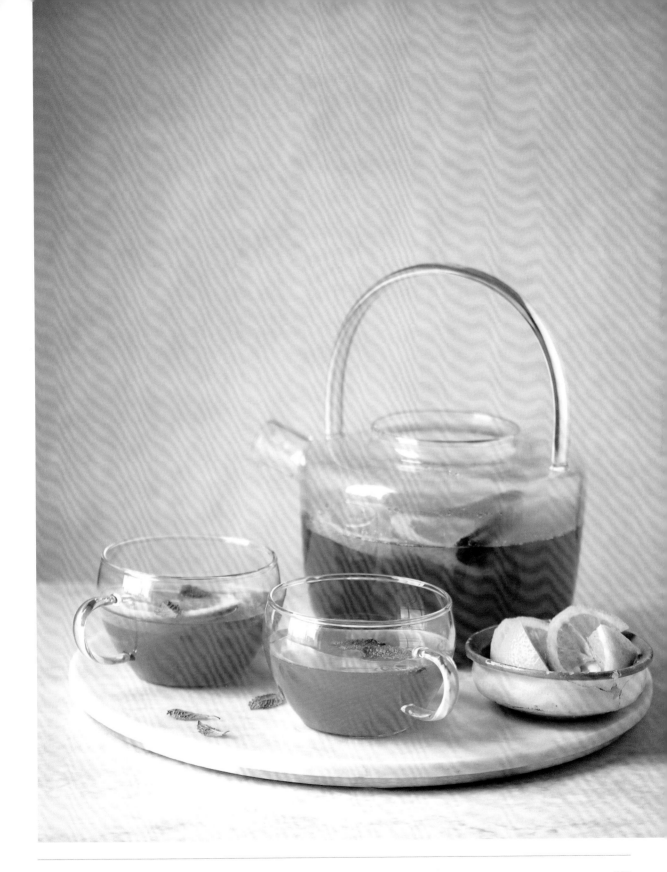

VANILLA DATE HEMP SEED SMOOTHIE ❶

V, VEG, DF, GF

🍴 Meal Prep 🥄 Cooking for Friends and Family
🔒 10 Ingredients or Less 🕐 Under 1 hour

This smoothie has such a sweet caramel flavour and is packed with healthy omega-3 and omega-6 fatty acids from the hemp seeds, plus natural sweetness from the Zamli dates with plenty of antioxidants. Hemp seeds have high nutritional value (see page 66).

SERVES 2

2 bananas
115g (½ cup, or 11) Zamli dates (or Medjool or plain will work if you can't get Zamli), pitted
1 tsp honey (or a vegan alternative, see page 88)
4 tbsp hulled hemp seeds
260ml (1 cup + 1 tbsp) plant milk
¼ tsp vanilla extract
¼ tsp ground ginger
140ml (½ cup + 1 tbsp) water

TO SERVE (OPTIONAL)
Ice cubes
Date syrup

1. Blend all of the ingredients in a blender.
2. Pour into 2 glasses, with ice if preferred. Squeeze a swirl of date syrup on top of each smoothie if you like. Yummy.

GOLDEN DELICIOUS GREEN SMOOTHIE ❷

V, VEG, DF, GF

❄ Freezable 🍴 Meal Prep 🥄 Cooking for Friends and Family 🔒 10 Ingredients or Less 🕐 Under 30 minutes

Using green Golden Delicious apples and spirulina, this smoothie is scrumptious, and packed with health benefits from the apples (quercetin), spinach (carotenoids), mint (carnosol) and superfood powders especially. Spirulina comes from algae and it's consumption has been cited in some studies as effectively reducing anti-inflammatory and pain-related infectious diseases, even with a potential to support brain health. Quercetin is found in apples, and is especially in the skins, which is why you blend this smoothie with the apple skins on.

SERVES 2–4

1 Galia melon, peeled and cubed (you can buy pre-chopped melon if easier)
2 Golden Delicious apples, cored and chopped
2 small bananas, peeled
2 handfuls of spinach
1 tsp spirulina, moringa or chlorella powder
1 tsp honey (or a vegan alternative, see page 88) (optional)
10g (¼oz) fresh mint (optional)

TO SERVE (OPTIONAL)
Ice cubes
Fresh mint leaves

1. Blend all of the ingredients in a blender – I have a vacuum option so that the smoothie retains all of its vibrancy.
2. Fill 2–4 glasses with ice cubes, pour over the juice and top with a sprig of fresh mint per glass – so delicious!

TURMERIC KICK JUICE ❸

V, VEG, DF, GF

❋ Freezable   🍴 Meal Prep   🌿 Cooking for Friends and Family
🛍 10 Ingredients or Less   ⏱ Under 30 minutes

SERVES 4–6

20–30g (1oz) fresh turmeric
85g (3oz) fresh ginger
6 large oranges (I use
    seedless Navel oranges,
    but any large oranges will
    work), peeled
6 Gala apples
½ cucumber
20 frozen mango cubes
    (115g/4oz)
½ tsp ground black pepper
Ice cubes, to serve (optional)

By now, I am sure you know how powerful turmeric is as a natural anti-inflammatory spice, fighting those free radicals in our system. But be careful when using it as it does leave its mark in other ways too as it stains hands and clothing if not handled carefully. Turmeric, in combination with ginger, and the antioxidants found in oranges, apples and black pepper, makes this a powerful anti-inflammatory drink.

—

1. Juice all of the ingredients apart from the frozen mango and black pepper.
2. Blend the juice with the frozen mango and black pepper.
3. Serve the juice as it is, or with ice. It will keep in the fridge for 3 days but is best drunk fresh. You could freeze some in ice-cube trays if you are unable to drink it all at once.

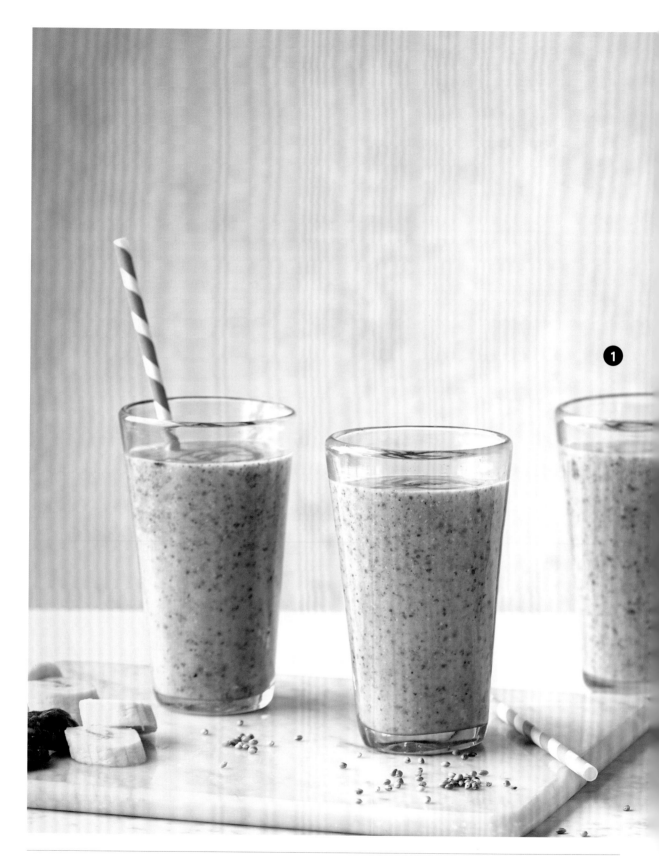

EAT WELL WITH ARTHRITIS

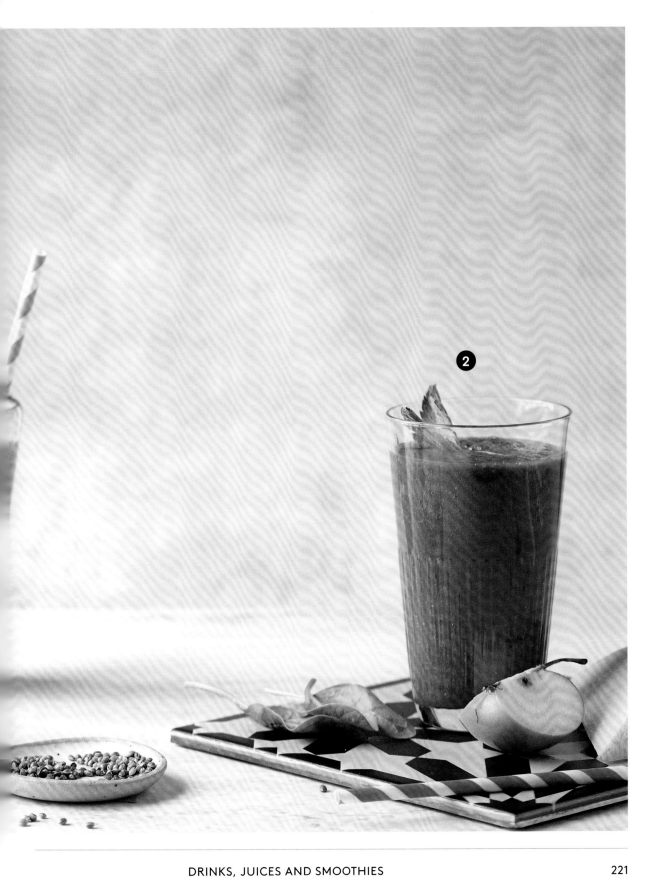

GREEN DREAM JUICE ❹

V, VEG, DF, GF

❄ Freezable 🍴 Meal Prep 🥄 Cooking for Friends and Family 🔒 10 Ingredients or Less 🕐 Under 30 minutes

This drink is so refreshing and nourishing with the sweetness of the pineapple and apple juices combined with the cooling cucumber and spicy ginger. You only need to drink a small amount of this, as it is high in natural sugars and low in fibre, so perhaps it is better as a weekend treat to have alongside a gut-nourishing breakfast! Mint leaves increase the polyphenol content due to their carnosol.

—

SERVES 1

1 pineapple (970g/2¼lb), leaves
   and hard outer skin removed
3 Royal Gala apples
50g (2oz) fresh ginger
1 lime
6–7 celery sticks
½ cucumber
20g (¾oz) fresh mint leaves

TO SERVE (OPTIONAL)
Ice cubes
Sprig of fresh mint

1. Cut the skin off the pineapple and place in a juicer. Add the rest of the ingredients and juice.
2. Fill 4 glasses with ice cubes, pour over the juice and top with a sprig of mint. You can also store the juice in the fridge and consume within 24 hours for freshness – just shake before drinking.

SUNSHINE JUICE ❺

V, VEG, DF, GF

❄ Freezable 🍴 Meal Prep 🥄 Cooking for Friends and Family 🔒 10 Ingredients or Less 🕐 Under 30 minutes

A juice experiment that worked the first time around! I'm always experimenting in the kitchen and using the juicing machine is no different. I am so pleased with how this juice turned out – looking literally as bright as sunshine! It will brighten your mood, and it's packed with an anti-inflammatory punch too.

—

SERVES 2–4

4 Conference pears
3 Royal Gala apples
2 large oranges, peeled
1 white grapefruit, peeled
6g (⅛oz) fresh turmeric
Sprinkle of black pepper
Ice cubes, to serve

1. Place all of the ingredients (apart from the black pepper) into a juicer and juice. Stir in the black pepper – you won't be able to taste it, but it increases the absorption of the curcumin in the turmeric.
2. Serve with ice in 2 pint glasses or for a smaller serving for 4 people, pour into half-pint glasses.

BOLD BEETROOT JUICE ❻

V, VEG, DF, GF

✳ Freezable ⏱ Meal Prep 🥄 Cooking for
Friends and Family 🛍 10 Ingredients or Less
🕐 Under 30 minutes

Beetroot dilates blood vessels, turning them into
superhighways for your nutrient- and oxygen-
rich blood (see page 56). Nutritionist Victoria Jain
recommends this juice as a great option for those
living with RA and beetroot supplementation
has also been shown to improve thumb blood
flow, and anti-inflammatory status, in people
with Raynaud's (often associated with arthritic
conditions such as RA, scleroderma, lupus or
Sjogren's syndrome).

—

SERVES 2/MAKES 570ML/2¼ CUPS

3 Golden Delicious apples (300g/10oz)
3 raw beetroots (200g/7oz)
8 carrots (600g/1lb 5oz)
25g (1oz) fresh ginger
2 handfuls of spinach (optional)

1. Place all of the ingredients into a juicer and juice.
2. Serve straightaway, or chill in the fridge for up to
   30 minutes before drinking.

ANTI-INFLAMMATORY POWER JUICE ❼

V, VEG, DF, GF

✳ Freezable ⏱ Meal Prep 🥄 Cooking for
Friends and Family 🛍 10 Ingredients or Less
🕐 Under 30 minutes

Spicy and sweet, this juice packs an anti-
inflammatory punch! It's really refreshing in
the mornings, or as a booster in the afternoon.
Remember, if the vegetables are organic, or
produced locally, they are likely to have more
of the health benefits and good gut bugs. Serve
with ice and a slice of cucumber on a hot day.

—

SERVES 2

70g (2½oz) fresh ginger
6 Gala apples (690g/1lb 9oz)
½ cucumber (200g/7oz)
6 carrots (660g/1lb 7oz)

TO SERVE (OPTIONAL)
Ice cubes
Cucumber slices

1. Add all of the ingredients to a juicer and juice.
2. Fill 2 glasses with ice cubes, pour over the
   juice and add a slice of cucumber to each
   glass, if liked.

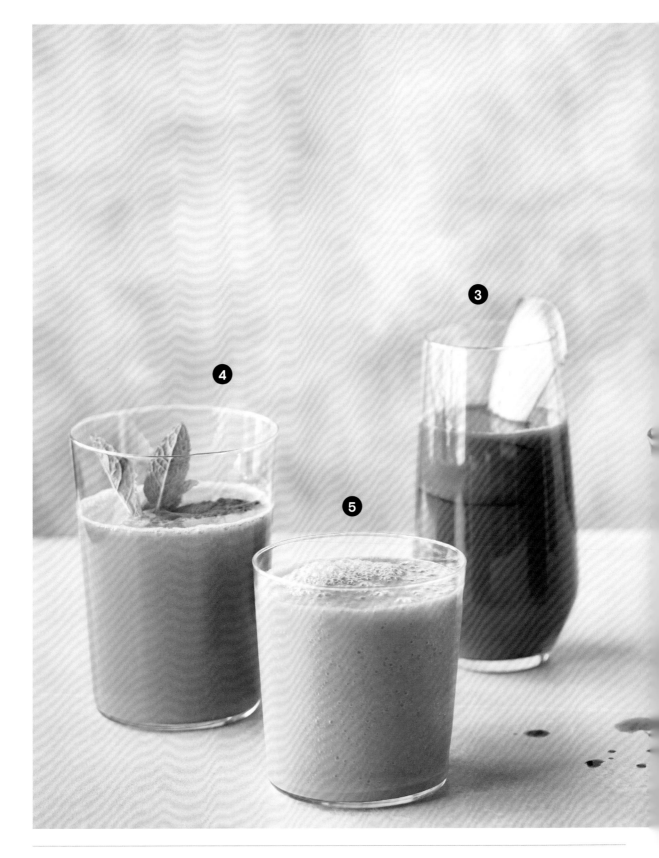

EAT WELL WITH ARTHRITIS

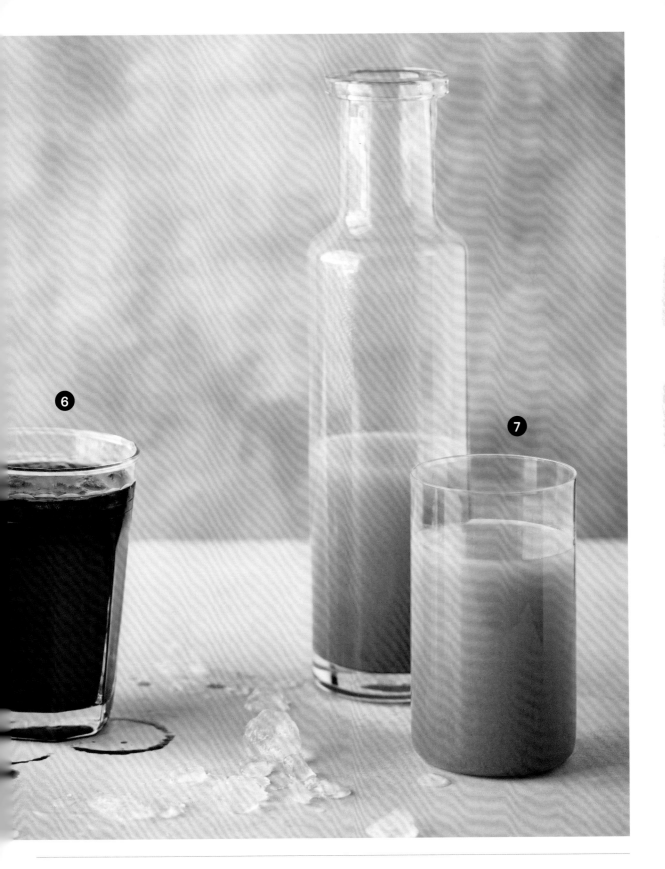

CALM AND ENERGISING MATCHA

V, VEG, DF, GF   🏷 10 Ingredients or Less   ⏱ Under 30 minutes

SERVES 1

½–1 tsp matcha
    green tea powder
2–3 tbsp warm/tepid water
250ml (1 cup) plant milk
    (latte) or water (tea),
    hot or cold
Traditional Japanese
    tea-ceremony utensils
    (optional, but worth
    investing if you do enjoy
    it and would like to keep
    making it at home):
Chakoshi: small matcha
    sieve; as matcha is so
    finely milled it does often
    clump
Chashaku: thin bamboo
    spoon; alternative:
    teaspoon
Chawan: small tea bowl;
    alternative: large, wide
    tea mug or small bowl
Chasen: special bamboo
    whisk; alternative: small
    baking whisk

I love making a matcha tea, and it's packed with antioxidant and anti-inflammatory polyphenol content (see page 68). Matcha also has a lower caffeine content than coffee, so the caffeine is released slowly in the body, allowing for alertness without the jitters, so it creates a calming effect, alleviating stress. Regular consumption of matcha may have a positive effect on both physical and mental health, which I can vouch for!

If trying it for the first time, try using a sweeter plant milk like soya, or oat milk, otherwise it might be a bit bitter. Almond milk is my milk of choice, as it has no sugar in it.

—

1. To prepare your matcha in the traditional Japanese way, measure the matcha tea powder into your chakoshi, and sieve gently, using a chashaku, into the chawan.
2. Add the 2–3 tablespoons of warm/tepid water into the chawan with the matcha (now sieved) and gently whisk using a chasen from left to right, to form a smooth and silky consistency, removing any clumping.
3. Heat the 250ml (1 cup) plant milk in a frother machine, or the water in a small saucepan, no higher than 70°C (158°F). (Skip this part if you're having a cold matcha.)
4. Add the cold or hot liquid to the chawan or pour into your glass/mug of choice.
5. You then could add a few sprinkles of matcha green tea powder on the top for decoration, or ice if it is cold.
6. Drink straightaway, and ideally before 11am, to be on the safe side when it comes to sleep and caffeine content. One matcha a day, if you can afford it, or a few times a week feels good.

Tip:
Most coffee shops and restaurants sell matcha now, and so before investing, perhaps try one while you are out. I would recommend trying it more than once though, as I didn't like the first 3 matcha lattes I had, and it was only when I reached the fifth one that I started to enjoy it. So, persevere with your taste buds, as they do adjust – and hopefully you will come to love matcha as much as I do.

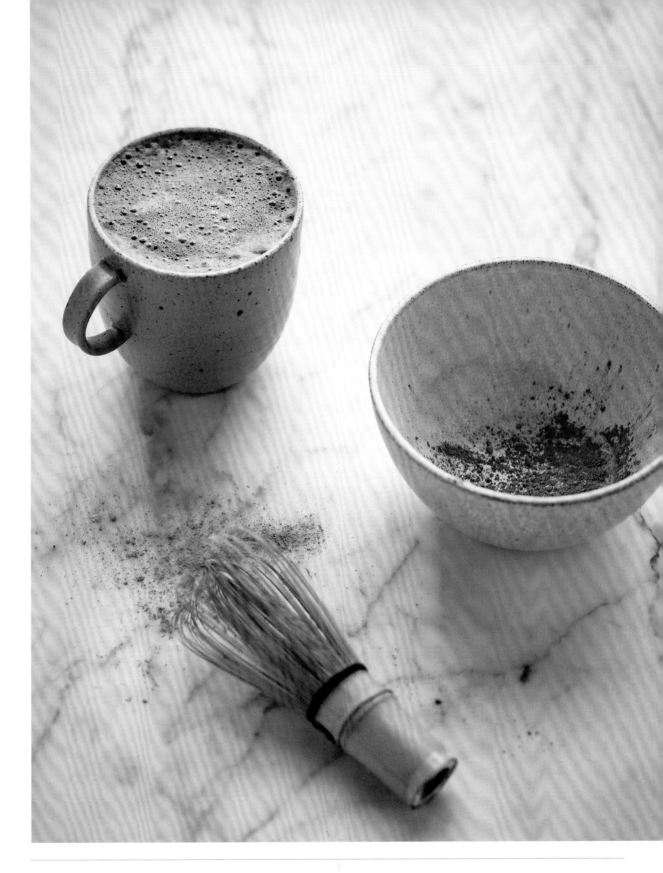

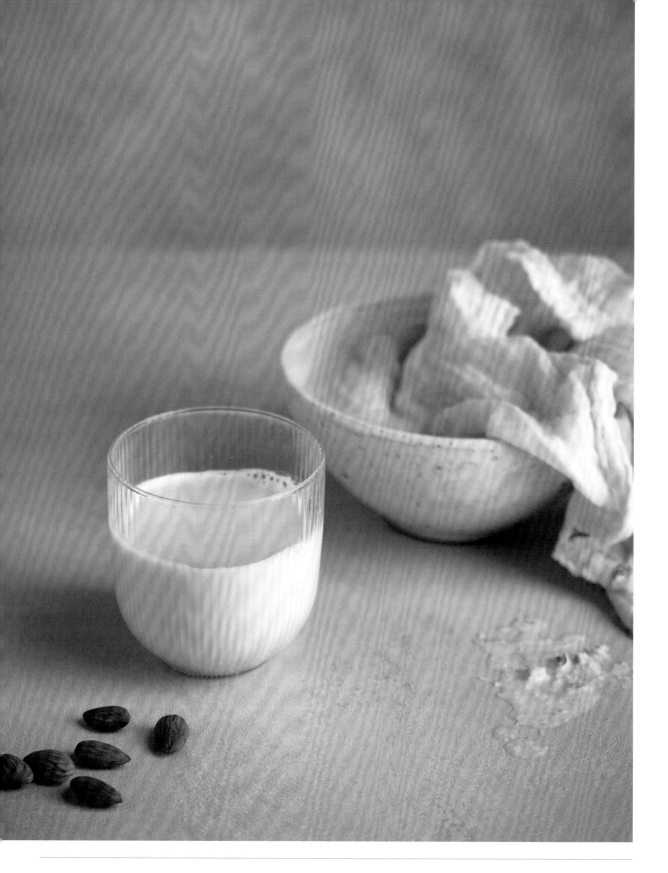

EAT WELL WITH ARTHRITIS

HOMEMADE ALMOND MYLK

V, VEG, DF, GF

❄ Freezable ‖ Meal Prep 🍃 Cooking for Friends and Family
🔒 10 Ingredients or Less 🕐 Under 30 minutes (not including overnight soaking)

MAKES 1.25 LITRES (5⅓ CUPS)

150g (1 cup) almonds
1.4 litres (5½ cups
   + ⅛ cup) water
3 dates, pitted
Pinch of salt
You will also need:
   Nut milk bag, to strain

I'm always having almond milk at home, and when I discovered how few ingredients there are in the good stuff (such as Plenish drinks, or Innocent), I bought a nut milk strainer and thought I'd have a go at making my own. This keeps in the fridge for around 3–4 days and will save spending on shop-bought products. For more on the health benefits of almonds, see page 54.

1. Soak the almonds in a container with 1 litre (4 cups) of water in the fridge for 12–24 hours.
2. Blend the almonds and the soaking liquid with another 400ml (1½ cups + ⅛ cup) of water, the dates and salt. Blend in two batches if you have a smaller food processor. Strain through the nut milk bag into a jar (for pouring) and squeeze the residue where you can.
3. Pour into sterilised glass container(s), seal and store in the fridge for 3–4 days. Use for smoothies, drinks, overnight oats, porridge and more.

MINT CHOC CHIP SMOOTHIE

V, VEG, DF, GF

✳ Freezable 🍴 Meal Prep 🥄 Cooking for Friends and Family
🏷 10 Ingredients or Less 🕐 Under 30 minutes

SERVES 1

1 banana, peeled
200ml (¾ cup) plant milk
1 tbsp raw cacao powder
100ml (¼ cup +
   3 tbsp) water
8 sprigs of fresh mint,
   leaves picked
½ tsp honey (optional)

TO SERVE
Ice cubes
Sprig of fresh mint

I have recreated the refreshingly sweet flavour of mint chocolate chip ice cream in this smoothie. You'll need fresh mint, and if you grow it in your garden or at home – even better! For the health benefits of mint and the polyphenol carnosol, go to page 66.

—

1. Blend all of the ingredients in a blender.
2. Add some ice to a glass, pour over the smoothie and top with a sprig of mint.

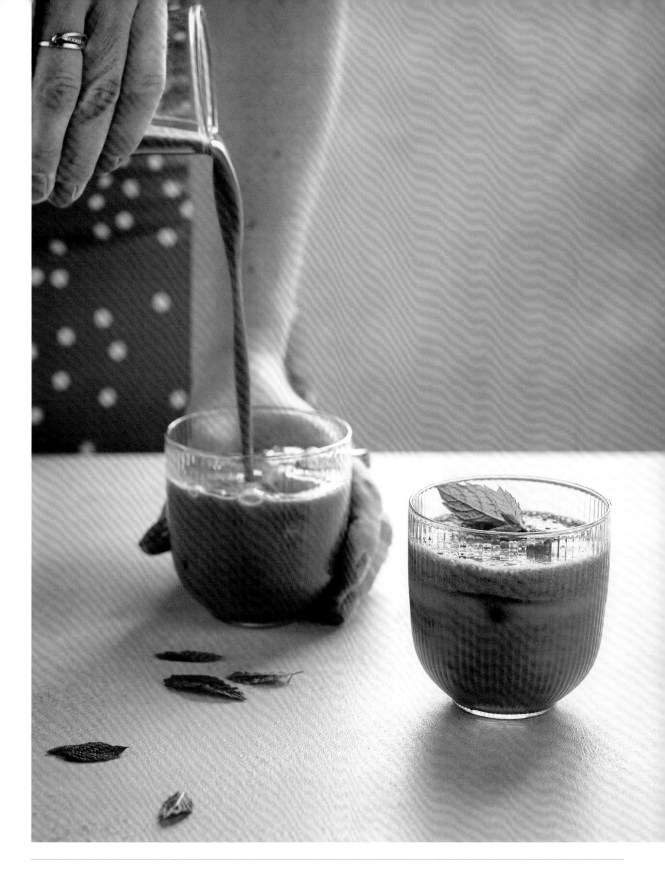

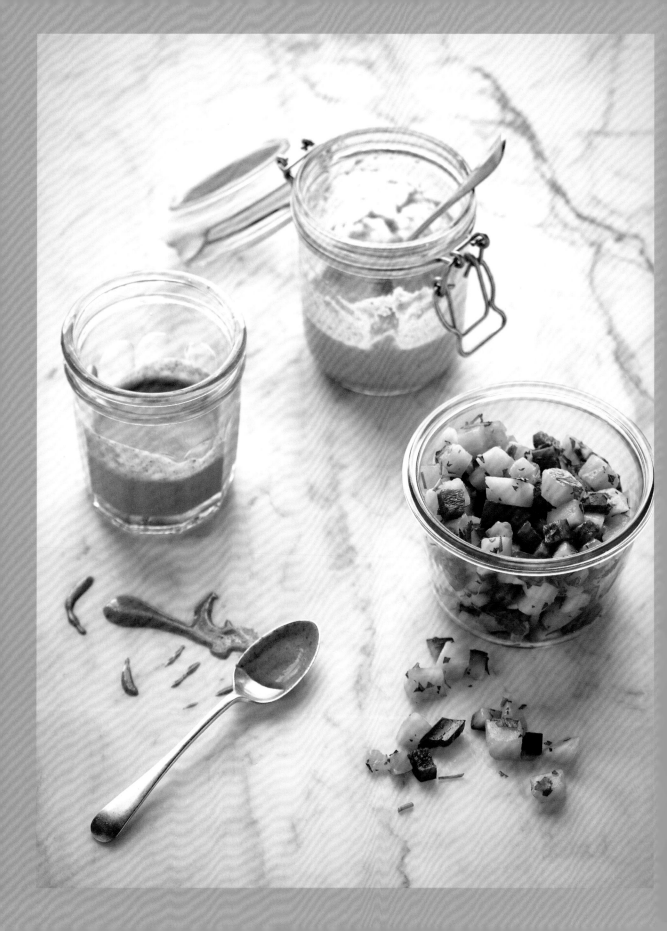

SAUCES, JAMS AND DIPS

RASPBERRY JAM

V, VEG, DF, GF

⦚ Meal Prep 🥄 Cooking for Friends and Family
🔒 10 Ingredients or Less 🕐 Under 1 hour

This jam is so delicious! It keeps in the fridge for around one month and it is perfect to put on top of your morning porridge, or for use in the Bakewell Tart Overnight Oats on page 101 or the Matcha pudding on page 184. Chia seeds have plenty of healthy fats and are surprisingly high in calcium too. Raspberries are also packed with anti-inflammatory components such as the flavonoid anthocyanin, vitamin C and quercetin.

SERVES 6 (MAKES AROUND 300G/10OZ)

285g (1⅓ cups) raspberries
2 tbsp chia seeds
3 tbsp honey (or a vegan alternative, see page 88)
3 drops almond extract (or vanilla extract)
50ml (¼ cup) water
1 tbsp lemon juice

1. Add all of the ingredients to a saucepan and cook gently for 10 minutes until the jam starts to bubble.
2. Turn down the heat and simmer for a further 20–25 minutes until thick and jammy. Add more honey towards the end of cooking if you'd like it sweeter.
3. Set aside to cool, then transfer to a sterilised jar. Store in the fridge or enjoy straightaway.

CHIPOTLE SAUCE

V, VEG, DF, GF

⦚ Meal Prep ⦚ 'Fakeaway' 🥄 Cooking for Friends and Family 🔒 10 Ingredients or Less 🕐 Under 30 minutes

Cooked tomatoes are typically higher in the phytonutrient lycopene than raw tomatoes, and in fact, as a tip for other recipes, if you cook them in olive oil, the lycopene content is even higher. Lycopene is a carotenoid that is responsible for the red to pink colours seen in tomatoes, pink grapefruit and other foods too. Lycopene has antioxidant and anti-inflammatory properties and could ease inflammation in arthritic conditions like osteoarthritis. Some are suspicious of tomatoes (see page 76), but there is little evidence to support it being problematic to us (just yet anyway). However, if you do feel that it is impacting you, then try doing a Trigger Tracker for it on pages 34–37.

SERVES 2

2 tsp tomato purée
4 tsp mayonnaise
   (or vegan mayo)
1 tsp chipotle powder
½ tsp garlic paste
Juice of ½ lime
¼ tsp ground coriander
1 tsp extra virgin olive oil
Sea salt and black pepper

1. Add all of the ingredients to a small bowl and stir well.

CHOCOLATE SAUCE

V, VEG, DF, GF

🍴 Meal Prep ∥ 'Fakeaway' 🥣 Cooking for Friends and Family 🔒 10 Ingredients or Less ⏱ Under 30 minutes

This is perfect with fruit salads or desserts. A great topping for the Matcha and Berry Compote with Pistachio Crumb and Chocolate Sauce (see page 235) or the Coconut Banana 'Cookie' Bites on page 201. It contains resveratrol from the cacao powder, and plenty of healthy fats from the nut butter.

MAKES 4 SERVINGS

3 tbsp nut butter (almond, macadamia or hazelnut)
1 tbsp raw cacao powder
1 tsp date syrup
1 tbsp honey (or a vegan alternative, see page 88)
4 tbsp plant milk
2 tbsp water
Pinch of sea salt

1. Gently melt all the ingredients together in a small saucepan on a low–medium heat for 2–3 minutes until it thickens and is smooth and silky. You can add more water or plant milk if you'd like a thinner sauce.
2. Eat straightaway, or cool and store in the fridge for 3–5 days. It will thicken when cold, so heat gently in a pan with a splash of water to loosen if re-heating.

MANGO SALSA

V, VEG, DF, GF

🍴 Meal Prep 🥣 Cooking for Friends and Family 🔒 10 Ingredients or Less ⏱ Under 30 minutes

This salsa contains fresh coriander, basil, pepper, mango, all uncooked to retain their health benefits even more. Coriander is packed with polypehnols, and vitamin K too, which plays a pivotal role in maintenance of the bone strength. Mango is my favourite fruit; if you can catch it when it is in season (usually June to August), grown in places such as India and Pakistan (chaunsa mango, alphonso mango, and other varieties). Find it in your local corner shop – it's super honey-flavoured and delicious. Mango is rich in polyphenols and dietary fibre, find out more on page 68.

SERVES 4–6

1 mango
½ red bell pepper
¼ cucumber
Handful of fresh mint leaves
5–6 sprigs of fresh coriander
½ lime juice (optional, but helps with storing)
Sea salt and black pepper

1. Peel and chop the mango and cut the pepper into chunks.
2. Cut the cucumber into small triangles.
3. Remove the stalks on the mint and coriander, and chop.
4. Combine all of the ingredients with sea salt and black pepper.
5. This will keep in the fridge for a few hours, so you can prepare it in the morning to eat in the evening, but it's better eaten fresh, or it can become soggy and a little sour.

CLASSIC SALAD DRESSING

V, VEG, DF, GF

🍴 Meal Prep 🥣 Cooking for Friends and Family
🔒 10 Ingredients or Less ⏱ Under 30 minutes

An easy salad dressing to replace any processed ones. Try it with the Easy Frittata on page 116. Uncooked extra virgin olive oil is the best form to consume it in, which means getting it into salad dressings (like this recipe!). For more information on the benefits of extra virgin olive oil go to page 64.

—

MAKES 255ML (1 CUP)

12 tbsp extra virgin olive oil
2 tbsp apple cider vinegar
1 tbsp balsamic vinegar
2 tbsp honey (or maple syrup, if vegan)
½ tsp black pepper
Pinch of sea salt

1. Put all of the ingredients in a jar and shake well to prevent the dressing from separating. It will keep in the fridge for 3–5 days.

CASHEW PARSLEY SAUCE

V, VEG, DF, GF

🍴 Meal Prep 🥣 Cooking for Friends and Family
🔒 10 Ingredients or Less ⏱ Under 30 minutes

Enjoy this nutty sauce with the fishcakes on page 116, or it also works nicely with white fish recipes. The parsley brings the polyphenol content in the form of carnosol, and the cashew nuts bring the healthy fats, fibre and other anti-inflammatory properties.

—

MAKES 160ML (⅔ CUP)

65g (⅓ cup + 1 tbsp) cashews
2 heaped tbsp curly leaf parsley
Squeeze of lemon juice (½–1 tsp)
½ tsp Dijon mustard
90ml (⅓ cup + 1 tbsp) plant milk
Sea salt and black pepper

1. Soak the cashews in boiling water for 15 minutes. Drain.
2. Combine the soaked cashews with the parsley, lemon juice, Dijon mustard, plant milk and a sprinkle of salt and pepper to taste. Blend until smooth and no nut pieces remain. You may add a dash of water here to play with the consistency.
3. Heat the sauce in a pan to warm it through or serve it at room temperature to cool down your dish. It will keep in the fridge for 3 days.

CHILLI APRICOT CHUTNEY

V, VEG, DF, GF

🍴 Meal Prep 🥄 Cooking for Friends and Family
🕐 Under 1 hour

This goes so well with the Hasselback Potatoes on page 163 and is a great alternative to shop-bought chutneys. It contains quite a bit of sugar though, so use sparingly. Cardamom pods are packed with antioxidant and anti-inflammatory properties, and interestingly, a recent study found that cardamom seeds and fruit could help improve oral health. This is important when it comes to inflammatory conditions; one study reported that those with rheumatoid arthritis are four times more likely to have gum disease than those without it.

MAKES 2 LARGE JARS

A drizzle of extra virgin olive oil
1 red onion, finely sliced
6 garlic cloves, finely sliced
2 tsp brown mustard seeds
3 tomatoes, finely sliced
20g (¾oz) fresh ginger, peeled and finely sliced
½ tsp ground cinnamon
4 large red chillies, finely sliced (deseeded, if you prefer)
Seeds from 3 cardamom pods
300g (1½ cups) sulphur dioxide-free dried apricots, sliced
200ml (¾ cup) apple cider vinegar
260g (1¼ cups) unrefined natural caster sugar
150ml (⅔ cup) water

1. Pour the oil into a medium saucepan on a medium heat and, once hot, cook the onion, garlic and mustard seeds for 5 minutes. Add the tomatoes, ginger, cinnamon, chillies and cardamom seeds and cook for 5 minutes.
2. Stir in the dried apricots with the vinegar, sugar and water. Simmer for 45 minutes until reduced, stirring occasionally.
3. Leave to cool, then transfer to sterilised jars and keep in the fridge for up to 4 months.

CASHEW CHEESE

V, VEG, DF, GF

🍴 Meal Prep 🥄 Cooking for Friends and Family
🫙 10 Ingredients or Less 🕐 Under 30 minutes
(not including overnight soaking)

This recipe is perfect with the Hasselback Potatoes on page 163, however, you could add it to salads, on top of sourdough with walnuts and spinach, as it imitates the consistency of cream cheese without the dairy. Cashew nuts are rich in fibre (good for the gut, see page 60), protein, and healthy fats. There are also the health benefits from the EVOO, which contains a number of polyphenols and monounsaturated healthful fats, see page 64 for more detail.

MAKES 445G

200g (1⅓ cups) cashew nuts
3 tbsp nutritional yeast flakes
1 tsp garlic powder
1 tsp onion powder
2 tbsp extra virgin olive oil
100ml (¼ cup + 3 tbsp) water
Squeeze of lemon juice
Sea salt and black pepper

1. Soak the cashew nuts in 360ml (1½ cups) of water for 3–5 hours or for 12 hours overnight if you can.
2. Drain the cashew nuts and add to a food processor with the nutritional yeast, garlic powder, onion powder, extra virgin olive oil and sea salt and black pepper to taste (a pinch of each should suffice). With the processor running, drizzle in the water slowly and mix until the cashew cheese is smooth and thick. For a creamier taste, you could swap 50ml (¼ cup) of the water for 50ml (¼ cup) of plant milk.
3. Add the lemon juice to taste, and a dash more water, plant milk and salt or pepper if needed.
4. Store in an airtight container in the fridge for up to 5 days.

VEGAN PESTO, THREE WAYS

V, VEG, DF, GF ✳ Freezable (in ice-cube trays) 🍴 Meal Prep 🥣 Cooking for Friends and Family 🎒 10 Ingredients or Less 🕐 Under 30 minutes

Use the pestle and mortar setting on your food processor to easily whip up any of these three pestos. Packing in extra virgin olive oil (see page 64 for its health benefits), carnosol from the basil, and various nuts packed with omega-3 health benefits too. Use for the pizza on page 166 or enjoy with the fishcakes on page 116.

Classic Vegan Pesto

—

SERVES 2–4

10g (½ cup) fresh basil
80g (½ cup) pine nuts
2 tbsp nutritional yeast flakes
5 tbsp extra virgin olive oil
1 garlic clove (roasted if you have time, see page 89)
2–3 tbsp plant milk (depending on how thick you'd like it to be)
Squeeze of lemon juice
½ tsp apple cider or balsamic vinegar
Sea salt and black pepper

1. Blend all of the ingredients together well using the pestle and mortar setting on your food processor (it's kinder to your hands). Use immediately or store in the fridge for 3–5 days.

Walnut Vegan Pesto

—

SERVES 2–4

80g (⅔ cup) walnuts
30g (2½ cups) basil
6 tbsp extra virgin olive oil
2 tbsp nutritional yeast flakes
1 tsp plant milk
½ tsp balsamic vinegar
Squeeze of lemon juice
¼ tsp pink Himalayan salt
¼ tsp black pepper
2 large roasted garlic cloves (see page 89)

1. Blend all the ingredients together well using the pestle and mortar setting on your food processor. Use immediately or store in the fridge for 3–5 days.

Saucy Vegan Pesto

—

SERVES 2–4

10g (handful) of fresh basil
85g (½ cup) pine nuts
2 tbsp nutritional yeast
4 tbsp extra virgin olive oil
½ tsp garlic paste or 1 garlic clove
    (roasted if you have time, see page 89)
3 tbsp plant milk
Drizzle of lemon juice
Sea salt and black pepper

1. Blend all of the ingredients together well using the pestle and mortar setting on your food processor. Use immediately or store in the fridge for 3–5 days.

A FINAL WORD – BE YOUR OWN ADVOCATE

You may not know everything there is to know about arthritis, rheumatology, inflammation, medicine (conventional, complementary, alternative or otherwise), or the totality of health and beyond, and nobody expects you to. By reading this book, you know more than you did before, and you have shown courage in taking this step towards bettering your health.

What should be at the heart of this is you – because this is your journey, and it is personal. Make the time now to get to know yourself, because it is the one investment that will bring you endless returns. Whether it's knowing your triggers, the pain relief that really hits the spot, a certain type of exercise that helps untangle a knotting knee, or a recipe that nourishes you from the inside out, learning about what helps you, hinders you and, above all, makes you feel happy, should be the takeaway from this book.

It's not just about eating well with arthritis, it is about looking after yourself with arthritis, and only you can know what the best route along this road is for you. The changes that you are making may not make sense to everyone, but that does not matter: hold on to the fact that *you are in control of making these changes*, whether they are big or small, a handful or a book-full. Whether you manage those changes every day, or not, you are trying, and you are learning. Become your own advocate, your own champion, as you step forward.

Listen to your body and trust yourself because you are your own best expert.

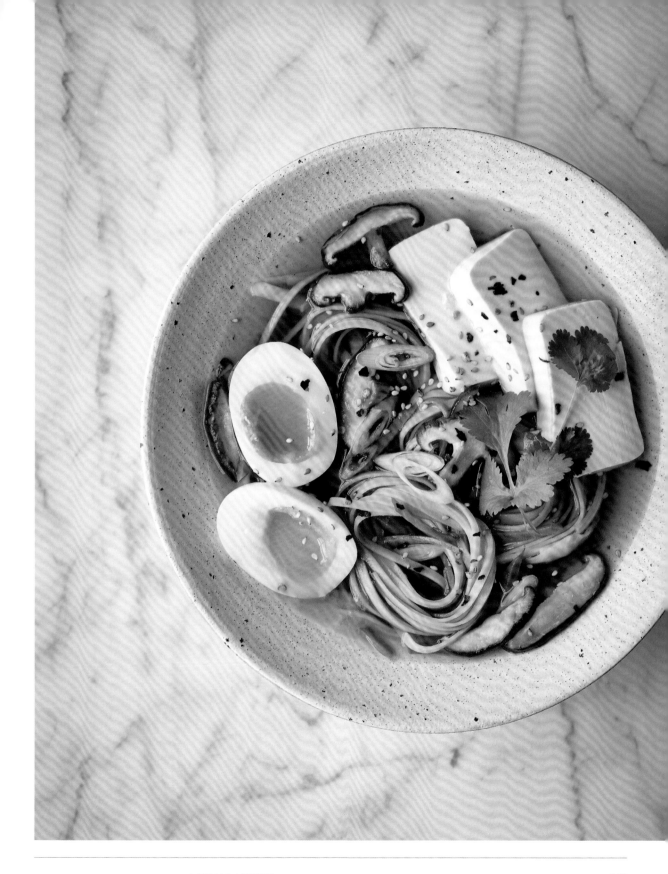

REFERENCES

Introduction

1. Vighi, G., Marcucci, F., Sensi, L., Di Cara, G., & Frati, F. (2008). Allergy and the gastrointestinal system. *Clinical & Experimental Immunology*, 153 Suppl 1, 3–6. https://doi.org/10.1111/j.1365-2249.2008.03713.x.
2. Simons, G., Mason, A., Falahee, M., Kumar, K., Mallen, C.D., Raza, K., & Stack, R.J. (2017). Qualitative Exploration of Illness Perceptions of Rheumatoid Arthritis in the General Public. *Musculoskeletal Care*, 15(1), 13–22. https://doi.org/10.1002/msc.1135.
3. National Rheumatoid Arthritis Society. YouGov, 2035 Adults Surveyed, 17 June 2019, https://twitter.com/NRAS_UK/status/1140547640813346816.
4. Arthritis Foundation (2022). How Arthritis Hurts. Different types of arthritis can cause different kinds of pain. arthritis.org. https://www.arthritis.org/health-wellness/healthy-living/managing-pain/understanding-pain/sources-of-arthritis-pain#:~:text=There%20are%20more%20than%20100,changing%20pain%20in%20different%20ways.
5. Pahwa, R., Goyal, A., Bansal, P., et al. (2020) *Chronic Inflammation*. In:Treasure Island (FL): StatPearls Publishing. https://www.ncbi.nlm.nih.gov/books/NBK493173/.

Chapter 1:
Living with Arthritis

1. World Health Organization. (14 July 2022). Musculoskeletal health. https://www.who.int/news-room/fact-sheets/detail/musculoskeletal-conditions.
2. Cieza, A., Causey, K., Kamenov, K., Hanson, S.W., Chatterji, S., & Vos, T. (2021). Global estimates of the need for rehabilitation based on the Global Burden of Disease study 2019: a systematic analysis for the Global Burden of Disease Study 2019. *The Lancet*, 396(10267), 2006. https://doi.org/10.1016/S0140-6736(20)32340-0.
3. Vojdani, A., Pollard, K.M., & Campbell, A.W. (2014). Environmental Triggers and Autoimmunity. *Autoimmune Diseases*, 2014, 798029. https://doi.org/10.1155/2014/798029.
4. Pande, I. (2006). An update on gout. *Indian Journal of Rheumatology*, 1(2), 60–65. https://doi.org/10.1016/S0973-3698(10)60005-2.
5. Goldring, M.B., & Otero, M. (2011). Inflammation in osteoarthritis. *Current Opinion in Rheumatology*, 23(5), 471–478. https://doi.org/10.1097/BOR.0b013e328349c2b1.
6. van den Bosch M.H.J. (2019). Inflammation in osteoarthritis: is it time to dampen the alarm in this debilitating disease?. *Clinical and Experimental Immunology*, 195(2), 153–166. https://doi.org/10.1111/cei.13237.
7. Ansari, M.Y., Ahmad, N., & Haqqi, T.M. (2020). Oxidative stress and inflammation in osteoarthritis pathogenesis: Role of polyphenols. *Biomedicine & Pharmacotherapy*, 129, 110452. https://doi.org/10.1016/j.biopha.2020.110452.
8. Kunnumakkara, A.B., Sailo, B.L., Banik, K., Harsha, C., Prasad, S., Gupta, S.C., Bharti, A.C., & Aggarwal, B.B. (2018). Chronic diseases, inflammation, and spices: how are they linked?. *Journal of Translational Medicine*, 16(1), 14. https://doi.org/10.1186/s12967-018-1381-2.
9. O'Brien, A., Backman, C. (2010). Chapter 16 - Inflammatory arthritis. Rheumatology, Churchill Livingstone, 2010, 211-233, https://doi.org/10.1016/B978-0-443-06934-5.00016-4. v
10. Robinson, W.H., Lepus, C.M., Wang, Q., Raghu, H., Mao, R., Lindstrom, T.M., & Sokolove, J. (2016). Low-grade inflammation as a key mediator of the pathogenesis of osteoarthritis. *Nature Reviews Rheumatology*, 12(10), 580–592. https://doi.org/10.1038/nrrheum.2016.136.
11. Pahwa, R., Goyal, A., & Jialal, I. (2022). Chronic inflammation. In StatPearls. StatPearls Publishing.
12. Furman, D., Campisi, J., Verdin, E., Carrera-Bastos, P., Targ, S., Franceschi, C., Ferrucci, L., Gilroy, D.W., Fasano, A., Miller, G.W., Miller, A.H., Mantovani, A., Weyand, C.M., Barzilai, N., Goronzy, J.J., Rando, T.A., Effros, R.B., Lucia, A., Kleinstreuer, N., & Slavich, G.M. (2019). Chronic inflammation in the etiology of disease across the life span. *Nature Medicine*, 25(12), 1822–1832. https://doi.org/10.1038/s41591-019-0675-0.
13. Collins. 2022. 'Exposome'. Collins Dictionary. https://www.collinsdictionary.com/dictionary/english/exposome.
14. Kato, J., & Svensson, C.I. (2015). Role of Extracellular Damage-Associated Molecular Pattern Molecules (DAMPs) as Mediators of Persistent Pain. *Progress in Molecular Biology and Translational Science*, 131, 251–279. https://doi.org/10.1016/bs.pmbts.2014.11.014.
15. Bach-Faig, A., Berry, E.M., Lairon, D., Reguant, J., Trichopoulou, A., Dernini, S., Medina, F.X., Battino, M., Belahsen, R., Miranda, G., & Serra-Majem, L. (2011). Mediterranean diet pyramid today. Science and cultural updates. *Public Health Nutrition*, 14(12A), 2274–2284. https://doi.org/10.1017/S1368980011002515.
16. Khanna, S., Jaiswal, K.S., & Gupta, B. (2017). Managing Rheumatoid Arthritis with Dietary Interventions. *Frontiers in Nutrition*, 4, 52. https://doi.org/10.3389/fnut.2017.00052.
17. Tomasello, G., Mazzola, M., Leone, A., Sinagra, E., Zummo, G., Farina, F., Damiani, P., Cappello, F., Gerges Geagea, A., Jurjus, A., Bou Assi, T., Messina, M., & Carini, F. (2016). Nutrition, oxidative stress and intestinal dysbiosis: Influence of diet on gut microbiota in inflammatory bowel diseases. *Biomedical Papers of the Medical Faculty of the University Palacky*, Olomouc, Czechoslovakia, 160(4), 461–466. https://doi.org/10.5507/bp.2016.052.
18. Casas, R., Sacanella, E., Urpí-Sardà, M., Corella, D., Castañer, O., Lamuela-Raventos, R. M., Salas-Salvadó, J., Martínez-González, M., Ros, E., & Estruch, R. (2016). Long-Term Immunomodulatory Effects of a Mediterranean Diet in Adults at High Risk of Cardiovascular Disease in the PREvención con DIeta MEDiterránea (PREDIMED) Randomized Controlled Trial. The Journal of Nutrition, 146(9), 1684–1693. https://doi.org/10.3945/jn.115.229476.
19. Santangelo, C., Vari, R., Scazzocchio, B., De Sancti, P., Giovannini, C., D'Archivio, M., & Masella, R. (2018). Anti-inflammatory Activity of Extra Virgin Olive Oil Polyphenols: Which Role in the Prevention and Treatment of Immune-Mediated Inflammatory Diseases?. *Endocrine, Metabolic & Immune Disorders: Drug Targets*, 18(1), 36–50. https://doi.org/10.2174/1871530317666171114114321.
20. Oliviero, F., Scanu, A., Zamudio-Cuevas, Y., Punzi, L., & Spinella, P. (2018). Anti-inflammatory effects of polyphenols in arthritis. *Journal of the Science of Food and Agriculture*, 98(5), 1653–1659. https://doi.org/10.1002/jsfa.8664.
21. Behl, T., Upadhyay, T., Singh, S., Chigurupati, S., Alsubayiel, A.M., Mani, V., Vargas-De-La-Cruz, C., Uivarosan, D., Bustea, C., Sava, C., Stoicescu, M., Radu, A.F., & Bungau, S.G. (2021). Polyphenols Targeting MAPK Mediated Oxidative Stress and Inflammation in Rheumatoid Arthritis. *Molecules*, 26(21), 6570. https://doi.org/10.3390/molecules26216570.
22. Maity, S., & Wairkar, S. (2022). Dietary polyphenols for management of rheumatoid arthritis: Pharmacotherapy and novel delivery systems. *Phytotherapy Research*, 36(6), 2324–2341. https://doi.org/10.1002/ptr.7444.
23. Direito, R., Rocha, J., Sepodes, B., & Eduardo-Figueira, M. (2021). Phenolic Compounds Impact on Rheumatoid Arthritis, Inflammatory Bowel Disease and Microbiota Modulation. *Pharmaceutics*, 13(2), 145. https://doi.org/10.3390/pharmaceutics13020145.
24. Khan, H., Sureda, A., Belwal, T., Çetinkaya, S., Süntar, İ., Tejada, S., Devkota, H.P., Ullah, H., & Aschner, M. (2019). Polyphenols in the treatment of autoimmune diseases. *Autoimmunity Reviews*, 18(7), 647–657. https://doi.org/10.1016/j.autrev.2019.05.001.
25. Devore, E., Kang, J., Breteler, M., & Grodstein, F. (2012). Dietary Intakes of Berries and Flavonoids in Relation to Cognitive Decline. *Annals of Neurology*. 72, 135-43. 10.1002/ana.23594.
26. Ng, T-P., Chiam, P-C., Lee, T., Chua, H-C., Lim, L., & Kua, E-H. (2006). Curry Consumption and Cognitive Function in the Elderly. *American Journal of Epidemiology*, 164(9), 898–906. https://doi.org/10.1093/aje/kwj267.
27. Hughes, R.L., & Holscher, H.D. (2021). Fueling Gut Microbes: A Review of the Interaction between Diet, Exercise, and the Gut Microbiota in Athletes. *Advances in Nutrition*, 12(6), 2190–2215. https://doi.org/10.1093/advances/nmab077.
28. Rausch Osthoff, A-K., Niedermann, K., Braun, J., Adams, J., Brodin, N., Dagfinrud, H., Duruoz, T., Esbensen, B.A., Günther, K-P., Hurkmans, E., Juhl, C.B., Kennedy, N., Kiltz, U., Knittle, K., Nurmohamed, M., Pais, S., Severijns, G., Swinnen, T.W., Pitsillidou, I.A., Warburton, L., Yankov, Z., & Vliet Vlieland, T.P.M. (2018). 2018 EULAR recommendations for physical activity in people with inflammatory arthritis and osteoarthritis. *Annals of the Rheumatic Diseases*, 77(9), 1251–1260. https://doi.org/10.1136/annrheumdis-2018-213585.
29. Dimitrov, S., Hulteng, E., & Hong, S. (2017). Inflammation and exercise: inhibition of monocytic intracellular TNF production by acute exercise via β_2-adrenergic activation. *Brain, Behavior, and Immunity*, 61, 60–68. https://doi.org/10.1016/j.bbi.2016.12.017.
30. Burini, R.C., Anderson, E., Durstine, J.L., & Carson, J.A. (2020). Inflammation, physical activity, and chronic disease: an evolutionary perspective. *Sports Medicine and Health Science*, 2(1), 1-6. https://doi.org/10.1016/j.smhs.2020.03.004.
31. Benatti, F.B., & Pedersen, B.K. (2015). Exercise as an anti-inflammatory therapy for rheumatic diseases-myokine regulation. *Nature Reviews Rheumatology*, 11(2), 86–97. https://doi.org/10.1038/nrrheum.2014.193.
32. Balchin, C., Tan, A.L., Golding, J., Bissell, L-A., Wilson, O.J., McKenna, J., & Stavropoulos-Kalinoglou, A. (2022). Acute effects of exercise on pain symptoms, clinical inflammatory markers and inflammatory cytokines in people with rheumatoid arthritis: a systematic literature review. *Therapeutic Advances in Musculoskeletal Disease*, 14, 1759720X221114104. https://doi.org/10.1177/1759720X221114104.
33. Cerdá, B., Pérez, M., Pérez-Santiago, J.D., Tornero-Aguilera, J.F., González-Soltero, R., & Larrosa, M. (2016). Gut Microbiota Modification: Another Piece in the Puzzle of the Benefits of Physical Exercise in Health?. *Frontiers in Physiology*, 7, 51. https://doi.org/10.3389/fphys.2016.00051.
34. Codella, R., Luzi, L., & Terruzzi, I. (2018). Exercise has the guts: how physical activity may positively modulate gut microbiota in chronic and immune-based diseases. *Digestive and Liver Disease: Official journal of the Italian Society of Gastroenterology and the Italian Association for the Study of the Liver*, 50(4), 331–341. https://doi.org/10.1016/j.dld.2017.11.016.
35. Modarresi Chahardehi, A., Masoumi, S.A., Bigdeloo, M., Arsad, H., & Lim, V. (2022). The effect of exercise on patients with rheumatoid arthritis on the modulation of inflammation. *Clinical and Experimental Rheumatology*, 40(7), 1420–1431. https://doi.org/10.55563/clinexprheumatol/fohyoy.
36. University of California - San Diego. (2017, January 12). Exercise … It does a body good: 20 minutes can act as anti-inflammatory: One moderate exercise session has a cellular response that may help suppress inflammation in the body. ScienceDaily. Retrieved 20 August 2020 from www.sciencedaily.com/releases/2017/01/170112115722.htm.
37. Clarke, J. (2021). Exercise exerts anti-inflammatory effects on muscle via the JAK-STAT pathway. *Nature Reviews Rheumatology*, 17, 127. https://doi.org/10.1038/s41584-021-00581-7.
38. Loprinzi, P.D., Cardinal, B.J., (2011). Association between objectively-measured physical activity and sleep, NHANES 2005–2006. *Mental Health and Physical Activity*, 4(2), 65-69, https://doi.org/10.1016/j.mhpa.2011.08.001.
39. Pascoe, M.C., Thompson, D.R., & Ski, C.F. (2017). Yoga, mindfulness-based stress reduction and stress-related physiological measures: A meta-analysis. *Psychoneuroendocrinology*, 86, 152–168. https://doi.org/10.1016/j.psyneuen.2017.08.008.
40. Haaz, S., & Bartlett, S.J. (2011). Yoga for arthritis: a scoping review. *Rheumatic diseases clinics of North America*, 37(1), 33–46. https://pubmed.ncbi.nlm.nih.gov/21220084/.
41. Stefanaki, C. (2019). Chapter 3 - The Gut Microbiome Beyond the Bacteriome—The Neglected Role of Virome and Mycobiome in Health and Disease. Microbiome and Metabolome in Diagnosis, Therapy, and other Strategic Applications, 27-32, https://doi.org/10.1016/B978-0-12-815249-2.00003-8.
42. Walker, M. (2018). *Why We Sleep: The New Science of Sleep and Dreams*. London: Penguin Random House.
43. Colten, H. R., Altevogt, B. M. (eds.) & Institute of Medicine (US) Committee on Sleep Medicine and Research. (2006). Sleep Disorders and Sleep Deprivation: An Unmet Public Health Problem. National Academies Press (US).
44. Lyon, L. (2019). Is an epidemic of sleeplessness increasing the incidence of Alzheimer's disease?. *Brain: A Journal of Neurology*, 142(6), e30. https://doi.org/10.1093/brain/awz087.
45. Morin, C.M., LeBlanc, M., Daley, M., Gregoire, J.P., & Mérette, C. (2006). Epidemiology of insomnia: prevalence, self-help treatments, consultations, and determinants of help-seeking behaviors. *Sleep Medicine*, 7(2), 123–130. https://doi.org/10.1016/j.sleep.2005.08.008.

46. Smith, M.T., & Haythornthwaite, J.A. (2004). How do sleep disturbance and chronic pain inter-relate? Insights from the longitudinal and cognitive-behavioral clinical trials literature. *Sleep Medicine Reviews*, 8(2), 119–132. https://doi.org/10.1016/S1087-0792(03)00044-3.
47. Hughes, M., Chalk, A., Sharma, P., Dahiya, S., & Galloway, J. (2021). A cross-sectional study of sleep and depression in a rheumatoid arthritis population. *Clinical Rheumatology*, 40(4), 1299–1305. https://doi.org/10.1007/s10067-020-05414-8.
48. Bryant, P.A., Trinder, J., & Curtis, N. (2004). Sick and tired: does sleep have a vital role in the immune system?. *Nature Reviews Immunology*, 4(6), 457–467. https://doi.org/10.1038/nri1369.
49. Youm, Y-H., Nguyen, K.Y., Grant, R.W., et al. (2015). The ketone metabolite β-hydroxybutyrate blocks NLRP3 inflammasome-mediated inflammatory disease. *Nature Medicine* 21, 263–269. https://doi.org/10.1038/nm.3804.
50. Farrow, M.R., & Washburn, K. (2019). A Review of Field Experiments on the Effect of Forest Bathing on Anxiety and Heart Rate Variability. *Global Advances in Health and Medicine*, 8, 2164956119848654. https://doi.org/10.1177/2164956119848654.
51. Igarashi, M., Song, C., Ikei, H., & Miyazaki, Y. (2015). Effect of Stimulation by Foliage Plant Display Images on Prefrontal Cortex Activity: A Comparison with Stimulation using Actual Foliage Plants. *Journal of Neuroimaging*, 25(1), 127–130. https://doi.org/10.1111/jon.12078.
52. Lewis, D. (2009), Galaxy Stress Research. Mindlab International, Sussex University, UK.
53. Smith, M.A., Thompson, A., Hall, L.J., Allen, S.F., & Wetherell, M.A. (2018). The physical and psychological health benefits of positive emotional writing: investigating the moderating role of Type D (distressed) personality. *British Journal of Health Psychology*, 23(4), 857–871. https://doi.org/10.1111/bjhp.12320.
54. Kaimal, G., Ray, K., & Muniz, J. (2016). Reduction of Cortisol Levels and Participants' Responses Following Art Making. *Art Therapy: Journal of the American Art Therapy Association*, 33(2), 74–80. https://doi.org/10.1080/07421656.2016.1166832.
55. Kaimal, G., Ayaz, H., Herres, J., Dieterich-Hartwell, R., Makwana, B., Kaiser, D.H., Nasser, J.A. (2017). Functional near-infrared spectroscopy assessment of reward perception based on visual self-expression: coloring, doodling, and free drawing. *The Arts in Psychotherapy*, 55(85), 85–92. doi: 10.1016/j.aip.2017.05.004.
56. Mosley, M. (2020), *Fast Asleep: How to get a really good night's rest*, London: Short Books.
57. Leubner, D., & Hinterberger, T. (2017). Reviewing the Effectiveness of Music Interventions in Treating Depression. *Frontiers in Psychology*, 8, 1109. https://doi.org/10.3389/fpsyg.2017.01109.
58. Ekholm, O., Juel, K., & Bonde, L.O. (2016). Associations between daily musicking and health: Results from a nationwide survey in Denmark. *Scandinavian Journal of Public Health*, 44(7), 726–732. https://doi.org/10.1177/1403494816664252.
59. Saeed, S.A., Cunningham, K., & Bloch, R.M. (2019). Depression and Anxiety Disorders: Benefits of Exercise, Yoga, and Meditation. *American Family Physician*, 99(10), 620–627.
60. Brandel, M.G., Lin, C., Hennel, D., Khazen, O., Pilitsis, J.G., & Ben-Haim, S. (2022). Mindfulness Meditation in the Treatment of Chronic Pain. Neurosurgery Clinics of North America, 33(3), 275–279. https://doi.org/10.1016/j.nec.2022.02.005.
61. Statovci, D., Aguilera, M., MacSharry, J., & Melgar, S. (2017). The Impact of Western Diet and Nutrients on the Microbiota and Immune Response at Mucosal Interfaces. *Frontiers in Immunology*, 8, 838. https://doi.org/10.3389/fimmu.2017.00838.
62. Tan, M., He, F.J., & MacGregor, G.A. (2020). Obesity and covid-19: the role of the food industry. *BMJ* (Clinical research ed.), 369, m2237. https://doi.org/10.1136/bmj.m2237.
63. Artemniak-Wojtowicz, D., Kucharska, A. M., & Pyrżak, B. (2020). Obesity and chronic inflammation crosslinking. *Central European Journal of Immunology*, 45(4), 461–468. https://doi.org/10.5114/ceji.2020.103418.
64. Saltiel, A.R., & Olefsky, J.M. (2017). Inflammatory mechanisms linking obesity and metabolic disease. *The Journal of Clinical Investigation*, 127(1), 1–4. https://doi.org/10.1172/JCI92035.
65. Daïen, C.I., & Sellam, J. (2015). Obesity and inflammatory arthritis: impact on occurrence, disease characteristics and therapeutic response. *Rheumatic & Musculoskeletal Diseases*, 1(1), e000012. https://doi.org/10.1136/rmdopen-2014-000012.
66. Müller-Ladner, U., Frommer, K., Karrasch, T., Neumann, E., & Schäffler, A. (2021). Der Einfluss von Adipositas auf die Krankheitsaktivität bei entzündlich rheumatischen Erkrankungen [The effect of obesity on disease activity of inflammatory rheumatic diseases]. *Zeitschrift für Rheumatologie*, 80(4), 353–361. https://doi.org/10.1007/s00393-021-00987-4.
67. Anderson, S.C., Cryan, J.F., Dinan, T. (2019). *The Psychobiotic Revolution*, Washington: National Geographic Partners, LLC.
68. Foster, H. (2019, October), The diet to tame inflammation. *Women's Health*, pp. 48–50.
69. Jacka, F.N., Ystrom, E., Brantsaeter, A.L., Karevold, E., Roth, C., Haugen, M., Meltzer, H.M., Schjolberg, S., & Berk, M. (2013). Maternal and Early Postnatal Nutrition and Mental Health of Offspring by Age 5 Years: A Prospective Cohort Study. *Journal of the American Academy of Child & Adolescent Psychiatry*, 52(10), 1038–1047. https://doi.org/10.1016/j.jaac.2013.07.002.
70. Jacka, F. N., Mykletun, A., Berk, M., Bjelland, I., & Tell, G. S. (2011). The Association Between Habitual Diet Quality and the Common Mental Disorders in Community-Dwelling Adults: The Hordaland Health Study. *Psychosomatic Medicine*, 73(6), 483–490. https://doi.org/10.1097/PSY.0b013e318222831a.
71. Giugliano, D., Ceriello, A., & Esposito, K. (2006). The Effects of Diet on Inflammation: Emphasis on the Metabolic Syndrome. *Journal of the American College of Cardiology*, 48(4), 677–685. https://doi.org/10.1016/j.jacc.2006.03.052.
72. Esposito, K., Nappo, F., Marfella, R., Giugliano, G., Giugliano, F., Ciotola, M., Quagliaro, L., Ceriello, A., & Giugliano, D. (2002). Inflammatory Cytokine Concentrations Are Acutely Increased by Hyperglycemia in Humans: Role of Oxidative Stress. *Circulation*, 106(16), 2067–2072. https://doi.org/10.1161/01.cir.0000034509.14906.ae.
73. Jones, J.L., Park, Y., Lee, J., Lerman, R.H., & Fernandez, M.L. (2011). A Mediterranean-style, low-glycemic-load diet reduces the expression of 3-hydroxy-3-methylglutaryl-coenzyme A reductase in mononuclear cells and plasma insulin in women with metabolic syndrome. *Nutrition Research*, 31(9), 659–664. https://doi.org/10.1016/j.nutres.2011.08.011.
74. Aparicio-Soto, M., Sánchez-Hidalgo, M., Rosillo, M.Á., Castejón, M.L., & Alarcón-de-la-Lastra, C. (2016). Extra virgin olive oil: a key functional food for prevention of immune-inflammatory diseases. *Food & Function*, 7(11), 4492–4505. https://doi.org/10.1039/c6fo01094f.
75. World Health Organization. (2018, September). Launch of new global estimates on levels of physical activity in adults. https://www.who.int/news/item/05-09-2018-launch-of-new-global-estimates-on-levels-of-physical-activity-in-adults.
76. Fellows Brands Press Release. (2018, April). Brits sedentary for up to nine hours a day in the workplace alone, study finds. https://assets.fellowes.com/press/181018-UK-sedentary-research.pdf.
77. George, M.D., Giles, J.T., Katz, P.P., England, B.R., Mikuls, T.R., Michaud, K., Ogdie-Beatty, A. R., Ibrahim, S., Cannon, G.W., Caplan, L., Sauer, B.C., & Baker, J. F. (2017). Impact of Obesity and Adiposity on Inflammatory Markers in Patients With Rheumatoid Arthritis. *Arthritis Care & Research*, 69(12), 1789–1798. https://doi.org/10.1002/acr.23229.
78. Phillips, C.M., Dillon, C.B., & Perry, I.J. (2017). Does replacing sedentary behaviour with light or moderate to vigorous physical activity modulate inflammatory status in adults?. *International Journal of Behavioral Nutrition and Physical Activity*, 14(1), 138. https://doi.org/10.1186/s12966-017-0594-8.
79. Jankord, R., & Jemiolo, B. (2004). Influence of Physical Activity on Serum IL-6 and IL-10 Levels in Healthy Older Men. *Medicine & Science in Sports & Exercise*, 36(6), 960–964. https://doi.org/10.1249/01.mss.0000128186.09416.18.
80. Irwin, M.R., Olmstead, R., Carrillo, C., Sadeghi, N., Fitzgerald, J.D., Ranganath, V.K., & Nicassio, P.M. (2012). Sleep Loss Exacerbates Fatigue, Depression, and Pain in Rheumatoid Arthritis. *Sleep*, 35(4), 537–543. https://doi.org/10.5665/sleep.1742.
81. Finan, P.H., Goodin, B.R., & Smith, M.T. (2013). The Association of Sleep and Pain: An Update and a Path Forward. *The Journal of Pain*, 14(12), 1539–1552. https://doi.org/10.1016/j.jpain.2013.08.007.
82. Haack, M., Simpson, N., Sethna, N., Kaur, S., & Mullington, J. (2020). Sleep deficiency and chronic pain: potential underlying mechanisms and clinical implications. *Neuropsychopharmacology*, 45(1), 205–216. https://doi.org/10.1038/s41386-019-0439-z.
83. Koffel, E., Kroenke, K., Bair, M.J., Leverty, D., Polusny, M.A., & Krebs, E.E. (2016). The bidirectional relationship between sleep complaints and pain: Analysis of data from a randomized trial. *Health Psychology*, 35(1), 41–49. https://doi.org/10.1037/hea0000245.
84. Besedovsky, L., Lange, T., & Born, J. (2012). Sleep and immune function. *Pflugers Archiv - European Journal of Physiology*, 463(1), 121–137. https://doi.org/10.1007/s00424-011-1044-0.
85. Burgess, H.J., Burns, J.W., Buvanendran, A., Gupta, R., Chont, M., Kennedy, M., & Bruehl, S. (2019). Associations Between Sleep Disturbance and Chronic Pain Intensity and Function: A Test of Direct and Indirect Pathways. *The Clinical Journal of Pain*, 35(7), 569–576. https://doi.org/10.1097/AJP.0000000000000711.
86. Smith, M.T., Edwards, R.R., McCann, U.D., & Haythornthwaite, J.A. (2007). The Effects of Sleep Deprivation on Pain Inhibition and Spontaneous Pain in Women. *Sleep*, 30(4), 494–505. https://doi.org/10.1093/sleep/30.4.494.
87. Roehrs, T., & Roth, T. (2005). Sleep and Pain: Interaction of Two Vital Functions. *Seminars in Neurology*, 25(1), 106–116. https://doi.org/10.1055/s-2005-867079.
88. Irwin, M., Mascovich, A., Gillin, J.C., Willoughby, R., Pike, J., & Smith, T.L. (1994). Partial sleep deprivation reduces natural killer cell activity in humans. *Psychosomatic Medicine*, 56(6), 493–498. https://doi.org/10.1097/00006842-199411000-00004.
89. Yahia, N., Brown, C., Potter, S., Szymanski, H., Smith, K., Pringle, L., Herman, C., Uribe, M., Fu, Z., Chung, M., & Geliebter, A. (2017). Night eating syndrome and its association with weight status, physical activity, eating habits, smoking status, and sleep patterns among college students. *Eating and Weight Disorders*, 22(3), 421–433. https://doi.org/10.1007/s40519-017-0403-z.
90. O'Reardon, J.P., Ringel, B.L., Dinges, D.F., Allison, K.C., Rogers, N.L., Martino, N.S., & Stunkard, A.J. (2004). Circadian Eating and Sleeping Patterns in the Night Eating Syndrome. *Obesity Research*, 12(11), 1789–1796. https://doi.org/10.1038/oby.2004.222.
91. Fujiwara, Y., Machida, A., Watanabe, Y., Shiba, M., Tominaga, K., Watanabe, T., Oshitani, N., Higuchi, K., & Arakawa, T. (2005). Association Between Dinner-to-Bed time and Gastro-Esophageal Reflux Disease. *The American Journal of Gastroenterology*, 100(12), 2633–2636. https://doi.org/10.1111/j.1572-0241.2005.00354.x.
92. Gill, S., & Panda, S. (2015). A Smartphone App Reveals Erratic Diurnal Eating Patterns in Humans that Can Be Modulated for Health Benefits. *Cell Metabolism*, 22(5), 789–798. https://doi.org/10.1016/j.cmet.2015.09.005.
93. Pittenger, C., Duman, R. Stress, Depression, and Neuroplasticity: A Convergence of Mechanisms. *Neuropsychopharmacology*, 33, 88–109 (2008). https://doi.org/10.1038/sj.npp.1301574.
94. Danese, A., Moffitt, T.E., Harrington, H., et al. (2009). Adverse Childhood Experiences and Adult Risk Factors for Age-Related Disease: Depression, Inflammation, and Clustering of Metabolic Risk Markers. *Archives of Pediatrics & Adolescent Medicine*, 163(12), 1135–1143. https://doi.org/10.1001/archpediatrics.2009.214.
95. Lépine, J-P., & Briley, M. (2004). The epidemiology of pain in depression. *Human Psychopharmacology*, 19 Suppl 1, S3–S7. https://doi.org/10.1002/hup.618.
96. Public Health England. (2018). PHE Fingertips Tool Musculoskeletal Diseases Profile. Public Health England.
97. Carnegie Mellon University. (2 April 2012). How stress influences disease: study reveals inflammation as the culprit. ScienceDaily. Retrieved 21 July 2020 from www.sciencedaily.com/releases/2012/04/120402162546.htm.
98. Liu, Y-Z., Wang, Y-X., & Jiang, C-L. (2017). Inflammation: The Common Pathway of Stress-Related Diseases. *Frontiers in Human Neuroscience*, 11, 316. https://doi.org/10.3389/fnhum.2017.00316.
99. Lee, J., Taneja, V., & Vassallo, R. (2012). Cigarette Smoking and Inflammation: Cellular and Molecular Mechanisms. *Journal of Dental Research*, 91(2), 142–149. https://doi.org/10.1177/0022034511421200.
100. NHS, UK. (October 2018). What are the health risks of smoking? https://www.nhs.uk/common-health-questions/lifestyle/what-are-the-health-risks-of-smoking/#:~:text=Every%20year%20around%2078%2C000%20people,term%20damage%20to%20your%20health.
101. Pezzolo, E., & Naldi, L. (2019). The relationship between smoking, psoriasis and psoriatic arthritis. *Expert Review of Clinical Immunology*, 15(1), 41–48. https://doi.org/10.1080/1744666X.2019.1543591.
102. Adams, S. (14 December 2010). Smoking 'causes a third of severe rheumatoid arthritis cases'. *The Telegraph*. https://www.telegraph.co.uk/news/health/news/8198868/Smoking-causes-a-third-of-severe-rheumatoid-arthritis-cases.html.
103. Di Giuseppe, D., Discacciati, A., Orsini, N., & Wolk, A. (2014). Cigarette smoking and risk of rheumatoid arthritis: a dose-response meta-analysis. *Arthritis Research & Therapy*, 16(2), R61. https://doi.org/10.1186/ar4498.
104. Hedström, A.K., Stawiarz, L., Klareskog, L., & Alfredsson, L. (2018). Smoking and susceptibility to rheumatoid arthritis in a Swedish population-based case-control study. *European Journal of Epidemiology*, 33(4), 415–423. https://doi.org/10.1007/s10654-018-0360-5.
105. Colrain, I.M., Nicholas, C.L., & Baker, F.C. (2014). Alcohol and the sleeping brain. *Handbook of Clinical Neurology*, 125, 415–431. https://doi.org/10.1016/B978-0-444-62619-6.00024-0.
106. Bishehsari, F., Magno, E., Swanson, G., Desai, V., Voigt, R.M., Forsyth, C.B., & Keshavarzian,

A. (2017). Alcohol and Gut-Derived Inflammation. *Alcohol Research: Current Reviews,* 38(2), 163-171. https://www.ncbi.nlm.nih.gov/pmc/articles/PMC5513683/.

107. Muthuri, S.G., Zhang, W., Maciewicz, R.A., Muir, K., & Doherty, M. (2015). Beer and wine consumption and risk of knee or hip osteoarthritis: a case control study. *Arthritis Research & Therapy*, 17(1), 23. https://www.ncbi.nlm.nih.gov/pmc/articles/PMC4355424/.

108. Shield, K.D., Parry, C., & Rehm, J. (2013). Chronic diseases and conditions related to alcohol use. *Alcohol Research: Current Reviews*, 35(2), 155-173.

109. Roehrs, T., & Roth, T. (2008). Caffeine: sleep and daytime sleepiness. *Sleep Medicine Reviews.* 12(2): 153-162. https://doi.org/10.1016/j.smrv.2007.07.004.

110. Dunwiddie, T.V., & Masino, S.A. (2001). The role and regulation of adenosine in the central nervous system. *Annual Review of Neuroscience*, 24, 31-55. https://pubmed.ncbi.nlm.nih.gov/11283304/.

111. Ferré S. (2008). An update on the mechanisms of the psychostimulant effects of caffeine. *Journal of Neurochemistry,* 105(4), 1067-1079. https://doi.org/10.1111/j.1471-4159.2007.05196.x.

112. Drake, C., Roehrs, T., Shambroom, J., & Roth, T. (2013). Caffeine Effects on Sleep Taken 0, 3, or 6 Hours before Going to Bed. *Journal of Clinical Sleep Medicine*, 9(11), 1195-1200. https://doi.org/10.5664/jcsm.3170.

113. Ganesh, J. (11 January 2019). Sleep expert Matthew Walker on the secret to a good night's rest. *Financial Times*. https://www.ft.com/content/e6ccdcac-133d-11e9-a581-4ff78404524e.

Chapter 2:
How to Navigate Life with Chronic Pain
Section 1:
How to Overcome Your Pain: What is Pain, and How Can You Manage it for a Better Quality of Life? with Dr Deepak Ravindran

1. Ravindran, D. (2021). *The Pain-Free Mindset: 7 Steps to Taking Control and Overcoming Chronic Pain*, London: Ebury Publishing, 309.

2. Goldberg, D.S., & McGee, S.J. (2011). Pain as a global public health priority. *BMC Public Health*, 11, 770. https://doi.org/10.1186/1471-2458-11-770.

3. Raffaeli, W., Tenti, M., Corraro, A., Malafoglia, V., Ilari, S., Balzani, E., & Bonci, A. (2021). Chronic Pain: What Does It Mean? A Review on the Use of the Term Chronic Pain in Clinical Practice. Journal of Pain Research, 14, 827-835. https://doi.org/10.2147/JPR.S303186.

Section 2:
Cooking Without Pain: The Best Life Hacks, Tools and Adaptations for the Kitchen, with Cheryl Crow

1. Gainer, R.D. (2008). History of ergonomics and occupational therapy. [Abstract]. Work (Reading, Mass.), 31(1), 5-9, https://pubmed.ncbi.nlm.nih.gov/18820415/.

Chapter 3:
Anti-Inflammatory Components

1. Franzago, M., Santurbano, D., Vitacolonna, E., & Stuppia, L. (2020). Genes and Diet in the Prevention of Chronic Diseases in Future Generations. *International Journal of Molecular Sciences*, 21(7), 2633. https://doi.org/10.3390/ijms21072633.

2. Martinez, J.E., Kahana, D.D., Ghuman, S., Wilson, H.P., Wilson, J., Kim, S.J., Lagishetty, V., Jacobs, J.P., Sinha-Hikim, A.P., & Friedman, T.C. (2021). Unhealthy Lifestyle and Gut Dysbiosis: A Better Understanding of the Effects of Poor Diet and Nicotine on the Intestinal Microbiome. *Frontiers in Endocrinology*, 12, 667066. https://doi.org/10.3389/fendo.2021.667066.

3. Martel, J., Chang, S-H., Ko, Y-F., Hwang, T-L., Young, J.D., & Ojcius, D.M. (2022). Gut barrier disruption and chronic disease. *Trends in Endocrinology & Metabolism*: TEM, 33(4), 247-265. https://doi.org/10.1016/j.tem.2022.01.002.

4. Ballway, J.W., & Song, B-J. (2021). Translational Approaches with Antioxidant Phytochemicals against Alcohol-Mediated Oxidative Stress, Gut Dysbiosis, Intestinal Barrier Dysfunction, and Fatty Liver Disease. *Antioxidants*, 10(3), 384. https://doi.org/10.3390/antiox10030384.

5. Nahar L., Xiao J., Sarker S.D. (2020) Introduction of Phytonutrients. In: Xiao, J., Sarker, S., Asakawa, Y. (eds) *Handbook of Dietary Phytochemicals*. Springer, Singapore.

6. Gupta, C., & Prakash, D. Phytonutrients as therapeutic agents. *Journal of Complementary and Integrative Medicine*, 11.3: 151-169. https://doi.org/10.1515/jcim-2013-0021.

7. Carrera-Quintanar, L., López Roa, R.I., Quintero-Fabián, S., Sánchez-Sánchez, M.A., Vizmanos, B., & Ortuño-Sahagún, D. (2018). Phytochemicals That Influence Gut Microbiota as Prophylactics and for the Treatment of Obesity and Inflammatory Diseases. *Mediators of Inflammation*. https://doi.org/10.1155/2018/9734845.

8. Mahapatra, D.K., & Bharti, S.K. (eds.). (2019). *Medicinal Chemistry with Pharmaceutical Product Development* (1st ed.). Apple Academic Press. https://doi.org/10.1201/9780429487842.

9. Hussain, T., Tan, B., Yin, Y., Blachier, F., Tossou, M. C. B., & Rahu, N. (2016). Oxidative Stress and Inflammation: What Polyphenols Can Do for Us?. *Oxidative Medicine and Cellular Longevity*, 2016, 7432797. https://doi.org/10.1155/2016/7432797.

10. Yu, G., Xiang, W., Zhang, T., Zeng, L., Yang, K., & Li, J. (2020). Effectiveness of Boswellia and Boswellia extract for osteoarthritis patients: a systematic review and meta-analysis. *BMC Complementary Medicine and Therapies*, 20(1), 225. https://doi.org/10.1186/s12906-020-02985-6.

11. Matsumoto, Y., Sugioka, Y., Tada, M., Okano, T., Mamoto, K., Inui, K., Habu, D., & Koike, T. (2018). Monounsaturated fatty acids might be key factors in the Mediterranean diet that suppress rheumatoid arthritis disease activity: The TOMORROW study. *Clinical Nutrition*, 37(2), 675-680. https://doi.org/10.1016/j.clnu.2017.02.011.

12. Esposito, K., Marfella, R., Ciotola, M., et al. (2004). Effect of a Mediterranean-Style Diet on Endothelial Dysfunction and Markers of Vascular Inflammation in the Metabolic Syndrome: A Randomized Trial. *JAMA*, 292(12), 1440-1446. https://doi.org/10.1001/jama.292.12.1440.

13. Chrysohoou, C., Panagiotakos, D.B., Pitsavos, C., Das, U.N., & Stefanadis, C. (2004). Adherence to the Mediterranean diet attenuates inflammation and coagulation process in healthy adults: The Attica Study. *Journal of the American College of Cardiology*, 44(1), 152-158. https://doi.org/10.1016/j.jacc.2004.03.039.

14. Lu, B., Driban, J.B., Xu, C., Lapane, K.L., McAlindon, T.E., & Eaton, C.B. (2017). Dietary Fat Intake and Radiographic Progression of Knee Osteoarthritis: Data From the Osteoarthritis Initiative. *Arthritis Care & Research*, 69(3), 368-375. https://doi.org/10.1002/acr.22952.

15. Hathaway, D., Pandav, K., Patel, M., Riva-Moscoso, A., Singh, B.M., Patel, A., Min, Z.C., Singh-Makkar, S., Sana, M. K., Sanchez-Dopazo, R., Desir, R., Fahem, M.M.M., Manella, S., Rodriguez, I., Alvarez, A., & Abreu, R. (2020). Omega 3 Fatty Acids and COVID-19: A Comprehensive Review. *Infection & Chemotherapy*, 52(4), 478-495. https://doi.org/10.3947/ic.2020.52.4.478.

16. Méndez, L., & Medina, I. (2021). Polyphenols and Fish Oils for Improving Metabolic Health: A Revision of the Recent Evidence for Their Combined Nutraceutical Effects. *Molecules*, 26(9), 2438. https://doi.org/10.3390/molecules26092438.

17. Gammone, M.A., Riccioni, G., Parrinello, G., & D'Orazio, N. (2018). Omega-3 Polyunsaturated Fatty Acids: Benefits and Endpoints in Sport. *Nutrients*, 11(1), 46. https://doi.org/10.3390/nu11010046.

18. Boyer, J., & Liu, R.H. (2004). Apple phytochemicals and their health benefits. *Nutrition Journal*, 3, 5. https://doi.org/10.1186/1475-2891-3-5.

19. Anand David, A.V., Arulmoli, R., & Parasuraman, S. (2016). Overviews of Biological Importance of Quercetin: A Bioactive Flavonoid. *Pharmacognosy Reviews*, 10(20), 84-89. https://doi.org/10.4103/0973-7847.194044.

20. Gardi, C., Bauerova, K., Stringa, B., Kuncirova, V., Slovak, L., Ponist, S., Drafi, F., Bezakova, L., Tedesco, I., Acquaviva, A., Bilotto, S., & Russo, G. L. (2015). Quercetin reduced inflammation and increased antioxidant defense in rat adjuvant arthritis. *Archives of Biochemistry and Biophysics*, 583, 150-157. https://doi.org/10.1016/j.abb.2015.08.008.

21. García-Mediavilla, V., Crespo, I., Collado, P. S., Esteller, A., Sánchez-Campos, S., Tuñón, M.J., & González-Gallego, J. (2007). The anti-inflammatory flavones quercetin and kaempferol cause inhibition of inducible nitric oxide synthase, cyclooxygenase-2 and reactive C-protein, and down-regulation of the nuclear factor kappaB pathway in Chang Liver cells. *European Journal of Pharmacology*, 557(2-3), 221-229. https://doi.org/10.1016/j.ejphar.2006.11.014.

22. Vijayalakshmi, A., Ravichandiran, V., Velraj, M., Nirmala, S., & Jayakumari, S. (2012). Screening of flavonoid 'quercetin' from the rhizome of Smilax china Linn. for anti-psoriatic activity. *Asian Pacific Journal of Tropical Biomedicine*, 2(4), 269-275. https://doi.org/10.1016/S2221-1691(12)60021-5.

23. Javadi, F., Ahmadzadeh, A., Eghtesadi, S., Aryaeian, N., Zabihiyeganeh, M., Rahimi Foroushani, A., & Jazayeri, S. (2017). The Effect of Quercetin on Inflammatory Factors and Clinical Symptoms in Women with Rheumatoid Arthritis: A Double-Blind, Randomized Controlled Trial. *Journal of the American College of Nutrition*, 36(1), 9-15. https://doi.org/10.1080/07315724.2016.1140093.

24. Al-Khayri, J.M., Sahana, G.R., Nagella, P., Joseph, B.V., Alessa, F.M., & Al-Mssallem, M.Q. (2022). Flavonoids as Potential Anti-Inflammatory Molecules: A Review. *Molecules*, 27(9), 2901. https://doi.org/10.3390/molecules27092901.

25. Imada, K., Tsuchida, A., Ogawa, K., Sofat, N., Nagase, H., Ito, A., & Sato, T. (2016). Anti-arthritic actions of ß-cryptoxanthin against the degradation of articular cartilage in vivo and in vitro. *Biochemical and Biophysical Research Communications*, 476(4), 352-358. https://doi.org/10.1016/j.bbrc.2016.05.126.

26. Drinkwater, J.M., Tsao, R., Liu, R., Defelice, C., & Wolyn, D.J. (2015). Effects of cooking on rutin and glutathione concentrations and antioxidant activity of green asparagus (Asparagus officinalis) spears. *Journal of Functional Foods*, 12, 342-353. https://doi.org/10.1016/j.jff.2014.11.013.

27. Gürbüz, N., Uluisik, S., Frary, A., Frary, A., & Doganlar, S. (2018). Health benefits and bioactive compounds of eggplant. *Food Chemistry,* 268, 602-610. https://doi.org/10.1016/j.foodchem.2018.06.093.

28. Sidhu, S.,J., Zafar, T.A. (2018). Bioactive compounds in banana fruits and their health benefits, *Food Quality and Safety*, 2(4), 183-188. https://doi.org/10.1093/fqsafe/fyy019.

29. Shinde, T., Perera, A.P., Vemuri, R., Gondalia, S.V., Beale, D.J., Karpe, A.V., Shastri, S., Basheer, W., Southam, B., Eri, R., & Stanley, R. (2020). Synbiotic supplementation with prebiotic green banana resistant starch and probiotic Bacillus coagulans spores ameliorates gut inflammation in mouse model of inflammatory bowel diseases. *European Journal of Nutrition.* https://www.ncbi.nlm.nih.gov/pmc/articles/PMC7669818/.

30. Abdel Aal, N., Kamil, R., Tayal, D., Hamed, R., & Abd El-Azeim, A. (2022). Efficacy of Mediterranean diet on pain and knee range of motion in patients with rheumatoid arthritis: A randomized controlled trial. *International Journal of Health Sciences*, 8718-8731. https://doi.org/10.53730/ijhs.v6nS4.10933. Singletary, K. W. (2018). Basil: A Brief Summary of Potential Health Benefits, *Nutrition Today.* 53 (2), 92-97 doi: 10.1097/NT.0000000000000267.

31. Eftekhar, N., Moghimi, A., & Boskabady, M. H. (2018). The Effects of Ocimum basilicum Extract and Its Constituent, Rosmarinic Acid on Total and Differential Blood WBC, Serum Levels of NO, MDA, Thiol, SOD, and CAT in Ovalbumin Sensitized Rats. *Iranian Journal of Pharmaceutical Research*, 17(4), 1371-1385.

32. Stavropoulos, A., Manthou, E., Nakopoulou, T., Georgakouli, K., Jamurtas, A. (2017). AB1215-HPR Effects of beetroot juice supplementation in endothelial function and markers of inflammation among patients with rheumatoid arthritis. *Annals of the Rheumatic Diseases*, 76:1536-1537. https://ard.bmj.com/content/76/Suppl_2/1536.3

33. Shepherd, A.I., Costello, J.T., Bailey, S.J., Bishop, N., Wadley, A.J., Young-Min, S., Gilchrist, M., Mayes, H., White, D., Gorczynski, P., Saynor, Z.L., Massey, H., & Eglin, C.M. (2019). 'Beet' the cold: beetroot juice supplementation improves peripheral blood flow, endothelial function, and anti-inflammatory status in individuals with Raynaud's phenomenon. *Journal of Applied Physiology* (Bethesda, Md.: 1985), 127(5), 1478-1490. https://doi.org/10.1152/japplphysiol.00292.2019.

34. Chávez-Mendoza, C., Sanchez, E., Muñoz-Marquez, E., Sida-Arreola, J.P., & Flores-Cordova, M.A. (2015). Bioactive Compounds and Antioxidant Activity in Different Grafted Varieties of Bell Pepper. *Antioxidants*, 4(2), 427-446. https://doi.org/10.3390/antiox4020427.

35. Mullins, A.P., & Arjmandi, B.H. (2021). Health Benefits of Plant-Based Nutrition: Focus on Beans in Cardiometabolic Diseases. *Nutrients*, 13(2), 519. https://doi.org/10.3390/nu13020519.

36. Reverri, E.J., Randolph, J.M., Steinberg, F.M., Kappagoda, C.T., Edirisinghe, I., & Burton-Freeman, B.M. (2015). Black Beans, Fiber, and Antioxidant Capacity Pilot Study: Examination of Whole Foods vs. Functional Components on Postprandial Metabolic, Oxidative Stress, and Inflammation in Adults with Metabolic Syndrome. *Nutrients*, 7(8), 6139-6154. https://doi.org/10.3390/nu7085273.

37. Shahi, A., Aslani, S., Ataollahi, M., et al. (2019). The role of magnesium in different inflammatory diseases. *Inflammopharmacol*, 27, 649-661. https://doi.org/10.1007/s10787-019-00603-7.

38. Nutrition Data. Beans, black, mature seeds, cooked, boiled, without salt. https://nutritiondata.self.com/facts/legumes-and-legume-products/4284/2.

39. Umar, S., Golam Sarwar, A.H., Umar, K., Ahmad, N., Sajad, M., Ahmad, S., Katiyar, C.K., & Khan, H.A. (2013). Piperine ameliorates oxidative stress, inflammation and histological outcome in collagen induced arthritis. *Cellular Immunology*, 284(1-2), 51-59. https://doi.org/10.1016/j.cellimm.2013.07.004.

40. Murunikkara, V., Pragasam, S.J., Kodandaraman, G., Sabina, E.P., & Rasool, M. (2012). Anti-inflammatory Effect of Piperine in Adjuvant-induced Arthritic Rats-a Biochemical Approach. *Inflammation*, 35(4), 1348-1356. https://doi.org/10.1007/s10753-012-9448-3.

41. Sabina, E.P., Nagar, S., & Rasool, M. (2011). A Role of Piperine on Monosodium Urate Crystal-Induced Inflammation-An Experimental Model of Gouty Arthritis. *Inflammation*, 34(3), 184-192. https://doi.org/10.1007/s10753-010-9222-3.

42. Jati, G.A.K., Assihhah, N., Wati, A.A., & Salasia, S.I.O. (2022). Immunosuppression by

piperine as a regulator of the NLRP3 inflammasome through MAPK/NF-KB in monosodium urate-induced rat gouty arthritis. *Veterinary World*, 15(2), 288–298. https://doi.org/10.14202/vetworld.2022.288-298.
43. Fairweather-Tait, S.J., Southon S., (2003). Bioavailability of Nutrients, *Encyclopedia of Food Sciences and Nutrition*, Elsevier: 478-484. https://doi.org/10.1016/B0-12-227055-X/00096-1.
44. Hewlings, S.J., & Kalman, D.S. (2017). Curcumin: A Review of Its Effects on Human Health. *Foods*, 6(10), 92. https://doi.org/10.3390/foods6100092.
45. Govers, C., Berkel Kasikci, M., van der Sluis, A.A., & Mes, J.J. (2018). Review of the health effects of berries and their phytochemicals on the digestive and immune systems. *Nutrition Reviews*, 76(1), 29–46. https://doi.org/10.1093/nutrit/nux039.
46. Polak, R., Phillips, E.M., & Campbell, A. (2015). Legumes: Health Benefits and Culinary Approaches to Increase Intake. *Clinical Diabetes: A Publication of the American Diabetes Association*, 33(4), 198–205. https://doi.org/10.2337/diaclin.33.4.198.
47. Li, H. (2020). Evaluation of bioactivity of butternut squash (Cucurbita moschata D.) seeds and skin. *Food Science & Nutrition*, 8(7), 3252–3261. https://doi.org/10.1002/fsn3.1602.
48. Zaccari, F., & Galietta, G. (2015). α-Carotene and β-Carotene Content in Raw and Cooked Pulp of Three Mature Stage Winter Squash 'Type Butternut'. *Foods*, 4(3), 477–486. https://doi.org/10.3390/foods4030477.
49. Kasarello, K., Köhling, I., Kosowska, A., Pucia, K., Lukasik, A., Cudnoch-Jedrzejewska, A., Paczek, L., Zielenkiewicz, U., & Zielenkiewicz, P. (2022). The Anti-Inflammatory Effect of Cabbage Leaves Explained by the Influence of bol-miRNA172a on FAN Expression. *Frontiers in Pharmacology*, 13, 846830. https://doi.org/10.3389/fphar.2022.846830.
50. Seong, G-U., Hwang, I-W., & Chung, S-K. (2016). Antioxidant capacities and polyphenolics of Chinese cabbage (Brassica rapa L. ssp. Pekinensis) leaves. *Food Chemistry*, 199, 612–618. https://doi.org/10.1016/j.foodchem.2015.12.066.
51. Lee, Y., Kim, S., Yang, B., Lim, C., Kim, J-H., Kim, H., & Cho, S. (2018). Anti-inflammatory Effects of Brassica oleracea Var. capitata L. (Cabbage) Methanol Extract in Mice with Contact Dermatitis. *Pharmacognosy Magazine*, 14(54), 174–179. https://doi.org/10.4103/pm.pm_152_17.
52. Riccio, B.V.F., Spósito, L., Carvalho, G.C., Ferrari, P.C., & Chorilli, M. (2020). Resveratrol isoforms and conjugates: A review from biosynthesis in plants to elimination from the human body. *Archiv der Pharmazie*, 353(12), e2000146. https://doi.org/10.1002/ardp.202000146.
53. Nguyen, C., Savouret, J-F., Widerak, M., Corvol, M-T., & Rannou, F. (2017). Resveratrol, Potential Therapeutic Interest in Joint Disorders: A Critical Narrative Review. *Nutrients*, 9(1), 45. https://doi.org/10.3390/nu9010045.
54. Riveiro-Naveira, R.R., Loureiro, J., Valcárcel-Ares, M.N., López-Peláez, E., Centeno-Cortés, A., Vaamonde-García, C., Hermida-Carballo, L., Blanco, F.J., & López-Armada, M. J. (2014). Anti-inflammatory effect of resveratrol as a dietary supplement in an antigen-induced arthritis rat model. *Osteoarthritis and Cartilage*, 22. S290. 10.1016/j.joca.2014.02.539. https://www.oarsijournal.com/article/S1063-4584(14)00579-2/pdf.
55. Wei, Y., Jia, J., Jin, X., Tong, W., & Tian, H. (2018). Resveratrol ameliorates inflammatory damage and protects against osteoarthritis in a rat model of osteoarthritis. *Molecular Medicine Reports*, 17(1), 1493–1498. https://doi.org/10.3892/mmr.2017.8036.
56. Marouf, B.H., Hussain, S.A., Ali, Z.S., & Ahmmad, R.S. (2018). Resveratrol Supplementation Reduces Pain and Inflammation in Knee Osteoarthritis Patients Treated with Meloxicam: A Randomized Placebo-Controlled Study. *Journal of Medicinal Food*, 10.1089/jmf.2017.4176. https://pubmed.ncbi.nlm.nih.gov/30160612/.
57. Khojah, H.M., Ahmed, S., Abdel-Rahman, M.S., & Elhakeim, E.H. (2018). Resveratrol as an effective adjuvant therapy in the management of rheumatoid arthritis: a clinical study. *Clinical Rheumatology*, 37(8), 2035–2042. https://doi.org/10.1007/s10067-018-4080-8.
58. Kazemian, M., Abad, M., Haeri, M.R., Ebrahimi, M., & Heidari, R. (2015). Anti-diabetic effect of Capparis spinosa L. root extract in diabetic rats. *Avicenna Journal of Phytomedicine*, 5(4), 325–332. https://pubmed.ncbi.nlm.nih.gov/26445712/.
59. Nabavi, S.F., Maggi, F., Daglia, M., Habtemariam, S., Rastrelli, L., & Nabavi, S.M. (2016). Pharmacological Effects of Capparis spinosa L. *Phytotherapy Research*, 30(11), 1733–1744. https://doi.org/10.1002/ptr.5684.
60. Eddouks, M., Lemhadri, A., Hebi, M., El Hidani, A., Zeggwagh, N. A., El Bouhali, B., Hajji, L., & Burcelin, R. (2017). Capparis spinosa L. aqueous extract evokes antidiabetic effect in streptozotocin-induced diabetic mice. *Avicenna Journal of Phytomedicine*, 7(2), 191–198. https://www.ncbi.nlm.nih.gov/pmc/articles/PMC5355824/.
61. Tlili, N., Khaldi, A., Triki, S., & Munné-Bosch, S. (2010). Phenolic Compounds and Vitamin Antioxidants of Caper (Capparis spinosa). *Plant Foods for Human Nutrition* (Dordrecht, Netherlands), 65(3), 260–265. https://doi.org/10.1007/s11130-010-0180-6.
62. Panico, A.M., Cardile, V., Garufi, F., Puglia, C., Bonina, F., & Ronsisvalle, G. (2005). Protective effect of Capparis spinosa on chondrocytes. *Life Sciences*, 77(20), 2479–2488. https://doi.org/10.1016/j.lfs.2004.12.051.
63. Pattison, D.J., Symmons, D.P.M., Lunt, M., Welch, A., Bingham, S.A., Day, N.E., & Silman, A.J. (2005). Dietary ß-cryptoxanthin and inflammatory polyarthritis: results from a population-based prospective study. *The American Journal of Clinical Nutrition*, 82(2), 451–455. https://doi.org/10.1093/ajcn.82.2.451.
64. Bolling, B.W., Chen, C-Y. O., McKay, D.L., & Blumberg, J.B. (2011). Tree nut phytochemicals: composition, antioxidant capacity, bioactivity, impact factors. A systematic review of almonds, Brazils, cashews, hazelnuts, macadamias, pecans, pine nuts, pistachios and walnuts. *Nutrition Research Reviews*, 24(2), 244–275. https://doi.org/10.1017/S095442241100014X.
65. Cordaro, M., Siracusa, R., Fusco, R., D'Amico, R., Peritore, A.F., Gugliandolo, E., Genovese, T., Scuto, M., Crupi, R., Mandalari, G., Cuzzocrea, S., Di Paola, R., & Impellizzeri, D. (2020). Cashew (Anacardium occidentale L.) Nuts Counteract Oxidative Stress and Inflammation in an Acute Experimental Model of Carrageenan-Induced Paw Edema. *Antioxidants*, 9(8), 660. https://doi.org/10.3390/antiox9080660.
66. Moon, S. J., Jhun, J., Ryu, J., Kwon, J. Y., Kim, S-Y., Jung, K., Cho, M-L., & Min, J-K. (2021). The anti-arthritis effect of sulforaphane, an activator of Nrf2, is associated with inhibition of both B cell differentiation and the production of inflammatory cytokines. PloS one, 16(2), e0245986. https://doi.org/10.1371/journal.pone.0245986.
67. Silva Rodrigues, J.F., Silva E Silva, C., França Muniz, T., de Aquino, A.F., Neuza da Silva Nina, L., Fialho Sousa, N.C., Nascimento da Silva, L.C., de Souza, B., da Penha, T.A., Abreu-Silva, A.L., de Sá, J.C., Soares Fernandes, E., & Grisotto, M. (2018). Sulforaphane Modulates Joint Inflammation in a Murine Model of Complete Freund's Adjuvant-Induced Mono-Arthritis. *Molecules*, 23(5), 988. https://doi.org/10.3390/molecules23050988.
68. Monteiro do Nascimento, M.H., Ambrosio, F.N., Ferraraz, D.C., Windisch-Neto, H., Querobino, S.M., Nascimento-Sales, M., Alberto-Silva, C., Christoffolete, M.A., Franco, M.K.K.D., Kent, B., Yokaichiya, F., Lombello, C.B., & de Araujo, D.R. (2021). Sulforaphane-loaded hyaluronic acid-poloxamer hybrid hydrogel enhances cartilage protection in osteoarthritis models. *Materials Science & Engineering*: C, 128, 112345. https://doi.org/10.1016/j.msec.2021.112345.
69. Liang, J., Jahraus, B., Balta, E., Ziegler, J. D., Hübner, K., Blank, N., Niesler, B., Wabnitz, G. H., & Samstag, Y. (2018). Sulforaphane Inhibits Inflammatory Responses of Primary Human T-Cells by Increasing ROS and Depleting Glutathione. *Frontiers in Immunology*, 9, 2584. https://doi.org/10.3389/fimmu.2018.02584.
70. Kelley, D.S., Adkins, Y., & Laugero, K.D. (2018). A Review of the Health Benefits of Cherries. *Nutrients*, 10(3), 368. https://doi.org/10.3390/nu10030368.
71. Vírgen Gen, J.J., Guzmán-Gerónimo, R.I., Martínez-Flores, K., Martínez-Nava, G.A., Fernández-Torres, J., & Zamudio-Cuevas, Y. (2020). Cherry extracts attenuate inflammation and oxidative stress triggered by monosodium urate crystals in THP-1 cells. *Journal of Food Biochemistry*, e13403. https://doi.org/10.1111/jfbc.13403.
72. Zhang, Y., Neogi, T., Chen, C., Chaisson, C., Hunter, D.J., & Choi, H.K. (2012). Cherry Consumption and Decreased Risk of Recurrent Gout Attacks. *Arthritis & Rheumatism*, 64(12), 4004-4011. https://doi.org/10.1002/art.34677.
73. Chen, P-E., Liu, C-Y., Chien, W-H., Chien, C-W., & Tung, T-H. (2019). Effectiveness of Cherries in Reducing Uric Acid and Gout: A Systematic Review. Evidence-Based Complementary and Alternative Medicine 2019, 9896757. https://doi.org/10.1155/2019/9896757.
74. Kulczyński, B., Kobus-Cisowska, J., Taczanowski, M., Kmiecik, D., & Gramza-Michałowska, A. (2019). The Chemical Composition and Nutritional Value of Chia Seeds-Current State of Knowledge. *Nutrients*, 11(6), 1242. https://doi.org/10.3390/nu11061242.
75. Muñoz, A.,L., Cobos, A., Diaz, O., Aguilera, J.,M. (2013). Chia Seed (Salvia hispanica): An Ancient Grain and a New Functional Food. *Food Reviews International*, 29:4. 394-408. DOI: 10.1080/87559129.2013.818014.
76. Taga, M.S., Miller, E.E. & Pratt, D.E. (1984). Chia seeds as a source of natural lipid antioxidants. *Journal of the American Oil Chemists' Society*, 61, 928-931. https://doi.org/10.1007/BF02542169.
77. Koner, S., Dash, P., Priya, V., Rajeswari, D., V. (2019). 15 - Natural and Artificial Beverages: Exploring the Pros and Cons, *Natural Beverages*, 427-445, https://doi.org/10.1016/B978-0-12-816689-5.00015-8.
78. Suri, S., Passi, J.S., Goyat, J. (2016). Chia Seed (Salvia Hispanica L.) - A New Age Functional Food. 4th International Conference on Recent Innovations in Science Engineering and Management.
79. Alfredo, V-O, Gabriel, R., et al. (2009). Physicochemical properties of a fibrous fraction from chia (Salvia hispanica L.). *LWT - Food Science and Technology*, 42(1), 168-173, https://doi.org/10.1016/j.lwt.2008.05.012.
80. Pahan, S., & Pahan, K. (2020). Can cinnamon spice down autoimmune diseases?. *Journal of Clinical & Experimental Immunology*, 5(6), 252–258. https://www.ncbi.nlm.nih.gov/pmc/articles/PMC7720887/.
81. Shishehbor, F., Safar, M.,R., Rajaei, E., Haghighizadeh, M-H. (2018). Cinnamon Consumption Improves Clinical Symptoms and Inflammatory Markers in Women With Rheumatoid Arthritis. *Journal of the American College of Nutrition*, 37:8, 685-690, DOI: 10.1080/07315724.2018.1460733
82. Li, X., Wang, Y. (2020). Cinnamaldehyde Attenuates the Progression of Rheumatoid Arthritis through Down-Regulation of PI3K/AKT Signaling Pathway. *Inflammation*, 43, 1729-1741. https://doi.org/10.1007/s10753-020-01246-5.
83. Gruenwald, J., Freder, J., & Armbruester, N. (2010). Cinnamon and Health. *Critical Reviews in Food Science and Nutrition*, 50(9), 822-834. https://doi.org/10.1080/10408390902773052.
84. Rathi, B., Bodhankar, S., Mohan, V., & Thakurdesai, P. (2013). Ameliorative Effects of a Polyphenolic Fraction of Cinnamomum zeylanicum L. Bark in Animal Models of Inflammation and Arthritis. *Scientia Pharmaceutica*, 81(2), 567–589. https://doi.org/10.3797/scipharm.1301-16.
85. Lynch, S.R., & Cook, J.D. (1980). Interaction of vitamin C and iron. *Annals of the New York Academy of Sciences*, 355, 32–44. https://doi.org/10.1111/j.1749-6632.1980.tb21325.x.
86. Shen, C-L., Smith, B.J., Lo, D-F., Chyu, M-C., Dunn, D.M., Chen, C-H., & Kwun, I-S. (2012). Dietary polyphenols and mechanisms of osteoarthritis. *The Journal of Nutritional Biochemistry*, 23(11), 1367-1377. https://doi.org/10.1016/j.jnutbio.2012.04.001.
87. Okwu, D. E. (2008). A Review Citrus Fruits: A Rich Source Of Phytochemicals And Their Roles In Human Health. *International Journal of Chemical Sciences*,: 6(2), 451-471.
88. de Cássia Ortiz, A., Fideles, S.O.M., Reis, C.H.B., Bellini, M.Z., Pereira, E. de S.B.M., Pilon, J.P.G., de Marchi, M.Â., Detregiachi, C.R.P., Flato, U.A.P., Trazzi, B.F. de M., Pagani, B.T., Ponce, J.B., Gardizani, T.P., Veronez, F. de S., Buchaim, D.V., & Buchaim, R.L. (2022). Therapeutic Effects of Citrus Flavonoids Neohesperidin, Hesperidin and Its Aglycone, Hesperetin on Bone Health. *Biomolecules*, 12(5), 626. https://doi.org/10.3390/biom12050626.
89. Manchope, M., F., Ferraz, C. R., et al. (2022). Chapter 38 - Therapeutic Role of Naringenin to Alleviate Inflammatory Pain, Treatments, Mechanisms, and Adverse Reactions of Anesthetics and Analgesics,. *Academic Press*, 443-455, https://doi.org/10.1016/B978-0-12-820237-1.00038-7.
90. Miles, E.A., & Calder, P.C. (2021). Effects of Citrus Fruit Juices and Their Bioactive Components on Inflammation and Immunity: A Narrative Review. *Frontiers in Immunology*, 12, 712608. https://doi.org/10.3389/fimmu.2021.712608.
91. Montoya, T., Sánchez-Hidalgo, M., Castejón, M.L., Rosillo, M.Á., González-Benjumea, A., & Alarcón-de-la-Lastra, C. (2021). Dietary Oleocanthal Supplementation Prevents Inflammation and Oxidative Stress in Collagen-Induced Arthritis in Mice. *Antioxidants* ,10(5), 650. https://doi.org/10.3390/antiox10050650.
92. Lucas, L., Russell, A., & Keast, R. (2011). Molecular Mechanisms of Inflammation. Anti-Inflammatory Benefits of Virgin Olive Oil and the Phenolic Compound Oleocanthal. *Current Pharmaceutical Design*, 17(8), 754-768. https://doi.org/10.2174/138161211795428911.
93. Vilaplana-Pérez C, Auñón D, García-Flores, L.A., & Gil-Izquierdo A. (2014). Hydroxytyrosol and potential uses in cardiovascular diseases, cancer, and AIDS. *Frontiers in Nutrition*, 1:18. doi: 10.3389/fnut.2014.00018.
94. EFSA Panel on Dietetic Products, Nutrition and Allergies (NDA); Scientific Opinion on the substantiation of health claims related to polyphenols in olive and protection of LDL particles from oxidative damage (ID 1333, 1638, 1639, 1696, 2865), maintenance of normal blood HDL-cholesterol concentrations (ID 1639), maintenance of normal blood pressure (ID 3781), 'anti-inflammatory properties' (ID 1882), 'contributes to the upper respiratory tract health' (ID 3468), 'can help to maintain a normal function of gastrointestinal tract' (3779), and 'contributes to body defences against external agents' (ID 3467) pursuant to Article 13(1) of Regulation (EC) No 1924/2006. *EFSA Journal*: 2011; 9(4):2033 [25 pp.]. doi:10.2903/j.efsa.2011.2033.
95. Scotece, M., Gómez, R., Conde, J., Lopez, V., Gómez-Reino, J.J., Lago, F., Smith III, A.B., &

Gualillo, O. (2012). Further evidence for the anti-inflammatory activity of oleocanthal: inhibition of MIP-1α and IL-6 in J774 macrophages and in ATDC5 chondrocytes. *Life Sciences*, 91(23-24), 1229-1235. https://doi.org/10.1016/j.lfs.2012.09.012.
96. Carito, V., Ciafrè, S., Tarani, L., Ceccanti, M., Natella, F., Iannitelli, A., Tirassa, P., Chaldakov, G. N., Ceccanti, M., Boccardo, C., & Fiore, M. (2015). TNF-α and IL-10 modulation induced by polyphenols extracted by olive pomace in a mouse model of paw inflammation. *Annali dell'Istituto Superiore di Sanita*, 51(4), 382-386. https://doi.org/10.4415/ANN_15_04_21.
97. Rosillo, M.Á., Alcaraz, M.J., Sánchez-Hidalgo, M., Fernández-Bolaños, J.G., Alarcón-de-la-Lastra, C., & Ferrándiz, M.L. (2014). Anti-inflammatory and joint protective effects of extra-virgin olive-oil polyphenol extract in experimental arthritis. *The Journal of Nutritional Biochemistry*, 25(12), 1275-1281. https://doi.org/10.1016/j.jnutbio.2014.07.006.
98. Rosillo, M.A., Sánchez-Hidalgo, M., González-Benjumea, A., Fernández-Bolaños, J.G., Lubberts, E., & Alarcón-de-la-Lastra, C. (2015). Preventive effects of dietary hydroxytyrosol acetate, an extra virgin olive oil polyphenol in murine collagen-induced arthritis. *Molecular Nutrition & Food Research*, 59(12), 2537-2546. https://doi.org/10.1002/mnfr.201500304.
99. Silva, S., Sepodes, B., Rocha, J., Direito, R., Fernandes, A., Brites, D., Freitas, M., Fernandes, E., Bronze, M.R., & Figueira, M.E. (2015). Protective effects of hydroxytyrosol-supplemented refined olive oil in animal models of acute inflammation and rheumatoid arthritis. *The Journal of Nutritional Biochemistry*, 26(4), 360-368. https://doi.org/10.1016/j.jnutbio.2014.11.011.
100. Impellizzeri, D., Esposito, E., Mazzon, E., Paterniti, I., Di Paola, R., Morittu, V.M., Procopio, A., Britti, D., & Cuzzocrea, S. (2011). Oleuropein Aglycone, an Olive Oil Compound, Ameliorates Development of Arthritis Caused by Injection of Collagen Type II in Mice. *The Journal of Pharmacology and Experimental Therapeutics*, 339(3), 859-869. https://doi.org/10.1124/jpet.111.182808.
101. Rosillo, M.A., Sánchez-Hidalgo, M., Sánchez-Fidalgo, S., Aparicio-Soto, M., Villegas, I., & Alarcón-de-la-Lastra, C. (2016). Dietary extra-virgin olive oil prevents inflammatory response and cartilage matrix degradation in murine collagen-induced arthritis. *European Journal of Nutrition*, 55(1), 315-325. https://doi.org/10.1007/s00394-015-0850-0.
102. Ángeles Rosillo, M., Sánchez-Hidalgo, M., Castejón, M.L., Montoya, T., González-Benjumea, A., Fernández-Bolaños, J.G., Alarcón-de-la-Lastra, C. (2017). Extra-virgin olive oil phenols hydroxytyrosol and hydroxytyrosol acetate, down-regulate the production of mediators involved in joint erosion in human synovial cells. *Journal of Functional Foods*, 36, 27-33, https://doi.org/10.1016/j.jff.2017.06.041.
103. Dehghani, S., Alipoor, E., Salimzadeh, A., Yaseri, M., Hosseini, M., Feinle-Bisset, C., & Hosseinzadeh-Attar, M.J. (2018). The effect of a garlic supplement on the pro-inflammatory adipocytokines, resistin and tumor necrosis factor-alpha, and on pain severity, in overweight or obese women with knee osteoarthritis. *Phytomedicine: International Journal of Phytotherapy and Phytopharmacology*, 48, 70-75. https://doi.org/10.1016/j.phymed.2018.04.060.
104. Williams, F.M.K., Skinner, J., Spector, T. D., Cassidy, A., Clark, I.M., Davidson, R.M., & MacGregor, A.J. (2010). Dietary garlic and hip osteoarthritis: evidence of a protective effect and putative mechanism of action. *BMC Musculoskeletal Disorders*, 11, 280. https://doi.org/10.1186/1471-2474-11-280.
105. Borlinghaus, J., Albrecht, F., Gruhlke, M.C. H., Nwachukwu, I.D., & Slusarenko, A.J. (2014). Allicin: Chemistry and Biological Properties. *Molecules*, 19(8), 12591-12618. https://doi.org/10.3390/molecules190812591.
106. Nutrition Value. Garlic, raw. https://www.nutritionvalue.org/Garlic%2C_raw_nutritional_value.html
107. Semwal, R.B., Semwal, D.K., Combrinck, S., & Viljoen, A.M. (2015). Gingerols and shogaols: important nutraceutical principles from ginger. *Phytochemistry*, 117, 554-568. https://doi.org/10.1016/j.phytochem.2015.07.012.
108. Kumar, S., Saxena, K., et al. (2013). Anti-inflammatory action of ginger: a critical review in anemia of inflammation and its future aspects, *International Journal of Herbal Medicine*, 1 (4), 16-20. http://www.florajournal.com/archives/2013/vol1issue4/PartA/2.1.pdf.
109. Shishodia, S., Sethi, G., & Aggarwal, B. B. (2005). Curcumin: Getting Back to the Roots. *Annals of the New York Academy of Sciences*, 1056, 206-217. https://doi.org/10.1196/annals.1352.010.
110. Levy, A.S.A., Simon, O., Shelly, J., & Gardener, M. (2006). 6-Shogaol reduced chronic inflammatory response in the knees of rats treated with complete Freund's adjuvant. *BMC Pharmacology*, 6, 12. https://doi.org/10.1186/1471-2210-6-12.
111. Sharma, J.N., Srivastava, K.C., & Gan, E.K. (1994). Suppressive Effects of Eugenol and Ginger Oil on Arthritic Rats. *Pharmacology*, 49(5), 314-318. https://doi.org/10.1159/000139248.
112. Pragasam, S.J., Kumar, S., Bhoumik, M., Sabina, E. P., Rasool, M. (2011). 6-Gingerol, an active ingredient of ginger, suppresses monosodium ureate crystal-induced inflammation: an in vivo and in vitro evaluation. *Annals of Biological Research*, 2(3), 200-208.
113. Funk, J.L., Frye, J.B., Oyarzo, J.N., & Timmermann, B.N. (2009). Comparative Effects of Two Gingerol-Containing Zingiber officinale Extracts on Experimental Rheumatoid Arthritis. *Journal of Natural Products*, 72(3), 403-407. https://doi.org/10.1021/np8006183
114. Srivastava, K.C., & Mustafa, T. (1992). Ginger (Zingiber officinale) in rheumatism and musculoskeletal disorders. *Medical Hypotheses*, 39(4), 342-348. https://doi.org/10.1016/0306-9877(92)90059-l.
115. Rondanelli, M., Fossari, F., Vecchio, V., Gasparri, C., Peroni, G., Spadaccini, D., Riva, A., Petrangolini, G., Iannello, G., Nichetti, M., Infantino, V., & Perna, S. (2020). Clinical trials on pain lowering effect of ginger: a narrative review. Phytotherapy Research, 34(11), 2843-2856. https://doi.org/10.1002/ptr.6730.
116. Ahmed, S.H., Gonda, T., & Hunyadi, A. (2021). Medicinal chemistry inspired by ginger: exploring the chemical space around 6-gingerol. *RSC Advances*, 11(43), 26687-26699. https://doi.org/10.1039/d1ra04227k.
117. Khan, F., Nayab, M., & Ansari, A.N. (2021). Zanjabeel (Zingiber officinale Roscoe.): An Evidence-Based Review of Anti-nociceptive, Anti- inflammatory, Antioxidant, and Antimicrobial Properties. *Journal of Complementary and Alternative Medical Research*. 15. 26-35. 10.9734/JOCAMR/2021/v15i330269.
118. Aryaeian, N., Mahmoudi, M., Shahram, F., Poursani, S., Jamshidi, F., & Tavakoli, H. (2019). The effect of ginger supplementation on IL2, TNFα, and IL1β cytokines gene expression levels in patients with active rheumatoid arthritis: A randomized controlled trial. *Medical Journal of the Islamic Republic of Iran*, 33, 154. https://www.ncbi.nlm.nih.gov/pmc/articles/PMC7137811/.
119. Aryaeian, N., Shahram, F., Mahmoudi, M., Tavakoli, H., Yousefi, B., Arablou, T., & Jafari Karegar, S. (2019). The effect of ginger supplementation on some immunity and inflammation intermediate genes expression in patients with active Rheumatoid Arthritis. *Gene*, 698, 179-185. https://doi.org/10.1016/j.gene.2019.01.048.
120. Ramadan, G., Al-Kahtani, M.A., & El-Sayed, W.M. (2011). Anti-inflammatory and anti-oxidant properties of Curcuma longa (turmeric) versus Zingiber officinale (ginger) rhizomes in rat adjuvant-induced arthritis. *Inflammation*, 34(4), 291-301.
121. Prasad, S. & Aggarwal, B.B. (2014). Chronic Diseases Caused by Chronic Inflammation Require Chronic Treatment: Anti-inflammatory Role of Dietary Spices. *Journal of Clinical & Cellular Immunology.*
122. Rehman, R., Akram, M., Akhtar, N., et al. (2001). Zingiber officinale Roscoe (pharmacological activity). *Journal of Medicinal Plants Research*, 5(3): 344-348.
123. Zakeri, Z., Izadi, S., Bari, Z., Soltani, F., Narouie, B., Ghasemi-rad, M. (2011). Evaluating the effects of ginger extract on knee pain, stiffness and difficulty in patients with knee osteoarthritis. *Journal of Medicinal Plants Research*, 5(15), 3375-3379.
124. Feng, T., Su, J., Ding, Z.H., Zheng, Y.T., Li, Y., Leng, Y., & Liu, J.K. (2011). Chemical constituents and their bioactivities of 'Tongling White Ginger' (Zingiber officinale). *Journal of Agricultural and Food Chemistry*, 59(21), 11690-11695. https://doi.org/10.1021/jf202544w.
125. Altman, R.D., Marcussen, K.C. (2001). Effects of a ginger extract on knee pain in patients with osteoarthritis. *Arthritis and Rheumatism*, 44(11), 2531-8. https://doi.org/10.1002/1529-0131(200111)44:11<2531::aid-art433>3.0.co;2-j.
126. Haghighi, M., Khalvat, A., Toliat, T., Jallaei, S. (2005). Comparing the effects of ginger (Zingiber officinale) extract and ibuprofen on patients with osteoarthritis. *Archives of Iranian Medicine*, 8(4), 267-71.
127. Aryaeian, N., Mahmoudi, M., Shahram, F., Poursani, S., Jamshidi, F., & Tavakoli, H. The effect of ginger supplementation on IL2, TNFα, and IL1β cytokines gene expression levels in patients with active rheumatoid arthritis: A randomized controlled trial. *Medical Journal of the Islamic Republic of Iran*, 2019 December 27; 33(154). doi: 10.34171/mjiri.33.154. PMID: 32280660; PMCID: PMC7137811.
128. Yoshikawa, M., Hatakeyama, S., Chatani, N., Nishino, Y., & Yamahara, J. (1993). Yakugaku zasshi qualitative and quantitative analysis of ginger bioactive components using high performance liquid chromatography and gas chromatography, component variation in ginger quality evaluation and processing preparation. *Journal of the Pharmaceutical Society of Japan*, 113(4), 307-315. https://doi.org/10.1248/yakushi1947.113.4_307.
129. Al-Nahain, A., Jahan, R., & Rahmatullah, M. (2014). Zingiber officinale: A Potential Plant against Rheumatoid Arthritis. *Arthritis*, 2014, 159089. https://doi.org/10.1155/2014/159089.
130. Di Renzo, L., Merra, G., Botta, R., Gualtieri, P., Manzo, A., Perrone, M. A., Mazza, M., Cascapera, S., & De Lorenzo, A. (2017). Post-prandial effects of hazelnut-enriched high fat meal on LDL oxidative status, oxidative and inflammatory gene expression of healthy subjects: a randomized trial. *European Review for Medical and Pharmacological Sciences*, 21(7), 1610-1626.
131. Nutrition Data. Nuts, hazelnuts or filberts. https://nutritiondata.self.com/facts/nut-and-seed-products/3116/2 and https://www.nutritionvalue.org/Nuts%2C_hazelnuts_or_filberts_nutritional_value.html.
132. Rodriguez-Leyva, D., & Pierce, G.N. (2010). The cardiac and haemostatic effects of dietary hempseed. *Nutrition & Metabolism*, 7, 32. https://doi.org/10.1186/1743-7075-7-32.
133. Lockwood, G.B. (2009). Chapter 32 - The plant nutraceuticals. Trease and Evans' Pharmacognosy (Sixteenth Edition), W.B. Saunders, 459-470, https://doi.org/10.1016/B978-0-7020-2933-2.00032-0.
134. Cruz Rosas, E., Barbosa Correa, L., & das Graças Henriques, M. Chapter 28 - Anti-inflammatory Properties of Schinus terebinthifolius and Its Use in Arthritic Conditions. *Bioactive Food as Dietary Interventions for Arthritis and Related Inflammatory Diseases* (Second Edition). Academic Press. 489-505, https://doi.org/10.1016/B978-0-12-813820-5.00028-3.
135. Lee, C-J, Moon, S-J, Jeong, J-H., et al. (2018). Kaempferol targeting on the fibroblast growth factor receptor 3-ribosomal S6 kinase 2 signaling axis prevents the development of rheumatoid arthritis. *Cell Death & Diseasse*, 9, 401. https://doi.org/10.1038/s41419-018-0433-0.
136. Devi, K.P., Malar, D.S., Nabavi, S.F., Sureda, A., Xiao, J., Nabavi, S.M., & Daglia, M. (2015). Kaempferol and inflammation: From chemistry to medicine. *Pharmacological Research*, 99, 1-10. https://doi.org/10.1016/j.phrs.2015.05.002.
137. Pan, D., Li, N., Liu, Y., Xu, Q., Liu, Q., You, Y., Wei, Z., Jiang, Y., Liu, M., Guo, T., Cai, X., Liu, X., Wang, Q., Liu, M., Lei, X., Zhang, M., Zhao, X., & Lin, C. (2018). Kaempferol inhibits the migration and invasion of rheumatoid arthritis fibroblast-like synoviocytes by blocking activation of the MAPK pathway. *International Immunopharmacology*, 55, 174-182. https://doi.org/10.1016/j.intimp.2017.12.011.
138. Lin, F., Luo, X., Tsun, A., Li, Z., Li, D., & Li, B. (2015). Kaempferol enhances the suppressive function of Treg cells by inhibiting FOXP3 phosphorylation. *International Immunopharmacology*, 28(2), 859-865. https://doi.org/10.1016/j.intimp.2015.03.044.
139. Jiang, R., Hao, P., Yu, G., Liu, C., Yu, C., Huang, Y., & Wang, Y. (2019). Kaempferol protects chondrogenic ATDC5 cells against inflammatory injury triggered by lipopolysaccharide through down-regulating miR-146a. *International Immunopharmacology*, 69, 373-381. https://doi.org/10.1016/j.intimp.2019.02.014.
140. Zhuang, Z., Ye, G., & Huang, B. (2017). Kaempferol Alleviates the Interleukin-1β-Induced Inflammation in Rat Osteoarthritis Chondrocytes via Suppression of NF-κB. *Medical Science Monitor*, 23, 3925-3931. https://doi.org/10.12659/msm.902491.
141. Ganesan, K., & Xu, B. (2017). Polyphenol-Rich Lentils and Their Health Promoting Effects. *International Journal of Molecular Sciences*, 18(11), 2390. https://doi.org/10.3390/ijms18112390.
142. Girish, T.K., Pratape, V.M., Prasada Rao, U.J.S., (2012). Nutrient distribution, phenolic acid composition, antioxidant and alpha-glucosidase inhibitory potentials of black gram (Vigna mungo L.) and its milled by-products. *Food Research International*, 46(1), 370-377, https://doi.org/10.1016/j.foodres.2011.12.026.
143. Shubrook, S. (2021). Top 5 health benefits of maca. *BBC Good Food*. https://www.bbcgoodfood.com/howto/guide/health-benefits-maca-powder
144. Scepankova, H., Saraiva, J.A., Estevinho, L. M. (2017). Honey Health Benefits and Uses in Medicine. In: Alvarez-Suarez, J. (eds). *Bee Products - Chemical and Biological Properties*. Springer, Cham. https://doi.org/10.1007/978-3-319-59689-1_4.
145. Romário-Silva, D., Lazarini, J.G., Franchin, M., de Alencar, S.M., & Rosalen, P.L. (2022). Brazilian Organic Honey from Atlantic Rainforest Decreases Inflammatory Process in Mice. *Veterinary Sciences*, 9(6), 268. https://doi.org/10.3390/vetsci9060268.
146. Liu, M., Zhou, X., Zhou, L., Liu, Z., Yuan, J., Cheng, J., Zhao, J., Wu, L., Li, H., Qiu, H., & Xu, J. (2018). Carnosic acid inhibits inflammation response and joint destruction on osteoclasts, fibroblast-like synoviocytes, and collagen-induced arthritis rats. *Journal of Cellular Physiology*, 233(8), 6291-6303. https://doi.org/10.1002/jcp.26517.
147. Vázquez-Fresno, R., Rosana, A.R.R., Sajed, T., Onookome-Okome, T., Wishart, N.A., & Wishart, D.S. (2019). Herbs and Spices - Biomarkers of Intake Based on Human Intervention Studies - A

Systematic Review. *Genes & Nutrition*, 14, 18. https://doi.org/10.1186/s12263-019-0636-8.
148. Poeckel, D., Greiner, C., Verhoff, M., Rau, O., Tausch, L., Hörnig, C., Steinhilber, D., Schubert-Zsilavecz, M., & Werz, O. (2008). Carnosic acid and carnosol potently inhibit human 5-lipoxygenase and suppress pro-inflammatory responses of stimulated human polymorphonuclear leukocytes. *Biochemical Pharmacology*, 76(1), 91-97. https://doi.org/10.1016/j.bcp.2008.04.013.
149. Lo, A-H., Liang, Y-C., Lin-Shiau, S-Y., Ho, C-T., & Lin, J-K. (2002). Carnosol, an antioxidant in rosemary, suppresses inducible nitric oxide synthase through down-regulating nuclear factor-kappaB in mouse macrophages. *Carcinogenesis*, 23(6), 983-991. https://doi.org/10.1093/carcin/23.6.983.
150. Sanchez, C., Horcajada, M-N., Membrez Scalfo, F., Ameye, L., Offord, E., & Henrotin, Y. (2015). Carnosol Inhibits Pro-Inflammatory and Catabolic Mediators of Cartilage Breakdown in Human Osteoarthritic Chondrocytes and Mediates Cross-Talk between Subchondral Bone Osteoblasts and Chondrocytes. *PloS one*, 10(8), e0136118. https://doi.org/10.1371/journal.pone.0136118.
151. Ishitobi, H., Sanada, Y., Kato, Y., Ikuta, Y., Shibata, S., Yamasaki, S., Lotz, M.K., Matsubara, K., Miyaki, S., & Adachi, N. (2018). Carnosic acid attenuates cartilage degeneration through induction of heme oxygenase-1 in human articular chondrocytes. *European Journal of Pharmacology*, 830, 1-8. https://doi.org/10.1016/j.ejphar.2018.04.018.
152. Wang, J., Yang, G., Hua, Y-X, Sun, T., Gao, C., Xia, Q., Li, B. (2016). Carnosol ameliorates monosodium iodoacetate-induced osteoarthritis by targeting NF-κB and Nrf-2 in primary rat chondrocytes. *Journal of Applied Biomedicine*, 14(4): 307-314, https://doi.org/10.1016/j.jab.2016.05.001.
153. Schwager, J., Richard, N., Fowler, A., Seifert, N., & Raederstorff, D. (2016). Carnosol and Related Substances Modulate Chemokine and Cytokine Production in Macrophages and Chondrocytes. *Molecules*, 21(4), 465. https://doi.org/10.3390/molecules21040465.
154. Xia, G., Wang, X., Sun, H., Qin, Y., & Fu, M. (2017). Carnosic acid (CA) attenuates collagen-induced arthritis in db/db mice via inflammation suppression by regulating ROS-dependent p38 pathway. *Free Radical Biology & Medicine*, 108, 418-432. https://doi.org/10.1016/j.freeradbiomed.2017.03.023.
155. Dodd, F.L., Kennedy, D.O., Riby, L.M., & Haskell-Ramsay, C.F. (2015). A double-blind, placebo-controlled study evaluating the effects of caffeine and L-theanine both alone and in combination on cerebral blood flow, cognition and mood. *Psychopharmacology*, 232(14), 2563-2576. https://doi.org/10.1007/s00213-015-3895-0.
156. Nobre, A.C., Rao, A., & Owen, G.N. (2008). L-theanine, a natural constituent in tea, and its effect on mental state. *Asia Pacific Journal of Clinical Nutrition*, 17 Suppl 1, 167-168. https://pubmed.ncbi.nlm.nih.gov/18296328/.
157. Singh, R., Akhtar, N., & Haqqi, T.M. (2010). Green tea polyphenol epigallocatechin-3-gallate: Inflammation and arthritis. *Life Sciences*, 86(25-26), 907-918. https://doi.org/10.1016/j.lfs.2010.04.013.
158. Dietz, C., Dekker, M., & Piqueras-Fiszman, B. (2017). An intervention study on the effect of matcha tea, in drink and snack bar formats, on mood and cognitive performance. *Food Research International* (Ottawa, Ont.), 99(Pt 1), 72-83. https://doi.org/10.1016/j.foodres.2017.05.002.
159. Cristofori, F., Dargenio, V.N., Dargenio, C., Miniello, V.L., Barone, M., & Francavilla, R. (2021). Anti-Inflammatory and Immunomodulatory Effects of Probiotics in Gut Inflammation: A Door to the Body. *Frontiers in Immunology*, 12, 578386. https://doi.org/10.3389/fimmu.2021.578386.
160. Bungau, S.G., Behl, T., Singh, A., Sehgal, A., Singh, S., Chigurupati, S., Vijayabalan, S., Das, S., & Palanimuthu, V.R. (2021). Targeting Probiotics in Rheumatoid Arthritis. *Nutrients*, 13(10), 3376. https://doi.org/10.3390/nu13103376.
161. Pennisi, E., (May 2020). Meet the Psychobiome: mounting evidence that gut bacteria influence the nervous system inspires efforts to mine the microbiome for brain drugs. *Science*, https://www.science.org/content/article/meet-psychobiome-gut-bacteria-may-alter-how-you-think-feel-and-act [doi: 10.1126/science.abc6637]
162. Huang, R., Wang, K., & Hu, J. (2016). Effect of Probiotics on Depression: A Systematic Review and Meta-Analysis of Randomized Controlled Trials. *Nutrients*, 8(8), 483. https://doi.org/10.3390/nu8080483.
163. Chao, L., Liu, C., Sutthawongwadee, S., Li, Y., Lv, W., Chen, W., Yu, L., Zhou, J., Guo, A., Li, Z., & Guo, S. (2020). Effects of Probiotics on Depressive or Anxiety Variables in Healthy Participants Under Stress Conditions or With a Depressive or Anxiety Diagnosis: A Meta-Analysis of Randomized Controlled Trials. *Frontiers in Neurology*, 11, 421. https://doi.org/10.3389/fneur.2020.00421.
164. El Dib, R., Periyasamy, A.G., de Barros, J.L., França, C.G., Senefonte, F.L., Vesentini, G., Alves, M., Rodrigues, J., Gomaa, H., Gomes Júnior, J.R., Costa, L.F., Von Ancken, T.S., Toneli, C., Suzumura, E.A., Kawakami, C.P., Faustino, E.G., Jorge, E.C., Almeida, J.D., & Kapoor, A. (2021). Probiotics for the treatment of depression and anxiety: a systematic review and meta-analysis of randomized controlled trials. *Clinical Nutrition ESPEN*, 45, 75-90. https://doi.org/10.1016/j.clnesp.2021.07.027.
165. Johnson, D., Thurairajasingam, S., Letchumanan, V., Chan, K-G., & Lee, L-H. (2021). Exploring the Role and Potential of Probiotics in the Field of Mental Health: Major Depressive Disorder. *Nutrients*, 13(5), 1728. https://doi.org/10.3390/nu13051728.
166. Alli, S.R., Gorbovskaya, I., Liu, J.C.W., Kolla, N.J., Brown, L., & Müller, D. J. (2022). The Gut Microbiome in Depression and Potential Benefit of Prebiotics, Probiotics and Synbiotics: A Systematic Review of Clinical Trials and Observational Studies. *International Journal of Molecular Sciences*, 23(9), 4494. https://doi.org/10.3390/ijms23094494.
167. Nikolova, V.L., Cleare, A.J., Young, A.H., & Stone, J.M. (2021). Updated Review and Meta-Analysis of Probiotics for the Treatment of Clinical Depression: Adjunctive vs. Stand-Alone Treatment. *Journal of Clinical Medicine*, 10(4), 647. https://doi.org/10.3390/jcm10040647.
168. Gawlik-Kotelnicka, O., & Strzelecki, D. (2021). Probiotics as a Treatment for 'Metabolic Depression'? A Rationale for Future Studies. *Pharmaceuticals*, 14(4), 384. https://doi.org/10.3390/ph14040384.
169. Stohs, S.J., & Hartman, M.J. (2015). Review of the Safety and Efficacy of Moringa oleifera. *Phytotherapy Research*, 29(6), 796-804. https://doi.org/10.1002/ptr.5325.
170. Jan, B., Parveen, R., Zahiruddin, S., Khan, M.U., Mohapatra, S., & Ahmad, S. (2021). Nutritional constituents of mulberry and their potential applications in food and pharmaceuticals: A review. *Saudi Journal of Biological Sciences*, 28(7), 3909-3921. https://doi.org/10.1016/j.sjbs.2021.03.056.
171. El-Ramady, H., Abdalla, N., Badgar, K., Llanaj, X., Törös, G., Hajdú, P., Eid, Y., & Prokisch, J. (2022). Edible Mushrooms for Sustainable and Healthy Human Food: Nutritional and Medicinal Attributes. *Sustainability*, 14(9), 4941. https://doi.org/10.3390/su14094941.
172. Jedinak, A., Dudhgaonkar, S., Wu, Q., et al. (2011). Anti-inflammatory activity of edible oyster mushroom is mediated through the inhibition of NF-κB and AP-1 signaling. *Nutrition Journal*, 10(52). https://doi.org/10.1186/1475-2891-10-52.
173. Taofiq, O., Martins, A., Barreiro, F.M., et al. (2016). Anti-inflammatory potential of mushroom extracts and isolated metabolites. *Trends in Food Science & Technology*, 50, 193-210. https://doi.org/10.1016/j.tifs.2016.02.005.
174. Muszyńska, B., Grzywacz-Kisielewska, A., Kała, K., & Gdula-Argasińska, J. (2018). Anti-inflammatory properties of edible mushrooms: A review. *Food Chemistry*, 243, 373-381. https://doi.org/10.1016/j.foodchem.2017.09.149.
175. Jayachandran, M., Xiao, J., & Xu, B. (2017). A Critical Review on Health Promoting Benefits of Edible Mushrooms through Gut Microbiota. *International Journal of Molecular Sciences*, 18(9), 1934. https://doi.org/10.3390/ijms18091934.
176. Li, M., Yu, L., Zhao, J., Zhang, H., Chen, W., Zhai, Q., Tian, F. (2021). Role of dietary edible mushrooms in the modulation of gut microbiota. *Journal of Functional Foods*, 83, https://doi.org/10.1016/j.jff.2021.104538.
177. Dai, X., Stanilka, J.M., Rowe, C.A., Esteves, E.A., Nieves Jr.C., Spaiser, S.J., Christman, M.C., Langkamp-Henken, B., & Percival, S.S. (2015). Consuming Lentinula edodes (Shiitake) Mushrooms Daily Improves Human Immunity: A Randomized Dietary Intervention in Healthy Young Adults. *Journal of the American College of Nutrition*, 34(6), 478-487. https://doi.org/10.1080/07315724.2014.950391.
178. Kupcova, K., Stefanova, I., Plavcova, Z., Hosek, J., Hrouzek, P., & Kubec, R. (2018). Antimicrobial, Cytotoxic, Anti-Inflammatory, and Antioxidant Activity of Culinary Processed Shiitake Medicinal Mushroom (Lentinus edodes, Agaricomycetes) and Its Major Sulfur Sensory-Active Compound-Lenthionine. *International Journal of Medicinal Mushrooms*, 20(2), 165-175. https://doi.org/10.1615/IntJMedMushrooms.2018025455.
179. Elsayed, E.A., El Enshasy, H., Wadaan, M., & Aziz, R.A. (2014). Mushrooms: A Potential Natural Source of Anti-Inflammatory Compounds for Medical Applications. *Mediators of Inflammation*, 2014, 805841. https://doi.org/10.1155/2014/805841.
180. Tang, Y., Li, S., Yan, J., Peng, Y., Weng, W., Yao, X., et al. (2022). Bioactive Components and Health Functions of Oat. *Food Reviews International*, DOI: 10.1080/87559129.2022.2029477.
181. Yang, R., Zhou, Q., Wen, C., Hu, J., Li, H., Zhao, M., & Zhao, H. (2013). Mustard seed (Sinapis Alba Linn) attenuates imiquimod-induced psoriasiform inflammation of BALB/c mice. *The Journal of Dermatology*, 40(7), 543-552. https://doi.org/10.1111/1346-8138.12119.
182. Calder, P.C. (2017). Omega-3 fatty acids and inflammatory processes: from molecules to man. *Biochemical Society Transactions*, 45(5), 1105-1115. https://doi.org/10.1042/BST20160474.
183. Li, Y.R., Jia, Z., & Zhu, H. (2019). Dietary Supplementation with Anti-Inflammatory Omega-3 Fatty Acids for Cardiovascular Protection: Help or Hoax?. *Reactive Oxygen Species*, 7(20), 78-85. https://doi.org/10.20455/ros.2019.817.
184. Manchanda, S.C., & Passi, S.J. (2016). Selecting healthy edible oil in the Indian context. *Indian Heart Journal*, 68(4), 447-449. https://doi.org/10.1016/j.ihj.2016.05.004.
185. Lee, Y-H., Bae, S-C., & Song, G-G. (2012). Omega-3 Polyunsaturated Fatty Acids and the Treatment of Rheumatoid Arthritis: A Meta-analysis. *Archives of Medical Research*, 43(5), 356-362. https://doi.org/10.1016/j.arcmed.2012.06.011.
186. Goldberg, R.J., & Katz, J. (2007). A meta-analysis of the analgesic effects of omega-3 polyunsaturated fatty acid supplementation for inflammatory joint pain. *Pain*, 129(1-2), 210-223. https://doi.org/10.1016/j.pain.2007.01.020.
187. Kistner, K., Siklosi, N., Babes, A., Khalil, M., Selescu, T., Zimmermann, K., Wirtz, S., Becker, C., Neurath, M.F., Reeh, P.W., & Engel, M.A. (2016). Systemic desensitization through TRPA1 channels by capsazepine and mustard oil - a novel strategy against inflammation and pain. *Scientific Reports*, 6, 28621. https://doi.org/10.1038/srep28621.
188. Meydani, M. (2009). Potential health benefits of avenanthramides of oats. *Nutrition Reviews*, 67(12), 731-735, https://doi.org/10.1111/j.1753-4887.2009.00256.x
189. Nutrition Value. Black Olives. https://www.nutritionvalue.org/Olives%2C_black_75510020_nutritional_value.html.
190. Nutrition Value. Green Olives. https://www.nutritionvalue.org/Olives%2C_green_75510010_nutritional_value.html.
191. Bischoff, S.C. (2008). Quercetin: potentials in the prevention and therapy of disease. *Current Opinion in Clinical Nutrition and Metabolic Care*, 11(6), 733-740. https://doi.org/10.1097/MCO.0b013e32831394b8.
192. Guardia, T., Rotelli, A.E., Juarez, A.O., & Pelzer, L.E. (2001). Anti-inflammatory properties of plant flavonoids. Effects of rutin, quercetin and hesperidin on adjuvant arthritis in rat. *Il Farmaco* (Societa chimica italiana : 1989), 56(9), 683-687. https://doi.org/10.1016/s0014-827x(01)01111-9.
193. Mamani-Matsuda, M., Kauss, T., Al-Kharrat, A., Rambert, J., Fawaz, F., Thiolat, D., Moynet, D., Coves, S., Malvy, D., & Mossalayi, M. D. (2006). Therapeutic and preventive properties of quercetin in experimental arthritis correlate with decreased macrophage inflammatory mediators. *Biochemical Pharmacology*, 72(10), 1304-1310. https://doi.org/10.1016/j.bcp.2006.08.001.
194. Askari, G., Ghiasvand, R., Feizi, A., Ghanadian, S.M., & Karimian, J. (2012). The effect of quercetin supplementation on selected markers of inflammation and oxidative stress. *Journal of Research in Medical Sciences*, 17(7), 637-641. https://pubmed.ncbi.nlm.nih.gov/23798923/.
195. Javadi, F., Eghtesadi, S., Ahmadzadeh, A., Aryaeian, N., Zabihiyeganeh, M., Foroushani, A. R., & Jazayeri, S. (2014). The effect of quercetin on plasma oxidative status, C-reactive protein and blood pressure in women with rheumatoid arthritis. *International Journal of Preventive Medicine*, 5(3), 293-301. https://pubmed.ncbi.nlm.nih.gov/24829713/.
196. Slimestad, R., Fossen, T., & Vågen, I.M. (2007). Onions: A Source of Unique Dietary Flavonoids. *Journal of Agricultural and Food Chemistry*, 55(25), 10067-10080. https://doi.org/10.1021/jf0712503.
197. Mazarakis, N., Snibson, K., Licciardi, P.V., & Karagiannis, T.C. (2020). The potential use of l-sulforaphane for the treatment of chronic inflammatory diseases: A review of the clinical evidence. *Clinical Nutrition*, 39(3), 664-675. https://doi.org/10.1016/j.clnu.2019.03.022.
198. Ponder, A., Kulik, K., & Hallmann, E. (2021). Occurrence and Determination of Carotenoids and Polyphenols in Different Paprika Powders from Organic and Conventional Production. *Molecules*, 26(10), 2980. https://doi.org/10.3390/molecules26102980.
199. Hayman, M., Kam, P.C.A. (2008). Capsaicin: A review of its pharmacology and clinical applications. *Current Anaesthesia & Critical Care*, 19, 5-6, 338-343. https://doi.org/10.1016/j.cacc.2008.07.003.
200. Es-safi, I., Mechchate, H., Amaghnouje, A., Al Kamaly, O.M., Jawhari, F.Z., Imtara, H., Grafov, A., & Bousta, D. (2021). The Potential of Parsley Polyphenols and Their Antioxidant Capacity to Help in the Treatment of Depression and Anxiety: An In Vivo Subacute Study. *Molecules*, 26(7), 2009. https://doi.org/10.3390/molecules26072009.
201. Ajmera, P., Kalani, S., & Sharma, L. (2019). Parsley-benefits & side effects on health. *International Journal of Physiology, Nutrition and Physical Education*, 4(1), 1236-1242. https://www.journalofsports.com/pdf/2019/vol4issue1/PartAA/4-1-308-629.pdf.

202. Hamidi, M.S., Gajic-Veljanoski, O., & Cheung, A.M. (2013). Vitamin K and Bone Health. *Journal of Clinical Densitometry*, 16(4), 409–413, https://doi.org/10.1016/j.jocd.2013.08.017.
203. Loeser, R.F., Berenbaum, F., Kloppenburg, M. (2021). Vitamin K and osteoarthritis: is there a link?. *Annals of the Rheumatic Diseases*, 80, 547–549, https://ard.bmj.com/content/80/5/547.info.
204. Stock, M., & Schett, G. (2021). Vitamin K-Dependent Proteins in Skeletal Development and Disease. *International Journal of Molecular Sciences*, 22(17), 9328. https://doi.org/10.3390/ijms22179328.
205. Feskanich, D., Weber, P., Willett, W.C., Rockett, H., Booth, S.L., & Colditz, G.A. (1999). Vitamin K intake and hip fractures in women: a prospective study. *The American Journal of Clinical Nutrition*, 69(1), 74–79. https://doi.org/10.1093/ajcn/69.1.74.
206. Caraballo, P.J., Heit, J.A., Atkinson, E.J., Silverstein, M.D., O'Fallon, W.M., Castro, M.R., & Melton III, L.J. (1999). Long-term Use of Oral Anticoagulants and the Risk of Fracture. *Archives of Internal Medicine*, 159(15), 1750–1756. https://doi.org/10.1001/archinte.159.15.1750.
207. Chin, K-Y. (2020). The Relationship between Vitamin K and Osteoarthritis: A Review of Current Evidence. *Nutrients*, 12(5), 1208. https://doi.org/10.3390/nu12051208.
208. Boer, C.G., et al. (2021). Vitamin K antagonist anticoagulant usage is associated with increased incidence and progression of osteoarthritis. *Annals of the Rheumatic Diseases*, 80, 598–604. https://pubmed.ncbi.nlm.nih.gov/34412027/.
209. Ferrari, V., Gil, G., Heinzen, H., Zoppolo, R., & Ibáñez, F. (2022). Influence of Cultivar on Nutritional Composition and Nutraceutical Potential of Pecan Growing in Uruguay. *Frontiers in Nutrition*, 9, 868054. https://doi.org/10.3389/fnut.2022.868054.
210. Alvarez-Parrilla, E., Urrea-López, R. & de la Rosaa, L.A. (2018). Bioactive components and health effects of pecan nuts and their by-products: a review. *Journal of Food Bioactives*, 1, 56–92.
211. Chakraborty, A. J., Mitra, S., Tallei, T. E., Tareq, A. M., Nainu, F., Cicia, D., Dhama, K., Emran, T. B., Simal-Gandara, J., & Capasso, R. (2021). Bromelain a Potential Bioactive Compound: A Comprehensive Overview from a Pharmacological Perspective. *Life*, 11(4), 317. https://doi.org/10.3390/life11040317.
212. Pavan, R., Jain, S., Shraddha, & Kumar, A. (2012). Properties and Therapeutic Application of Bromelain: A Review. *Biotechnology Research International*, 2012, 976203. https://doi.org/10.1155/2012/976203.
213. Paterniti, I., Impellizzeri, D., Cordaro, M., Siracusa, R., Bisignano, C., Gugliandolo, E., Carughi, A., Esposito, E., Mandalari, G., & Cuzzocrea, S. (2017). The Anti-Inflammatory and Antioxidant Potential of Pistachios (Pistacia vera L.) In Vitro and In Vivo. *Nutrients*, 9(8), 915. https://doi.org/10.3390/nu9080915.
214. Case Western Reserve University. (1 September 2005). Pomegranate Fruit Shown To Slow Cartilage Deterioration In Osteoarthritis. ScienceDaily. www.sciencedaily.com/releases/2005/09/050901072114.htm.
215. Rasheed, Z. (2016). Intake of Pomegranate Prevents the Onset of Osteoarthritis: Molecular Evidences. *International Journal of Health Sciences*, 10(2), V–VIII. https://www.ncbi.nlm.nih.gov/pmc/articles/PMC4825888/.
216. Mahdavi, A.M., Seyedsadjadi, N., & Javadivala, Z. Potential effects of pomegranate (Punica granatum) on rheumatoid arthritis: A systematic review. *The International Journal of Clinical Practice*, 2021; 75:e13999. https://doi.org/10.1111/ijcp.13999.
217. Ghavipour, M., Sotoudeh, G., Tavakoli, E., et al. Pomegranate extract alleviates disease activity and some blood biomarkers of inflammation and oxidative stress in Rheumatoid Arthritis patients. *European Journal of Clinical Nutrition*, 71, 92–96 (2017). https://doi.org/10.1038/ejcn.2016.151.
218. Danesi, F., & Ferguson, L.R. (2017). Could Pomegranate Juice Help in the Control of Inflammatory Diseases?. *Nutrients*, 9(9), 958. https://doi.org/10.3390/nu9090958.
219. Giménez-Bastida, J.A., & Ávila-Gálvez, M.A., Espín, J.C. & González-Sarrías, A. (2021). Evidence for health properties of pomegranate juices and extracts beyond nutrition: a critical systematic review of human studies. *Trends in Food Science & Technology*, 114, 410–423. https://doi.org/10.1016/j.tifs.2021.06.014.
220. Syed, Q. A., Akram, M. & Shukat, R. (2019). Nutritional and Therapeutic Importance of the Pumpkin Seeds. *Biomedical Journal of Scientific & Technical Research*, 21, 3586. 10.26717/BJSTR.2019.21.003586.
221. Dotto, J.M. & Chacha, J.S. (2020). The potential of pumpkin seeds as a functional food ingredient: a review. *Scientific African*, 10, 575. 10.1016/j.sciaf.2020.e00575.
222. Peng, M., Lu, D., Liu, J., Jiang, B., & Chen, J. (2021). Effect of Roasting on the Antioxidant Activity, Phenolic Composition, and Nutritional Quality of Pumpkin (Cucurbita pepo L.) Seeds. *Frontiers in Nutrition*, 8, 647354. https://doi.org/10.3389/fnut.2021.647354.
223. Šamec, D., Loizzo, M. R., Gortzi, O., Çankaya, İ. T., Tundis, R., Suntar, İ., Shirooie, S., Zengin, G., Devkota, H.P., Reboredo-Rodríguez, P., Hassan, S., Manayi, A., Kashani, H., & Nabavi, S.M. (2022). The potential of pumpkin seed oil as a functional food – a comprehensive review of chemical composition, health benefits, and safety. *Comprehensive Reviews in Food Science and Food Safety*, 21(5), 4422–4446. https://doi.org/10.1111/1541-4337.13013.
224. Olivera, L., Best, I., Paredes, P., Perez, N., Chong, L., & Marzano, A. (2022). Nutritional Value, Methods for Extraction and Bioactive Compounds of Quinoa. In (Ed.), *Pseudocereals. IntechOpen*. https://doi.org/10.5772/intechopen.101891.
225. Gullón, B., Gullón, P., Tavaria, F. K., & Yáñez, R. (2016). Assessment of the prebiotic effect of quinoa and amaranth in the human intestinal ecosystem. *Food & Function*, 7(9), 3782–3788. https://doi.org/10.1039/c6fo00924g.
226. Lin, M., Han, P., Li, Y., Wang, W., Lai, D., & Zhou, L. (2019). Quinoa Secondary Metabolites and Their Biological Activities or Functions. *Molecules*, 24(13), 2512. https://doi.org/10.3390/molecules24132512.
227. Basu, A., Schell, J., & Scofield, R.H., (2018). Dietary fruits and arthritis. *Food & Function*, 9(1), 70–77. https://doi.org/10.1039/c7fo01435j.
228. Figueira, M.E., Câmara, M.B., Direito, R., Rocha, J., Serra, A.T., Duarte, C.M.M., Fernandes, A., Freitas, M., Fernandes, E., Marques, M.C., Bronze, M.R., & Sepodes, B. (2014). Chemical characterization of a red raspberry fruit extract and evaluation of its pharmacological effects in experimental models of acute inflammation and collagen-induced arthritis. *Food & Function*, 5(12), 3241–3251. https://doi.org/10.1039/c4fo00376d
229. Chen, Y., Yang, X., Li, H., & Fang, J. (2022). Red Raspberry Extract Decreases Depression-Like Behavior in Rats by Modulating Neuroinflammation and Oxidative Stress. *BioMed Research International*, 2022, 9943598. https://doi.org/10.1155/2022/9943598.
230. Jean-Gilles, D., Li, L., Ma, H., Yuan, T., Chichester III, C. O., & Seeram, N. P. (2012). Anti-inflammatory Effects of Polyphenolic-Enriched Red Raspberry Extract in an Antigen-Induced Arthritis Rat Model. *Journal of Agricultural and Food Chemistry*, 60(23), 5755–5762. https://doi.org/10.1021/jf203456w.
231. Sheik Abdul, N., & Marnewick, J.L. (2021). Rooibos, a supportive role to play during the COVID-19 pandemic?. *Journal of Functional Foods*, 86, 104684. https://doi.org/10.1016/j.jff.2021.104684.
232. Baba, H., Ohtsuka, Y., Haruna, H., Lee, T., Nagata, S., Maeda, M., Yamashiro, Y., & Shimizu, T. (2009). Studies of anti-inflammatory effects of Rooibos tea in rats. *Pediatrics International: Official Journal of the Japan Pediatric Society*, 51(5), 700–704. https://doi.org/10.1111/j.1442-200X.2009.02835.x.
233. Ghorbani, A., & Esmaeilizadeh, M. (2017). Pharmacological properties of Salvia officinalis and its components. Journal of Traditional and Complementary Medicine, 7(4), 433–440. https://doi.org/10.1016/j.jtcme.2016.12.014.
234. Phitak, T., Pothacharoen, P., Settakorn, J., Poompimol, W., Caterson, B., & Kongtawelert, P. (2012). Chondroprotective and anti-inflammatory effects of sesamin. *Phytochemistry*, 80, 77–88. https://doi.org/10.1016/j.phytochem.2012.05.016.
235. Khadem Haghighian, M., Alipoor, B., Malek Mahdavi, A., Eftekhar Sadat, B., Asghari Jafarabadi, M., & Moghaddam, A. (2015). Effects of sesame seed supplementation on inflammatory factors and oxidative stress biomarkers in patients with knee osteoarthritis. *Acta Medica Iranica*, 53(4), 207–213. https://pubmed.ncbi.nlm.nih.gov/25871017/.
236. Rafiee, S., Faryabi, R., Yargholi, A., Zareian, M.A., Hawkins, J., Shivappa, N., & Shirbeigi, L. (2021). Effects of Sesame Consumption on Inflammatory Biomarkers in Humans: A Systematic Review and Meta-Analysis of Randomized Controlled Trials. *Evidence-Based Complementary and Alternative Medicine*, 2021, 6622981. https://doi.org/10.1155/2021/6622981.
237. Singh R., Kumari, P., Kumar, S. (2017). 11 - Nanotechnology for enhanced bioactivity of bioactive phytomolecules. *Nutrient Delivery - Nanotechnology in the Agri-Food Industry*, Academic Press, 413–456, https://doi.org/10.1016/B978-0-12-804304-2.00011-1.
238. Li, J., Gang, D., Yu, X., et al. (2013). Genistein: the potential for efficacy in rheumatoid arthritis. *Clinical Rheumatology*, 32, 535–540. https://doi.org/10.1007/s10067-012-2148-4.
239. Polkowski, K., Mazurek, A.P. (2000). Biological properties of genistein. A review of in vitro and in vivo data. *Acta Polonaie Pharmaceutica*, 57(2):135–55. PMID: 10934794.
240. Li, J., et al. (2014). Genistein suppresses tumor necrosis factor α-induced inflammation via modulating reactive oxygen species/Akt/nuclear factor κB and adenosine monophosphate-activated protein kinase signal pathways in human synoviocyte MH7A cells. *Drug Design, Development and Therapy*, 8, 315–23. 17. doi:10.2147/DDDT.S52354.
241. Xu, J-X, Zhang, Y., Zhang, X-Z., Ma, Y-Y. (2011). Anti-angiogenic effects of genistein on synovium in a rat model of type II collagen-induced arthritis. *Zhong xi yi jie he xue bao* [Journal of Chinese Integrative Medicine]. 9(2), 186–193. doi: 10.3736/jcim20110212.
242. Liu, F-C., et al. (2019). Chondroprotective Effects of Genistein against Osteoarthritis Induced Joint Inflammation. *Nutrients*, 11(5), 1180. doi:10.3390/nu11051180.
243. Valsecchi, A.E., Franchi, S., Panerai, A. E., Sacerdote, P., Trovato, A.E., & Colleoni, M. (2008). Genistein, a natural phytoestrogen from soy, relieves neuropathic pain following chronic constriction sciatic nerve injury in mice: anti-inflammatory and antioxidant activity. *Journal of Neurochemistry*, 107, 230–240. doi:10.1111/j.1471-4159.2008.05614.x.
244. Zhang, Y., Dong, J., He, P., et al. (2012). Genistein Inhibit Cytokines or Growth Factor-Induced Proliferation and Transformation Phenotype in Fibroblast-Like Synoviocytes of Rheumatoid Arthritis. *Inflammation*, 35, 377–387. https://doi.org/10.1007/s10753-011-9365-x.
245. Shmagel, A., Onizuka, N., Langsetmo, L., Vo, T., Foley, R., Ensrud, K., & Valen, P. (2018). Low magnesium intake is associated with increased knee pain in subjects with radiographic knee osteoarthritis: data from the Osteoarthritis Initiative. *Osteoarthritis and Cartilage*, 26(5), 651–658. https://doi.org/10.1016/j.joca.2018.02.002.
246. Jennings, A., Welch, A. A., Spector, T., Macgregor, A., Cassidy, A. (2014). Intakes of anthocyanins and flavones are associated with biomarkers of insulin resistance and inflammation in women. *Journal of Nutrition*, 144, 202–208. doi: 10.3945/jn.113.184358.
247. Nielsen, F.H., Johnson, L.K., & Zeng, H. (2010). Magnesium supplementation improves indicators of low magnesium status and inflammatory stress in adults older than 51 years with poor quality sleep. *Magnesium Research*, 23(4), 158–168. https://pubmed.ncbi.nlm.nih.gov/21199787/
248. Chandrasekaran, N.C., Weir, C., Alfraji, S., Grice, J., Roberts, M.S., & Barnard, R.T. (2014). Effects of magnesium deficiency – more than skin deep. *Experimental Biology and Medicine*, 239(10), 1280–1291. https://doi.org/10.1177/1535370214537745.
249. Wienecke, E., & Nolden, C. (2016). Langzeit-HRV-Analyse zeigt Stressreduktion durch Magnesiumzufuhr [Long-term HRV analysis shows stress reduction by magnesium intake]. *MMW Fortschritte der Medizin*, 158(Suppl 6), 12–16. https://doi.org/10.1007/s15006-016-9054-7.
250. Cox, I.M., Campbell, M.J., & Dowson, D. (1991). Red blood cell magnesium and chronic fatigue syndrome. *Lancet*, 337(8744), 757–760. https://doi.org/10.1016/0140-6736(91)91371-z.
251. Imran, M., Ghorat, F., Ul-Haq, I., Ur-Rehman, H., Aslam, F., Heydari, M., Shariati, M.A., Okuskhanova, E., Yessimbekov, Z., Thiruvengadam, M., Hashempur, M.H., & Rebezov, M. (2020). Lycopene as a Natural Antioxidant Used to Prevent Human Health Disorders. *Antioxidants*, 9(8), 706. https://doi.org/10.3390/antiox9080706.
252. Khan, U.M., Sevindik, M., Zarrabi, A., Nami, M., Ozdemir, B., Kaplan, D.N., Selamoglu, Z., Hasan, M., Kumar, M., Alshehri, M.M., & Sharifi-Rad, J. (2021). Lycopene: Food Sources, Biological Activities, and Human Health Benefits. *Oxidative Medicine and Cellular Longevity*, 2021, 2713511. https://doi.org/10.1155/2021/2713511.
253. Fielding, J.M., Rowley, K.G., Cooper, P., & O'Dea, K. (2005). Increases in plasma lycopene concentration after consumption of tomatoes cooked with olive oil. *Asia Pacific Journal of Clinical Nutrition*, 14(2), 131–136.
254. Perdomo, F., Cabrera Fránquiz, F., Cabrera, J., & Serra-Majem, L. (2012). Influencia del procedimiento culinario sobre la biodisponibilidad del licopeno en el tomate [Influence of cooking procedure on the bioavailability of lycopene in tomatoes]. *Nutrición Hospitalaria*, 27(5), 1542–1546. https://doi.org/10.3305/nh.2012.27.5.5908.
255. Collins, E.J., Bowyer, C., Tsouza, A., & Chopra, M. (2022). Tomatoes: An Extensive Review of the Associated Health Impacts of Tomatoes and Factors That Can Affect Their Cultivation. *Biology*, 11(2), 239. https://doi.org/10.3390/biology11020239.
256. Khopde, S.M., Priyadarsini, K.I., Venkatesan, P., et al. (1999). Free radical scavenging ability and antioxidant efficiency of curcumin and its substituted analogue. *Biophysical Chemistry*, 80, 85–91.
257. Aggarwal, B.B., & Sung, B. (2009). Pharmacological basis for the role of curcumin in chronic diseases: an age-old spice with modern targets. *Trends in Pharmacological Sciences*, 30(2), 85–94. https://doi.org/10.1016/j.tips.2008.11.002.
258. Gupta, S.C., et al. (2013). Therapeutic roles of curcumin: lessons learned from clinical trials. *The AAPS Journal*, 15(1), 195–218. doi:10.1208/s12248-012-9432-8.

259. Makuch, S., Więcek, K., & Woźniak, M. (2021). The Immunomodulatory and Anti-Inflammatory Effect of Curcumin on Immune Cell Populations, Cytokines, and In Vivo Models of Rheumatoid Arthritis. *Pharmaceuticals*, 14(4), 309. https://doi.org/10.3390/ph14040309.
260. Razavi, B.M., Ghasemzadeh Rahbardar, M., & Hosseinzadeh, H. (2021). A review of therapeutic potentials of turmeric (Curcuma longa) and its active constituent, curcumin, on inflammatory disorders, pain, and their related patents. *Phytotherapy Research*, 35(12), 6489–6513. https://doi.org/10.1002/ptr.7224.
261. Memarzia, A., Khazdair, M.R., Behrouz, S., Gholamnezhad, Z., Jafarnezhad, M., Saadat, S., & Boskabady, M.H. (2021). Experimental and clinical reports on anti-inflammatory, antioxidant, and immunomodulatory effects of Curcuma longa and curcumin, an updated and comprehensive review. *BioFactors* (Oxford, England), 47(3), 311–350. https://doi.org/10.1002/biof.1716.
262. Zeng, L., Yang, T., Yang, K., Yu, G., Li, J., Xiang, W., & Chen, H. (2022). Efficacy and safety of curcumin and curcuma longa extract in the treatment of arthritis: a systematic review and meta-analysis of randomized controlled trial. *Frontiers in immunology*, 13, 891822.
263. Pourhabibi-Zarandi, F., Shojaei-Zarghani, S., & Rafraf, M. (2021). Curcumin and rheumatoid arthritis: a systematic review of literature. *The International Journal of Clinical Practice*, 75(10), e14280. https://doi.org/10.1111/ijcp.14280.
264. Kostoglou-Athanassiou, I., Athanassiou, L., & Athanassiou, P. (2020). The Effect of Omega-3 Fatty Acids on Rheumatoid Arthritis. *Mediterranean Journal of Rheumatology*, 31(2), 190–194. https://doi.org/10.31138/mjr.31.2.190.
265. Simopoulos, A.P. (2002). Omega-3 fatty acids in inflammation and autoimmune diseases. *Journal of the American College of Nutrition*, 21(6), 495–505. https://doi.org/10.1080/07315724.2002.10719248.

Chapter 4: Over 85 Anti-Inflammatory Recipes

Introduction and Tips

1. Epitideios, G. (16 December 2016). Toxicity of farmed salmon. European Parliament. https://www.europarl.europa.eu/doceo/document/E-8-2016-009527_EN.html#:~:text=The%20European%20Environment%20Agency%20states,a%20threat%20to%20consumers%27%20health.
2. Ma, Z., Du, B., Li, J., Yang, Y., & Zhu, F. (2021). An Insight into Anti-Inflammatory Activities and Inflammation Related Diseases of Anthocyanins: A Review of Both In Vivo and In Vitro Investigations. *International Journal of Molecular Sciences*, 22(20), 11076. https://doi.org/10.3390/ijms222011076.
3. Venlet, N.V., Hettinga, K.A., Schebesta, H., & Bernaz, N. (2021). Perspective: A Legal and Nutritional Perspective on the Introduction of Quinoa-Based Infant and Follow-on Formula in the EU. *Advances in Nutrition*, 12(4), 1100–1107. https://doi.org/10.1093/advances/nmab041.

Lunch

1. Dai, X., Stanilka, J.M., Rowe, C.A., Esteves, E.A., Nieves Jr., C., Spaiser, S.J., Christman, M.C., Langkamp-Henken, B., & Percival, S.S. (2015). Consuming Lentinula edodes (Shiitake) Mushrooms Daily Improves Human Immunity: A Randomized Dietary Intervention in Healthy Young Adults. *Journal of the American College of Nutrition*, 34(6), 478–487. https://doi.org/10.1080/07315724.2014.950391.
2. Kupcova, K., Stefanova, I., Plavcova, Z., Hosek, J., Hrouzek, P., & Kubec, R. (2018). Antimicrobial, Cytotoxic, Anti-Inflammatory, and Antioxidant Activity of Culinary Processed Shiitake Medicinal Mushroom (Lentinus edodes, Agaricomycetes) and Its Major Sulfur Sensory-Active Compound-Lenthionine. *International Journal of Medicinal Mushrooms*, 20(2), 165–175. https://doi.org/10.1615/IntJMedMushrooms.2018025455.
3. Lee, C. W., Ahn, Y-T., Zhao, R., Kim, Y. S., Park, S.M., Jung, D.H., Kim, J.K., Kim, H. W., Kim, S.C., & An, W.G. (2021). Inhibitory Effects of Porphyra tenera Extract on Oxidation and Inflammatory Responses. *Evidence-Based Complementary and Alternative Medicine*, 2021, 6650037. https://doi.org/10.1155/2021/6650037.
4. Jung, S-J., Jang, H-Y., Jung, E-S., Noh, S-O., Shin, S-W., Ha, K-C., Baek, H-I., Ahn, B-J., Oh, T-H., & Chae, S-W. (2020). Effects of Porphyra tenera Supplementation on the Immune System: A Randomized, Double-Blind, and Placebo-Controlled Clinical Trial. *Nutrients*, 12(6), 1642. https://doi.org/10.3390/nu12061642.
5. López-Jiménez, A., García-Caballero, M., Medina, M.Á., & Quesada, A.R. (2013). Anti-angiogenic properties of carnosol and carnosic acid, two major dietary compounds from rosemary. *European Journal of Nutrition*, 52(1), 85–95. https://doi.org/10.1007/s00394-011-0289-x.
6. Hsiao, A-F., Lien, Y-C., Tzeng, I-S., Liu, C-T., Chou, S-H., & Horng, Y-S. (2021). The efficacy of high- and low-dose curcumin in knee osteoarthritis: a systematic review and meta-analysis. *Complementary Therapies in Medicine*, 63, 102775. https://doi.org/10.1016/j.ctim.2021.102775.
7. Bagherniya, M., Darand, M., Askari, G., Guest, P. C., Sathyapalan, T., & Sahebkar, A. (2021). The Clinical Use of Curcumin for the Treatment of Rheumatoid Arthritis: A Systematic Review of Clinical Trials. *Advances in Experimental Medicine and Biology*, 1291, 251–263. https://doi.org/10.1007/978-3-030-56153-6_15.

Speedy Dinners

1. Than, K. (2007). Depressed? Go Play in the Dirt. Live Science. https://www.livescience.com/7270-depressed-play-dirt.html.

Meal Prep

1. Ranasinghe, R.A.S.N., Maduwanthi, S.D.T., & Marapana, R.A.U.J. (2019). Nutritional and Health Benefits of Jackfruit (Artocarpus heterophyllus Lam.): A Review. *International Journal of Food Science*, 2019, 4327183. https://doi.org/10.1155/2019/4327183.
2. Nutritionix. Jackfruit. https://www.nutritionix.com/food/jackfruit.
3. Ripani, U., Manzarbeitia-Arroba, P., Guijarro-Leo, S., Urrutia-Graña, J., & De Masi-De Luca, A. (2019). Vitamin C May Help to Reduce the Knee's Arthritic Symptoms. Outcomes Assessment of Nutriceutical Therapy. *Medical Archives*, 73(3), 173–177. https://doi.org/10.5455/medarh.2019.73.173-177.
4. Wojdyło, A., Nowicka, P., Grimalt, M., Legua, P., Almansa, M. S., Amorós, A., Carbonell-Barrachina, Á. A., & Hernández, F. (2019). Polyphenol Compounds and Biological Activity of Caper (Capparis spinosa L.) *Flowers Buds. Plants*, 8(12), 539. https://doi.org/10.3390/plants8120539.
5. Ferguson, J.A., Abbott, K.A., & Garg, M.L. (2021). Anti-inflammatory effects of oral supplementation with curcumin: a systematic review and meta-analysis of randomized controlled trials. *Nutrition Reviews*, 79(9), 1043–1066. https://doi.org/10.1093/nutrit/nuaa114.
6. Wilson, A., Yu, H-T., Goodnough, L.T., & Nissenson, A.R. (2004). Prevalence and outcomes of anemia in rheumatoid arthritis: a systematic review of the literature. *The American Journal of Medicine*, 116 Suppl 7A, 50S–57S. https://doi.org/10.1016/j.amjmed.2003.12.012.

Desserts

1. Abdulrazaq, M., Innes, J. K., & Calder, P. C. (2017). Effect of ω-3 polyunsaturated fatty acids on arthritic pain: a systematic review. *Nutrition*, 39-40, 57–66. https://doi.org/10.1016/j.nut.2016.12.003.
2. Rajaei, E., Mowla, K., Ghorbani, A., Bahadoram, S., Bahadoram, M., & Dargahi-Malamir, M. (2015). The Effect of Omega-3 Fatty Acids in Patients With Active Rheumatoid Arthritis Receiving DMARDs Therapy: Double-Blind Randomized Controlled Trial. *Global Journal of Health Science*, 8(7), 18–25. https://doi.org/10.5539/gjhs.v8n7p18.
3. Mateen, S., Rehman, M.T., Shahzad, S., Naeem, S.S., Faizy, A.F., Khan, A.Q., Khan, M.S., Husain, F.M., & Moin, S. (2019). Anti-oxidant and anti-inflammatory effects of cinnamaldehyde and eugenol on mononuclear cells of rheumatoid arthritis patients. *European Journal of Pharmacology*, 852, 14–24. https://doi.org/10.1016/j.ejphar.2019.02.031.
4. Wu, J-R., Zhong, W-J., Chen, Z-D., Zhu, B-Q., Jiang, Y-Y., & Wierzbicki, P.M. (2020). The protective impact of Trans-Cinnamaldehyde (TCA) against the IL-1b induced inflammation in in vitro osteoarthritis model by regulating PI3K/AKT pathways. *Folia Histochemica et Cytobiologica*, 58(4), 264–271. https://doi.org/10.5603/FHC.a2020.0025.
5. Rajaram, S., Connell, K.M., & Sabaté, J. (2010). Effect of almond-enriched high-monounsaturated fat diet on selected markers of inflammation: a randomised, controlled, crossover study. *British Journal of Nutrition*, 103(6), 907–912. https://doi.org/10.1017/S0007114509992480.
6. Kim, H., Castellon-Chicas, M.J., Arbizu, S., Talcott, S.T., Drury, N.L., Smith, S., & Mertens-Talcott, S.U. (2021). Mango (Mangifera indica L.) Polyphenols: Anti-Inflammatory Intestinal Microbial Health Benefits, and Associated Mechanisms of Actions. *Molecules*, 26(9), 2732. https://doi.org/10.3390/molecules26092732.

Snacks and Sides

1. Rajaram, S., Connell, K.M., & Sabaté, J. (2010). Effect of almond-enriched high-monounsaturated fat diet on selected markers of inflammation: a randomised, controlled, crossover study. *British Journal of Nutrition*, 103(6), 907–912. https://doi.org/10.1017/S0007114509992480

Drinks, Juices and Smoothies

1. Katengua-Thamahane, E., Marnewick, J.L., Ajuwon, O.R., et al. The combination of red palm oil and rooibos show anti-inflammatory effects in rats. *Journal of Inflammation*, 11, 41 (2014). https://doi.org/10.1186/s12950-014-0041-4.
2. Abu-Taweel, G.M., Mohsen G, A-M., Antonisamy, P., Arokiyaraj, S., Kim, H-J., Kim, S-J., Park, K.H., & Kim, Y.O. (2019). Spirulina consumption effectively reduces anti-inflammatory and pain related infectious diseases. *Journal of Infection and Public Health*, 12(6), 777–782. https://doi.org/10.1016/j.jiph.2019.04.014.
3. Trotta, T., Porro, C., Cianciulli, A., & Panaro, M.A. (2022). Beneficial Effects of Spirulina Consumption on Brain Health. *Nutrients*, 14(3), 676. https://doi.org/10.3390/nu14030676.
4. Prabakaran, G., Sampathkumar, P., Kavisri, M., & Moovendhan, M. (2020). Extraction and characterization of phycocyanin from Spirulina platensis and evaluation of its anticancer, antidiabetic and antiinflammatory effect. *International Journal of Biological Macromolecules*, 153, 256–263. https://doi.org/10.1016/j.ijbiomac.2020.03.009.
5. Azeez, T.B., & Lunghar, J. (2021). 6 - Antiinflammatory effects of turmeric (Curcuma longa) and ginger (Zingiber officinale), 127–146. 10.1016/B978-0-12-819218-4.00011-0.

Sauces, Jams and Dips

1. Story, E.N., Kopec, R.E., Schwartz, S.J., & Harris, G.K. (2010). An Update on the Health Effects of Tomato Lycopene. *Annual review of food science and technology*, 1, 189–210. https://doi.org/10.1146/annurev.food.102308.124120.
2. Zhan, J., Yan, Z., Kong, X., Liu, J., Lin, Z., Qi, W., Wu, Y., Lin, J., Pan, X., & Xue, X. (2021). Lycopene inhibits IL-1β-induced inflammation in mouse chondrocytes and mediates murine osteoarthritis. *Journal of Cellular and Molecular Medicine*, 25(7), 3573–3584. https://doi.org/10.1111/jcmm.16443.
3. Swathi, V., Rekha, R., Abhishek, J., Radha, G., Pallavi, S.K. & Praveen, G. Effect of chewing fennel and cardamom seeds on dental plaque and salivary pH – a randomized controlled trial. *International Journal of Pharmaceutical Sciences and Research*. 7(1), 406-12.doi: 10.13040/IJPSR.0975-8232.7 (1).406-12.
4. NRAS (National Rheumatoid Arthritis Society). Gum Disease. https://nras.org.uk/resource/gum-disease/.
5. Arthritis Foundation. Mouth Bacteria, Understanding Arthritis. https://www.arthritis.org/health-wellness/about-arthritis/understanding-arthritis/mouth-bacteria.
6. Tang, E.L.H., Rajarajeswaran, J., Fung, S. Y. et al. (2013). Antioxidant activity of Coriandrum sativum and protection against DNA damage and cancer cell migration. *BMC Complementary Medicine and Therapies*, 13, 347. https://doi.org/10.1186/1472-6882-13-347.
7. Akbari, S., & Rasouli-Ghahroudi, A.A. (2018). Vitamin K and Bone Metabolism: A Review of the Latest Evidence in Preclinical Studies. *BioMed Research International*, 2018, 4629383. https://doi.org/10.1155/2018/4629383.
8. Kim, H., Castellon-Chicas, M.J., Arbizu, S., Talcott, S.T., Drury, N.L., Smith, S., & Mertens-Talcott, S.U. (2021). Mango (Mangifera indica L.) Polyphenols: Anti-Inflammatory Intestinal Microbial Health Benefits, and Associated Mechanisms of Actions. *Molecules*, 26(9), 2732. https://doi.org/10.3390/molecules26092732.

INDEX

ACKNOWLEDGEMENTS

Grateful.

Let me start, and end, with the word grateful. Grateful is the word and the feeling I pull in whenever I have been working on this book, placing my hand on my heart as I say it. How privileged it is to have been able to write a second book, and thank you to the wonderful bunch of humans around me – without them, it would not have been possible.

To my mum and sister, thank you for being the other two legs on the three -legged stool, one that would not stand up without you. Your endless love and support, recipe-testing and reality-checks are very much appreciated. Thank you for being here for me in the worst and best of times. I love you both beyond words can say.

To Yellow Kite Books, what a joy it is to work with you all, and thank you to my editor Carolyn in particular for believing in me and the Arthritis Foodie mission. To Olivia and Vicky for their brilliant copyediting skills, and to Nassima, Hannah, Troy and Mark for a superb job on the shoot.

To my expert contributors, Dr Lauren Freid, Dr Deepak Ravindran, Cheryl Crow, VJ Hamilton and many others in this space who have supported both books and beyond: Dr Rupy Aujla, Dr Micah Yu, Dr Jenna Macciochi, and Dr Gemma Newman.

To the many authors, scientists and colleagues who I have learned from over the years, and who have encouraged, inspired and helped make this book possible.

Thank you to you, the Arthritis Foodie community, for staying with me on this journey, and providing a place of comfort and strength for me, but also for each other. For writing to each other on comments and in forums, for exchanging stories of support, and sharing the mission that nobody should ever feel alone with their condition.

To my nearest and dearest family, and closest friends. Thank you for your kindness and patience as I have navigated not only this condition, but the various shifts and turns, ups and downs, highs and lows of life. For being at the end of the phone or tasting my recipes. Thank you to my step-dad Stephen, for joining us on the healthy lifestyle ride, and eating plants (okay, maybe not all the time).

Finally, a note to my grandparents. How blessed to have been able to grow up with three sets of you all. To my Grandma Anne, I will never stop admiring your energy, joy and zest for life. Thank you for being a fabulous grandmother, and an even better friend. To Grandpa Johnson, for trying matcha green tea bags at the age of 90 and supporting this dream. Nanan Johnson, nobody will ever be able to cook Yorkshire puddings the way you did or bake an Apple Pie like you. I miss your big soft cuddles. To Grandma Pat, I have not yet made a 'healthy' buttercream chocolate yule log, but I will never not treasure yours just the way it is. Grandad Speight, I hope I have done your Nasi Goreng justice, and that people will love making it, as much as you once loved making it for your friends. Grandad Talbot, you probably would not choose to eat any of the healthy recipes in this book, but perhaps would opt for the most 'pud-DING'-like option and I promise I would not begrudge you the whiskey accompaniment. I miss you both, too.

Dad, I hope that you're somewhere with them and seeing all of this. Needless to say, I imagine that you are.

And I am grateful.

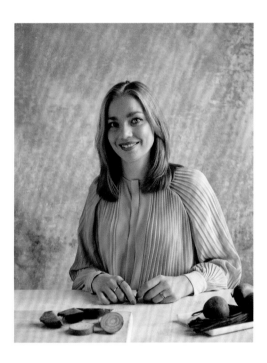

About the Author

Emily Johnson is the author of *Beat Arthritis Naturally: Supercharge your health with 65 recipes and lifestyle tips from Arthritis Foodie*. Emily launched the Instagram page @arthritisfoodie in September 2018 after struggling with seronegative arthritis for five years. The community has since grown to over 30K, with people looking to Emily for inspiration on living healthily with arthritis. Emily also works in marketing and is a social media influencer.

First published in Great Britain in 2023 by Yellow Kite
An imprint of Hodder & Stoughton
An Hachette UK company

1

Copyright © Emily Johnson 2023
Photography copyright © Nassima Rothacker 2023

A CIP catalogue record for this title is available from the British Library

Hardback ISBN 978 1 399 71245 3
eBook ISBN 978 1 399 71244 6

Editorial Director: Carolyn Thorne
Project Editor: Olivia Nightingall
Design: Studio Polka
Photography: Nassima Rothacker
Food Stylist: Troy Willis
Props Stylist: Hannah Wilkinson
Production Controller: Matt Everett

Colour origination by Alta Image London
Printed and bound in China by C&C Offset Printing Co., Ltd.

Hodder & Stoughton policy is to use papers that are natural, renewable and recyclable products and made from wood grown in sustainable forests. The logging and manufacturing processes are expected to conform to the environmental regulations of the country of origin.

Yellow Kite
Hodder & Stoughton Ltd
Carmelite House
50 Victoria Embankment
London
EC4Y 0DZ

www.yellowkitebooks.co.uk
www.hodder.co.uk